MEET ACUPOINTS
WITH FIGURES

画穴名 识内涵

汉英对照

针灸穴名释义

主编 ◎ 王 凡

全国百佳图书出版单位

中国中医药出版社

·北 京·

U0273244

图书在版编目（CIP）数据

画穴名，识内涵：针灸穴名释义：汉英对照 / 王
凡主编 . — 北京：中国中医药出版社，2024.8
ISBN 978 – 7 – 5132 – 8798 – 2

Ⅰ.①画…　Ⅱ.①王…　Ⅲ.①针灸疗法—穴位—汉、
英　Ⅳ.① R224.2

中国国家版本馆 CIP 数据核字（2024）第 101887 号

中国中医药出版社出版

北京经济技术开发区科创十三街 31 号院二区 8 号楼
邮政编码　100176
传真　010–64405721
北京联兴盛业印刷股份有限公司印刷
各地新华书店经销

开本 787 × 1092　1/16　印张 27　字数 634 千字
2024 年 8 月第 1 版　2024 年 8 月第 1 次印刷
书号　ISBN 978 – 7 – 5132 – 8798 – 2

定价　138.00 元
网址　www.cptcm.com

服 务 热 线　**010–64405510**
购 书 热 线　**010–89535836**
维 权 打 假　**010–64405753**

微信服务号　**zgzyycbs**
微商城网址　**https://kdt.im/LIdUGr**
官 方 微 博　**http://e.weibo.com/cptcm**
天猫旗舰店网址　**https://zgzyycbs.tmall.com**

如有印装质量问题请与本社出版部联系（010–64405510）

编 委 会

序

中华文化源远流长，标志着中华民族的数千年文明。中华文化的存续源于文字的发明创造。仓颉为了更好地记录和传递人类信息，思考如何创造一种符号来代表事物的形态和意义。他观察自然界万物，从日月星辰、山川河流、草原森林、鸟鱼动物以及人类生活中汲取灵感，创造出了最早的汉字。汉字的内涵和寓意是任何文字符号都无法比拟的，形象生动而又富有内涵的符号，形成了中华民族文化的载体，记录着几千年的中华文明。中华文化是华夏民族的灵魂，每一个文字和每一节音符都跳动着中华民族基因的火花。中华文化博大精深，囊括宇宙天地、人类古今，包括戏曲文化、民俗文化、宗教文化、酒文化、茶文化、饮食文化、民乐文化，等等。中医针灸文化作为中华文化的重要一脉，淋漓尽致地体现了中华文化的精髓、内涵和特点，可谓中华文化的精华和缩影。

中医针灸是中华民族与疾病作斗争的过程中形成的医学手段。针灸不仅在几千年来承担着维护中华民族健康的责任和使命，也是中华文化走向世界的先行者。2010年，中医针灸入选"人类非物质文化遗产代表作名录"，成为针灸数千年发展史上最辉煌的一页，意味着将针灸从医疗技术提升到了文化和艺术的更高境界。

中医针灸根植于中华文化，与中华文化息息相关，是中华文化的重要组成部分，同时也是中华文化的载体和光耀。针灸以经络腧穴为基本单位，构成其核心基础理论。古人对穴名的取义，可谓"仰则观象于天，俯则观法于地"，"近取诸身，远取诸物"，堪称中医针灸文化的缩影。穴名借用日月星辰、山川河流、交通要冲、植物动物等名称，隐喻了腧穴的分布特点、阴阳属性和主治功效。腧穴名称不仅仅是腧穴的文字符号，更蕴藏着深刻和广泛的内在涵义，是中华文化的结晶，彰显着中华文化的光耀。因此探究穴名内涵对于中医药文化的传承和发展有着重要的意义。

为了能够使国内外更多的中医专业学生、中医爱好者了解穴名文化，帮助读者领会其精髓真谛，学习知识的同时体会针灸文化之美，作者特编著了这本汉英双语的《画穴名，识内涵——针灸穴名释义》，图文并茂地介绍了穴名释义的源流发展和腧穴的命名特点，以及362个经穴名称的源流和内涵。难能可贵的是本书作者另辟新径，将艺术字设计应用于针灸穴名的阐释中，以汉字之象形，解腧穴之形象，令人印象深刻、豁然开朗。比如"列缺"的闪电设计，很容易让读者发挥想象，记住本穴为"络穴"的特定穴属性，及其像霹雳行空、消散阴霾一样能够清利头目、治疗头痛的功效。再比如"太白"以三星堆出土文物的设计，诠释了本穴五行属土的特性及其培土生金、同治肺脾的功效。采用图画文字的形式阐释穴位名称的深奥含义，可谓画龙点睛，难能可贵。

中医针灸已经走出国门，远播海外。但国际教材和文献中却丢弃了腧穴名称，取而代之的是数字符号，丢掉了腧穴名称的含义和价值实为可惜。著作者为了恢复腧穴的真实含义和价值，潜心研究中华文化、文字色彩和腧穴名称的内涵，并巧妙地有机结合，返璞归真，给予穴名以形象化，使得抽象化的文字符号更为形象生动，便于学习者记忆和理解。这部著作，对于中医院校学生，特别是非中文母语的留学生，可以形象化由浅入深理解腧穴的真实意义。本书可以作为国际和国内学者参考书常备案头枕边，随时翻阅，对于理解记忆穴位的定位和功效、提高针灸理论水平很有帮助。对于针灸爱好者来说，本书也是一本可贵的科普读本。

中华自信，文化自信，中医自信，针灸自信，传承真谛，传播精华。

非物质文化遗产"东氏针灸"代表性传承人
东贵荣博士
2024年4月23日

编写说明

　　腧穴名称是中医文化的载体，闪耀着中华民族智慧的光芒。其重要性与针灸技法一样，同属于"非物质文化遗产"的一部分，值得传承和发展。本书以诠释穴名内涵为己任，将意符文字设计应用到针灸穴名的阐释中，图文并茂地介绍腧穴命名的涵义，以及腧穴名称中蕴含着的阴阳五行等传统哲学思想、隐喻着的腧穴分布特点和作用特点。将针灸穴名的文化内涵以通俗易懂、鲜活有趣的方式介绍给读者，从而展现针灸之理、针灸之美、针灸之魂。随着中医药发展上升为国家战略以及"一带一路"的深入推进，越来越多的海外人士开始热衷于中医的学习。医学无国界、艺术无国界，穴名插画能够让非中文母语的学习者也可以直观地理解穴名背后所蕴含的中医文化信息。因此，本书特采用中英对照，以便更多的国际中医爱好者领略穴名文化的魅力。

　　本书共十四章。第一章为概述，介绍腧穴释义的源流发展，以及腧穴的由来和命名特点。第二章至第十五章为十四经362穴的腧穴释义。

　　本书特色是穴名插画，将穴名文字分解为笔画元素，主要根据穴名释义，结合腧穴的作用特点或者解剖特点，对笔画元素进行相应的绘画加工形成意符文字，从而形象地表达穴名的内涵。在文字设计时兼顾意象性、趣味性和美观性。插画下提供了简要的注释文字，说明插画创意的思路来源，以便读者能够见图明义、见图知用。

　　此外，各穴下列出处、别名、穴义、定位、主治、释义摘录。

　　别名参考《经穴释义汇解》《中国针灸穴位通鉴》和《针灸腧穴通考》。穴义参考了历代针灸穴名释义相关著作、期刊文献和《说文解字》等文字工具书，博采诸书之精华。遇到释义差别较大的穴位，以古代文献为主，并运用训诂学对穴位释义进行研究甄选。插画创意来源于腧穴的主治特点而非穴名释义的，穴义中将对腧穴的主治和临床应用进行简要的阐释，如上巨虚、下巨虚、内庭等穴。

　　历代释义摘录选录了一些公开出版书籍中的穴名释义原文。书目主要包括隋·杨上善《黄帝内经明堂类成》《黄帝内经太素》、清·程扶生《医经理解》、清·叶广祚《采艾编》、清·岳含珍《穴名解》、焦会元《(古法新解)会元针灸学》、张晟星《经穴释义汇解》、周楣声《针灸穴名释义》和高式国《针灸穴名解》。腧穴名称的形成年代离我们相去甚远，由于语言文化、字形语音的变迁，不同医家对于穴名的理解可谓仁者见仁智者见智。此处摘录不同观点之学说，供读者拓展思路、加深认知，以免理解和思维被一家之言所禁锢。无论古籍还是近现代作品，摘录内容中的异体字、古今字、通假字均统改为规范字，如"藏府"改为"脏腑"、"窌"改为"髎"等。

本书的穴名、英文代码、特定穴属性、定位和主治主要以国家标准《腧穴名称与定位》（GB/T 12346–2006、GB/T 12346–2021）和国家标准《腧穴主治》（GB/T 30233–2013）为依据。

除了别名和释义摘录，本书其他内容均提供了英文版本。中医术语的英文翻译主要参考 2022 年度《WHO international standard terminologies on traditional Chinese medicine》（ISBN 978–92–4–004232–2）。

本书第一章概论，由王凡编写，吴婕妤、肖然、金祺汇翻译；第二章至第五章、第十五章，由秦梦、王伽佑编写，吴婕妤、肖彬翻译；第六章至第九章由李华章、尹越、金祺汇编写，肖然、唐文超翻译；第十章至第十四章由李华章、徐静雯编写，周叙、程珂翻译。穴名出处、穴义由程珂审校考证；别名、释义摘录由邝守兰审校考证。插画由王凡、王莲芳、陆兆嘉、左丹烊、李伶晟、傅晨云设计制作。

目录

Catalog

第一章

概论

一 穴名的起源和发展

远古时期，人类在生产劳动中本能地发现，通过按压、锤击等方式刺激一些痛点，病患处会有"按者快然""按而痛止"的现象。这些部位被笼统地称为"砭灸处"，于是形成了腧穴的最早期雏形——"以痛为腧"。

随着实践经验的积累，人们逐渐认识到某些腧穴的特定治疗功能，一些有固定部位的"腧穴"便开始出现。在老官山汉墓出土的医简中，穴名主要是以"部位＋阴阳"的形式来表达的。比如"项钜阳"，"项"表明了"部位"，划定了身体所在的范围；"钜阳"是阴阳属性，表达了该部位的纵向区域。虽然这种定位并不精确，但在解剖学、生理学并不发达的时代，古人用自己的表达方式巧妙地对腧穴开始了最原始的命名。

最早有穴名记载的古籍是战国至秦汉时期成书的《黄帝内经》。该书记载了 173 个穴位，其中明确名称并沿用至今的腧穴已经达到 148 个之多，自此穴名实现了由面到点的历史演变。这些腧穴的命名取义很广，渗透了古代天文、气象、地理、人体、人事等多个方面。

成书于西汉末至东汉延平年间的《黄帝明堂经》，堪称我国第一部腧穴学专著，该书对汉以前散在医书中的腧穴进行了全面总结，包括腧穴的名称、部位、主治及刺灸法等。《黄帝明堂经》原书已佚，好在其内容被后世文献代代相承地辑录和保存了下来。最早引录《黄帝明堂经》的是晋代皇甫谧的《针灸甲乙经》，是我国现存最早的针灸学专著。该书收录了 349 个经穴，标志着针灸经穴的整理趋于完善。此后经穴数量变化甚微。至清代李学川《针灸逢源》一书，经穴穴名增至 361 个，此经穴命名和数量一直沿用到现代。2006 年颁布的国家标准《腧穴名称与定位》（GB/T 12346-2006），将原经外奇穴"印堂"归于督脉，至此经穴数量为 362 个。

由此可见，腧穴命名并非一人一时所为，其由来经历了一个从无到有、由面变点、逐渐增多的演变过程。是历代医家在当时的历史条件下，依据对自然的认知，上穷天文下极地理、宗阴阳五行之纲、考脏腑经络之形、依腧穴功用之效，历经数千年雕琢而成。

二　穴名释义的源流和发展

隋唐时期杨上善首开腧穴释名之先河。杨上善在《黄帝内经太素》第九卷十五络脉篇对十五经络穴穴名进行了注解。另外在《黄帝内经明堂》一书中，他对十四经穴也曾做过注解，可惜此书现存的内容只剩下手太阴一卷10穴（内少云门穴），其余部分均已散佚。

宋金元明时期鲜见腧穴释名的著作。明代张介宾的《类经》对腧穴穴名的含义作了综合性的概述。比如《类经·经络类》中指出："凡诸经腧穴，有曰天曰星者，皆所以应天也。有曰地曰山陵溪谷渊海泉泽都里者，皆所以应地也。又如穴名府者，为神之所集。穴名门户者，为神之所出入。穴名宅舍者，为神之所安。穴名台者，为神之所游行。此先圣之取义命名，皆有所因，用以类推，则庶事可见。"虽未逐穴注解，但对穴名释义的思考和总结为后世医家进一步认知腧穴提供了基本思路。

清代是穴名研究的高潮，出现了多部完整诠释经穴穴名的著作，对穴名的解释内容丰富，各有所长。

清代程知《医经理解·卷三》专设"穴名解"，对十四经腧穴穴名逐穴加以释义。程氏所言"欲世之学者，因名求义，因义得穴，以易于识取云尔"，道出了阐释穴名、探究其义的最直接原因。

清代叶广祚的《采艾编》是一本灸法专著，是岭南文化的代表。全书共四卷，第二卷对十二经穴的名称进行了非常简要的解释，如"眉冲，直眉头上，神庭曲差之间，眉上近中之处，直冲而上也"，"通天，上为脑，下为鼻，言气之通于颠也"。

清代齐鲁医家岳含珍编撰《经穴解》一书，对十四经穴的定位、针灸禁忌、穴名释义和主治作用进行了全面的论述。在注解腧穴时，岳氏擅长运用语言学，结合人体形态和经络理论解释穴名的由来。如承光穴，"承者，以下承上之象，光者，指百会穴而言也。百会在人顶上，有人君北辰之象，此穴在其左右之下，有人臣侍君之象，故曰承光"；内关穴，"内者，与外相对也，皆离肘而入掌骨节交经之处，有关象焉，故曰关"。另外，该书还匠心独运地将名称、含义、部位相似的腧穴放在一起进行对比、论述，以帮助读者进行鉴别。比如，为了区别冲门与腹股沟处其他诸穴，讲到"此穴乃脾经入腹之始，足三阴经并足阳明自股入腹者，横列数之。足少阴在里，其入腹之始穴为横骨穴，去中行各一寸。次则阳明经，入腹为气冲穴，去中行各二寸。次则足厥阴肝经，入腹为阴廉穴，去气冲穴二寸。次则足太阴脾经，入腹为冲门穴。以气冲已在中，去中行二寸之际，而此穴乃在去中行四寸半之际，反在气冲之外，以其近于胃经入腹穴之气冲也，故曰冲门"。

民国时期正值西学东渐。在此背景下成书的《（古法新解）会元针灸学》也颇具时代特色。作者焦会元开始尝试用中西融合的方式来解释穴名。如维道穴，"上通子宫带，下通连韧带，经和三焦"；承光穴，"目瞳似水精体，脾如磨电机，肾与命门如发电机，大小脑如收电机，脑后骨如平镜，能发返光，脑府诸阳环聚前脑，工于运用"。这些解释现在看来虽然有些牵强，但反映了作者用现代语言诠释中医的意识以及中医科学化的愿望。

中华人民共和国成立后，针灸事业日益发展，20 世纪 80 年代初在腧穴释名方面涌现出一批影响力较大的专著。高式国的《针灸穴名解》和周楣声的《针灸穴名释义》对十四经穴穴名进行了逐一考释，体例大致相同。前者注重古代文化，并结合自己在临床治疗中的经验体会；后者引用《诗经》《史记》《说文解字》等经典古籍，先解字、后解词，形成腧穴名称的"训诂学"研究体系。张晟星和戚淦合著《经穴释义汇解》，该书的经穴释义汇集古今数十家之说，取其精华、去其糟粕，参以己见编汇而成。其特点是释义简短精悍，并逐句引证文献资料。书中还附注了穴位别名和英译，英译采取直译的方式保留了穴名丰厚的文化内涵。另外值得一提的是王德深主编的《中国针灸穴位通鉴》（1994 年第 1 版），该书"穴名释义"部分全面搜集了每一个穴位从古至今历代医家的注解，可谓腧穴释名之集大成者，对腧穴名称的研究具有重要的参考价值。

三 腧穴的命名和分类

"名称者，别彼此而检虚实者也。自古至今，莫不用此而得，用彼而失。"（《尹文子·大道上》）中国文化自古十分重视事物的命名，而其孕育衍生出的针灸文化更是如此，每一个腧穴名称都有它的特殊含义，正如孙思邈在《千金翼方》中所说："凡诸孔穴，名不徒设，皆有深意。"

（一）腧穴命名的思维方法

腧穴命名的思维方法无外乎两种，取象比类法和写实记录法。

大部分腧穴命名采用的是取象比类法，即根据腧穴的解剖部位、阴阳五行、气血流注、功能作用等方面的特征，加之丰富的想象力，找寻天文、地理、动植物、建筑物、器物等与之相似的事物从而对腧穴进行命名的方法。"天地合气，命之曰人"（《素问·宝命全形论》），人得天地阴阳之气而生，而人体就是一个小宇宙，人体的功能就是天地阴阳之气交通往来的表现。这是"取象比类"法命名的哲学基础。从《医经理解》对穴名释义的概括可见一斑："海，言其所归。渊、泉，言其深。狭者为沟、渎。浅者为池、渚。市、府，言其所聚。里、道，言其所由。室、舍，言其所居。门、户，言其所出入。尊者为阙、堂。要会者为关、梁。丘、陵，言其骨肉之高起。髎，言其骨之空阔者也。俞，言其气之传输也。天，以言乎其上。地，以言乎其下也。"正因为如此，腧穴名称中蕴含着丰富的意义和内涵，了解穴名的意义，有利于了解古人的哲学思想，对深入了解穴位的分布特点、临床应用、气血流注有重要意义。

写实记录法，即真实记录腧穴的部位、功用等方面的特点。如巨骨、腕骨、京骨、乳中、大椎等因部位而得名；睛明、养老、迎香、光明、飞扬等由功用而得名。

两种方法可单独使用，也经常结合起来一起使用，如血海、听宫、风市、内关、哑门等。

（二）腧穴命名的分类

古人对穴名的取义，可谓"上察天文，下观地理，中通人事，远取诸物，近取诸身"。因此，现将腧穴命名用"法天""法地""法人"的三才思想归纳总结如下。

1. 法天 "天"有两层含义。首先，"天"代表天文、气象。我国古代天文学和气象学从原始社会就开始萌芽了。在江苏发现的"将军崖岩画"是距今至少四千年的岩画作品，上面清楚地描绘了太阳和带状星云，这可能是世界上现存最古老的星图。在河南安阳出土的殷墟甲骨文中，也已有风、云、雨、雷等丰富的气象记载。古人勤于观察日月星辰的位置及其变化，从而掌握规律，用来编制历法、为生产和生活服务。因此，古代天文气象对中国文化和医学产生了非常深远的影响。其次，"天"还包括天神，即主宰宇宙、日月、星辰、风雨之诸神。

（1）**天文气象** 以日月星辰等天文名词命名的穴位有紫宫、华盖、璇玑、天枢、曲垣、上星、日月、太乙、天宗、天溪、箕门、太白等；以气象名词命名的穴位有云门、列缺、丰隆等。这些穴位多分布于头、颈、胸等腰以上部位，以喻脉气通于天气。其中，紫宫、华盖、璇玑、曲垣、天宗等以星宿命名的穴位多集中分布于胸部和上背部。中国古代的天文学家将星官划分为三垣：上垣之太微垣、中垣之紫微垣和下垣之天市垣。而上述星宿隶属于紫微垣。紫微垣又被称为紫微宫，即皇宫的意思，为天帝所居。所以将此星名配之于人体心胸，以比类心为君主之官、肺为相傅之官。有趣的是，紫微垣作为星官，最早记录于《甘石星经》一书中，该书大致成书于战国时期，而这个时期恰好也是《黄帝内经》的成书年代。

（2）尚天神灵　有句俗语叫作"举头三尺有神明"，这种说法源自人们的祭祀活动。在人类的早期时代，人们对于很多自然现象感到神秘而恐惧，于是萌生了"神"的概念，认为神是天地万物的创造者及主宰者，无所不知，无所不能，因此便产生了对神灵的崇拜。有很多腧穴的命名取象于神灵，如"神"穴有神门、神堂、本神、神藏、神封、神道、神阙等；"灵"穴有灵道、青灵、承灵、灵墟、灵台等。中医认为"心者，君主之官也，神明出焉"（《素问·灵兰秘典论》），因此这些穴位大多分布在胸部和上背部，或者与"心藏神"的生理功能及主治作用相关，以喻心气藏聚之处或出入之通道。

2. 法地　古人"仰以观于天文，俯以察于地理"（《易经·系辞》），发现地表高低起伏，形成了山地、平原、河谷、沙丘、大川等地形地貌，这些地貌与人体的经络循行、穴位分布有很多的形似之处，于是用地理学名词来进行相关的描述。比如《灵枢·经水》中运用古代版图上清、渭、海、湖、汝、渑、淮、漯、江、河、济、漳十二条河流的大小、深浅来比喻十二经脉的气血运行状况。再如《素问·气穴论》中所言"肉之大会为谷，肉之小会为溪，肉分之间，溪谷之会，以行荣卫，以会大气"，就是以"溪""谷"来阐释气穴的概念。古人在为腧穴命名时也借助了大量的地理地貌名词来形容腧穴所在部位的解剖特点，如山、谷、丘、陵、海、溪、池、泽等。据统计，在《内经》出现的148个穴名中，以山川水道命名的最多，有37个。此外，在地面上生长的植物、生活的动物也是腧穴取名的重要素材。

（1）山谷丘陵　比如丘墟穴在足外踝的前下方，外踝突起如山丘，故以"丘墟"命名；大陵穴在掌侧，掌长肌腱与桡侧腕屈肌腱之间的凹陷中，此处起伏较大，掌骨高突犹如大山，故名为"大陵"；陷谷穴在第二、三跖骨结合部前方，穴处凹陷如山谷。再如外陵、梁丘、商丘、外丘、合谷、前谷、然谷、阳谷、率谷、承山、昆仑等，此类穴位大多分布于人体四肢靠近骨骼的部位。

（2）江河湖海　"海，言其所归。渊、泉，言其深。狭者为沟、渎。浅者为池、渚。"（《医经理解》）如血海有引血归经之功，比喻其功用犹如导洪流入江海；极泉位于手少阴心经的最高处，比喻经气犹如水流自极深之泉而下；清冷渊比喻手少阳三焦经之脉气血流注至此穴，似水注入深潭。类似的穴位还有小海、少海、照海、气海、尺泽、少泽、阳池、天池、曲池、阳溪、太溪、后溪、太渊、涌泉、曲泉、水泉、天泉、廉泉、四渎等。这些穴位大多分布在四肢部，其中不乏五输穴，穴名以海、泽、池、溪、渊、泉、冲等水道之名来比拟经气的流注运行。同时，穴名中还常常加以"大""小"之词来形容气血强弱，如小海、少海、少泽、太渊、太冲等。

（3）动物植物　动植物是自然界的重要组成部分。古人用取象比类的思维，以生活中常见的动植物命名具有相似特征的穴位，展现了丰富的想象力。如鸠尾穴，鸠是布谷鸟的别名，其尾常垂善蔽，此处以鸠尾来比类胸骨；鱼际穴在手掌拇指侧肌肉旁，此处肌肉肥厚，形如鱼腹。类似的穴位还有伏兔、犊鼻、攒竹、禾髎等。

3. 法人　"论理人形，列别脏腑，端络经脉，会通六合，气穴所发，各有处名。"（《素问·阴阳应象大论》）因此，"法人"首先是依据人体穴位处的解剖部位、相关脏腑器官、腧穴主治作用、阴阳五行属性对腧穴进行命名。其次，"法人"还包括人们所用的生活用品、所处的居所建筑等。

（1）解剖部位　如巨骨、腕骨、京骨、大椎直接以骨名来命名；太冲、人迎、带脉、急脉直接以脉名来命名；上、中、下脘以及肺俞、心俞、肝俞、脾俞、肾俞等背俞穴直接以其相应脏腑器官命名。在骨面上的空隙中或者骨骼边缘凹陷的穴位多以"髎"字命名，如八髎在骶骨背面的空隙中，肩髎穴在肩峰后下凹陷中，天髎穴在肩胛骨上角骨际的凹陷中，颧髎在颧骨下缘凹陷中。

穴名中还经常使用"上、下""头、足""手、足""前、后"等对偶词来体现穴位所处的部位。如上关、下关，上廉、下廉，头窍阴、足窍阴，头临泣、足临泣，手三里、足三里，前顶、后顶，前谷、后溪等。

（2）腧穴作用　光明主治眼疾；哑门为治哑疾之要穴；迎香能治鼻塞不闻香臭；周荣可以促进气血散布全身，有营养周身之用。类似的腧穴还有承浆、承光、飞扬、睛明、养老等。治疗风疾的穴位多以"风"命名，如治疗头风的风府、风池、翳风，治疗肩背风疾的风门、秉风，治疗下肢风疾的风市。还有一些"水"穴，如水道、水分、水泉。水道穴深部为小肠，靠近膀胱，多用于治疗小便不利等病证；水分穴能够分利清浊，使水液入膀胱、糟粕入大肠；水泉穴为足少阴肾经之郄穴，多用于治疗经水不调、小便不利等证。不难看出，上述"水"穴多与其"治水"的功效有关。

（3）阴阳五行　"阴阳学说"和"五行学说"都是中医学重要的哲学基础和思维方法，这些思维方法在腧穴的命名中也得以充分体现。

"阴阳"是宇宙中相互关联的事物或现象对立双方属性的概括，人体也是由阴阳结合而构成的有机整体，因此以"阳"命名的穴位多归属于阳经，如至阳、会阳、阳交、三阳络、阳陵泉、阳谷；以"阴"命名的穴位多归属于阴经，或与阴经相关，如会阴、阴交、三阴交、阴陵泉、阴谷、至阴。

"五行"即木、火、土、金、水五种物质及其运动变化。通过取象比类法和推演络绎法，"五行"将人体的脏腑器官与自然万物联系了起来。根据"五行学说"，五脏与五神的对应关系为：肺藏魄，心藏神，肝藏魂，脾藏意，肾藏志。因此，肺俞、心俞、肝俞、脾俞、肾俞的旁边分别有魄户、神堂、魂门、意舍和志室相伴。再比如，肺五行属"金"，五色对应"白"，五音对应"商"，故肺经穴中有侠白、少商之名。

（4）经络循行　经络循行犹如四通八达的道路，有直行，有分叉，相互之间还会发生交会。有的穴名体现了本经经络的循行，比如"曲差"体现了足太阳膀胱经在此曲折而行、参差不齐；"复溜"体现了足少阴肾经从足心斜走内踝后绕行，再斜走至本穴后恢复直行之正。有的穴名体现了经络的支离，如"支正"是手太阳小肠经络穴，小肠经络脉从此穴与正脉相别而行；"附分"体现了膀胱经第二侧线从此穴开始依附第一侧线直行而下，成为本经的一条分支。有的穴名则体现了两经或者多经的交会关系，多以"交""会"命名。如"三阴交"为足太阴经、足少阴经、足厥阴经之交会，"阳交"是足少阳经和阳维脉之交会，"交信"为足太阴与阴跷脉之交会，"会阴"为任脉、督脉、冲脉之所会。

（5）建筑居所　建筑居所大到行政划区，小到屋舍门窗，是人事活动的产物，也为人事活动提供了场所。"经筋犹山脉，经络犹河川，穴位则沿河两岸之城镇耳。"（《针灸穴名解》）生活中有亭台楼阁，人体中也有深宅大院。以建筑居所命名的腧穴非常多，其中"门"穴就有 22 个之多，还有大都、中都、阴都、胸乡、气街、府舍、中府、天府、灵台、步廊、神堂、玉堂、紫宫、库房、膺窗等等。其中"宫、府、堂、庭、廊"等以建筑命名的腧穴大多分布在胸廓部，更有意思的是它们的分布很有规律。比如沿着任脉的循行方向就像深入到了一座宫殿——推开"巨阙"大门，堂前之"中庭"映入眼帘，穿过会客议事之"玉堂"，步入君王居所之"紫宫"，庭堂两侧还有"步廊"——这是典型的中国古代庭院式建筑。这种布局设计不仅仅体现了中国古代建筑艺术，更反映了当时社会的宗法和礼教制度。胸廓内有心、肺两脏，心为"君"主之官，肺为"相"傅之官，胸廓犹如心肺之宅舍，因而此处腧穴以宫殿建筑命名，以合君主之仪。

（6）生活用品　在腧穴的命名中还出现了"钟""枕""箕""鼎""盆"等人们日常生活所需之物，多以取象比类法命名。例如，箕门穴取"箕"之象比类两腿分张之势，天鼎穴取"鼎"之象比类锁骨内侧端头、喉头突起和两耳形成的三足两耳之形，缺盆穴取"盆"之象比类锁骨上窝之状。

第二章

手太阴肺经穴

1 中府（肺募穴，手、足太阴经交会穴）

【出处】《黄帝明堂经》。

【别名】膺中俞。

【穴义】中，中焦；府，意为聚集。手太阴肺经起于中焦，其气血物质来源于脾胃化生水谷之精微，且本穴为肺之募穴，脏气输注聚集之处，故名"中府"。

【定位】在胸部，横平第1肋间隙，锁骨下窝外侧，前正中线旁开6寸。

【主治】①咳嗽，气喘，胸痛，胸满，胸中热；②肩背痛。

肺经起于中焦，故名"中"；穴为肺之募穴，脏气输注聚集之处，故名"府"。

【释义摘录】

《医经理解》："手太阴脉自中焦生，故谓中府。"

《古法新解会元针灸学》："中府者，肺之络系，府者从阳，由内而达于外。又名膺俞者，膊膺之部，气所过之俞穴，证各穴由胸而走手。"

《经穴释义汇解》："府，聚也。中府为手太阴肺脉之腧穴，肺手太阴之脉起于中焦，穴为中气所聚；又穴为肺之募。募，脏气结聚之所，府含募之意，故名中府。"

2 云门

【出处】《素问·水热穴论》。

【**别名**】无。

【**穴义**】云，云雾，比喻脉气；门，出入之门户。手太阴肺经之气上行至此穴，为本经最高之处，自此离胸入臂，气出如云，具有舒达抑郁之功，可用于宣肺止咳，化痰散结，犹如云雾气化飞升之门户，故名"云门"。

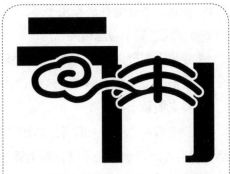

手太阴肺经之气出于本穴而散布于体表，犹如云雾气化飞升之门户。

【**定位**】肩胛骨喙突上方，锁骨下窝凹陷处，距前正中线6寸。

【**主治**】①咳嗽，气喘，心痛，胸满；②肩背痛。

【**释义摘录**】

《医经理解》："云门，夹气户旁二寸，言气出如云也。"

《经穴解》："穴名云门者，天之气为云，肺为五脏之华盖，而居五脏之上，有天之象焉，其所出气者，有云之象焉；自肺经而上行至此穴，为本经最高之所，将离胸而入臂之内，必有窍以通于臂，有门之象焉，故曰云门。"

《古法新解会元针灸学》："云门者，云应气也，上焦如雾，云遇冷下降，遇热升腾而散走；门者司守之门户，故名云门也。"

《针灸穴名释义》："肺之纹理有云气之象。《黄庭内景经》：'肺部之宫似华盖……素锦衣裳黄云带。'注：'肺在五脏之上，四垂为盖也。素锦衣裳，肺膜之色也。黄云带者，肺中之黄脉蔓延罗络，有象云气。'云门之义也与道家学说有关。"

《经穴释义汇解》："云，山川气也。云出天气，天气通于肺。肺者气之本，穴为手太阴脉气所发，为手太阴肺脉所出之门户，喻气出如云，故谓之云门。"

③ 天府

【**出处**】《素问·气穴论》。

【**别名**】无。

【**穴义**】天，指上部；府，府库。本穴为本经在臂部最高处，肺经循行自本穴离胸而入臂，统本经之气由臂下肘，灌注于本经诸穴，故名"天府"。以

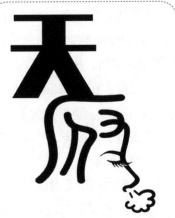

补法作用于本穴可治疗气虚不摄而导致的咳嗽上气、喘不得息诸症。

"府"命名，亦比喻补法作用于本穴，可使耗散之气集中于胸廓，治疗气虚不摄而导致的咳嗽上气、喘不得息诸症。

【定位】在臂内侧面，肱二头肌桡侧缘，腋前纹头下3寸处。

【主治】①鼻衄，咳嗽，气喘；②瘿气；③痹痛。

【释义摘录】

《经穴解》："穴名天府者，本经之脉初离胸而入臂，为本经诸穴最高之处，故曰天焉；曰府者，以统本经之气，而由臂下肘，灌注于本经诸穴者也。"

《古法新解会元针灸学》："天府者，平肩与云门相平，云气所聚象天，故名天府也。"

《经穴释义汇解》："穴为肺脉腧穴，天以候肺。穴在腋下三寸，臂臑内动脉中，居天位，应天府星名，故曰天府；又肺为上盖，为腑脏之天，肺气归于此穴，故名。"

《针灸穴名解》："古者朝廷制度，有天府、玉府、内府之设，天府即中央集权处也。故云'天府治中'，即治理内政得失也。补此穴可招致耗散之气，使之集中。宜施于虚不摄气之证，然必用补法。《甲乙经》谓治咳嗽上气，喘不得息，气逆不得卧。凡汗出身肿、恍惚善忘、胸缩诸症，俱具气不守中之象，故宜取此。以使集中，引致大气汇于胸廓，犹行政之治中。故称'天府'。"

4 侠白

【出处】《黄帝明堂经》。

【别名】无。

【穴义】侠，通"夹"；白，肺之色。本穴为手太阴肺经腧穴，肺色白；穴在臂内，夹于臑上白肉间，故名"侠白"。

【定位】在臂内侧面，肱二头肌桡侧缘，腋前纹头下4寸，或肘横纹上5寸处。

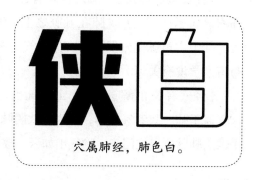

穴属肺经，肺色白。

【主治】①心痛，咳嗽，气喘，烦满；②干呕；③臂痛。

【释义摘录】

《黄帝内经明堂类成》："白，肺色也，此穴在臂，候肺两箱，故名侠白。"

《医经理解》："侠白，在天府下，去肘上五寸。肺为乾金，天象也。白者，金之色也，或谓其夹于臑上白肉间也。"

《经穴解》："穴名侠白者，白者金也。此穴在臑腋处，故曰侠白。"

《古法新解会元针灸学》："侠白者，肺色白，夹于赤白肉筋分间，故名侠白。"

《针灸穴名解》:"穴在上膊臑部内侧,白肉凸起之前方。垂手夹腋之处,故名'夹白'。"

5 尺泽（合穴）

【出处】《灵枢·本输》。

【别名】鬼受,肘中动脉。

【穴义】本穴定位从"尺",肘横纹至寸口约尺余长,本穴位于肘横纹中。功用从"泽"。泽,水液停聚的地方,本穴为合穴,比喻手太阴肺经经气至此如水入大泽,故名"尺泽"。

【定位】在肘区,肘横纹上,肱二头肌腱桡侧凹陷处。

【主治】①咳嗽,气喘,胸满,咳血,咽喉肿痛,肘臂痛;②小儿惊风;③干呕,泄泻。

【释义摘录】

《医经理解》:"尺泽,在肘中约纹罅中,其去掌后正得同身之尺也。"

《经穴解》:"穴名尺泽者,布肘而知尺,从腕上至此而长有尺也。肺经此穴,所入为合水,水之所聚为泽,故曰尺泽也。"

《古法新解会元针灸学》:"尺泽者,尺即寸关尺,泽为水平。由寸口至尺泽为一尺九分,至鱼际为一尺一寸,泽又象水,故名尺泽。"

《经穴释义汇解》:"泽,从水,水之钟也。喻手太阴脉气至此象水之归聚处;又因穴在肘横纹上偏桡动脉处,其去掌后,正得同身之尺,尺脉入泽,如水入大泽,故名尺泽。"

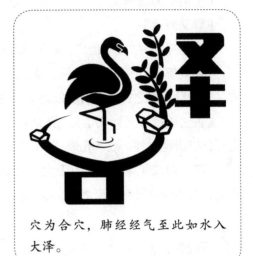

穴为合穴,肺经经气至此如水入大泽。

6 孔最（郄穴）

【出处】《黄帝明堂经》。

【别名】无。

【穴义】孔,孔隙。此穴为手太阴肺经之郄穴,郄即孔隙,是本经气血深聚之处。"孔"又有"通"的意思(《说文解字》)。最,

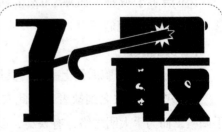

通窍之极也,形容本穴为通窍理血之要穴。

极，无比的。二字连用，即通窍之极也，形容本穴为通窍理血之要穴，临床常用于治疗咯血、衄血、热病无汗之证，故名"孔最"。

【定位】在前臂，腕掌侧远端横纹上7寸，尺泽与太渊连线上。

【主治】①热病无汗；②咳嗽，气喘，咯血，咽喉肿痛；③肘臂痛。

【释义摘录】

《医经理解》："其地最广，故谓其孔最大。"

《经穴解》："孔，窍也；最，高也。舒手而侧取，穴无高于此者，故曰孔最。且此穴又为过臂入肘之初穴，乃所以通上下之窍也。"

《古法新解会元针灸学》："孔最者，最主要之孔窍也。肺气通七窍最宜，起寸口上七寸，得诸经之气，故名孔最。"

《经穴释义汇解》："穴为手太阴之郄，去腕七寸。郄为孔隙，有孔穴的含义；最，聚也，穴为肺经气血汇聚之处，故名孔最。"

7 列缺（络穴；八脉交会穴，通任脉）

【出处】《灵枢·经脉》。

【别名】无。

【穴义】古称雷电之神为"列缺"。一则手太阴肺经自此穴别走阳明，脉气由此别裂而去，似闪电之形。二则雷电在大气中有通上彻下之能，"头痛寻列缺"，刺激本穴可使头目清爽，犹霹雳行空，阴霾消散而天朗气清，故名"列缺"。

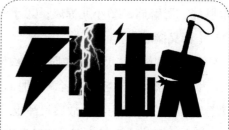

列缺，雷电之神。刺激本穴可使头目清爽，犹霹雷行空，阴霾消散而天朗气清。

【定位】在前臂，腕掌侧横纹上1.5寸，拇短伸肌腱与拇长展肌腱之间，拇长展肌腱沟的凹陷中。

【主治】①咳嗽，气喘；②齿痛，咽喉肿痛，口眼㖞斜；③头痛，颈项强痛；④半身不遂，手腕痛无力。

【释义摘录】

《医经理解》："腕后侧上一寸，其筋骨罅中，谓之列缺。言列于缺陷处也。"

《经穴解》："穴名列缺者，以此穴同经渠、太渊三穴，并列于寸口，而此穴独通于手阳明，而为手太阴之络，有缺焉，以通于阳明，故曰列缺。"

《古法新解会元针灸学》："高骨下缺，位列经穴，而生奇络。司肺细络，肺阴生阳，至缺处而交手阳明。脉斜至阳溪，即名反关脉。故高骨下缺，肺之络列穴，故名列缺。"

《经穴释义汇解》："列，分解也。缺，器破也；去也。列缺，古谓天上之裂缝：天门。手太阴属肺，肺为脏之盖，居诸脏之上。至高无上曰天，肺叶四垂，犹如天象。穴为手太阴之络，腕上一寸五分。手太阴自此分支别走阳明，脉气由此别裂而去，似天上之裂缝。又列缺指闪电，而闪电之形，有似天庭破裂，故名。"

8 经渠（经穴）

【出处】《灵枢·本输》。

【别名】无。

【穴义】经，动而不居；渠，沟渠。本穴为手太阴肺经之经穴，所行为经，形容经气在此流动不绝，如水流通的沟渠。且本穴主治以开瘀泻热、调理肺气为主，犹如水渠分洪灌溉之功用。故名"经渠"。

【定位】在前臂掌面桡侧，桡骨茎突与桡动脉之间凹陷处，腕横纹上 1 寸。

【主治】①咳嗽，气喘，胸痛，咽喉肿痛；②腕疼痛无力。

【释义摘录】

《黄帝内经明堂类成》："水出流注，入渠徐行，血气从井出已流注至此，徐引而行经。谓十二经脉也。渠，谓沟渠，谓十二经脉血气流于此穴，故曰经渠也。"

《医经理解》："寸口陷中，谓之经渠，盖太阴所经行之渠也。"

《经穴解》："穴名经渠者，渠乃盛水之所，本经至此而大见为关脉，如水之有渠，故曰经渠。"

《古法新解会元针灸学》："经渠，经长之沟渠也。阴阳所过如渠，故名经渠。"

《针灸穴名解》："犹分洪流为多渠也，故名'经渠'。"

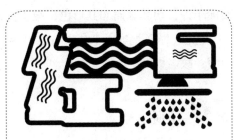

穴为经穴，经气在此流动不绝，如水流通的沟渠。

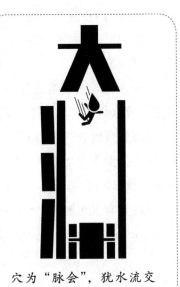

穴为"脉会"，犹水流交汇处，博大而深。

9 太渊（输穴、原穴，八会穴之脉会）

【出处】《灵枢·九针十二原》《灵枢·本输》。

【别名】太泉，鬼心。

【穴义】太，大也，极也；渊，指深涧。本穴为八会穴中"脉之大会"，犹水流交汇处，博大而深，故名"太渊"。

【定位】腕前区，桡骨茎突与舟状骨之间，拇长展肌腱尺侧凹陷中。

【主治】①咳嗽，气喘，咯血，咽喉肿痛；②无脉症；③手腕疼痛无力。

【释义摘录】

《医经理解》："渊，深也；太，大也，脉气所大会，故谓之太渊。"

《古法新解会元针灸学》："太渊者，脉之大会，阳阴之系统，渊源之出入，始于内而标于外，切其脉而知其形色，故名太渊也。"

《经穴释义汇解》："太，大也。渊，深也。穴在手掌后凹陷处，脉气所大会，博大而深，故名太渊。"

10 鱼际（荥穴）

【出处】《灵枢·本输》。

【别名】无。

【穴义】际，交界处。本穴位于手掌拇指桡侧赤白肉结合处，该处肌肉肥厚，形如鱼腹，故名"鱼际"。

【定位】在手外侧，第1掌骨桡侧中点赤白肉际处。

【主治】①咳嗽，咯血，咽干，咽喉肿痛；②身热，掌中热，头痛；③小儿疳积。

穴在手掌拇指桡侧赤白肉际处，该处肌肉肥厚，形如鱼腹。

【释义摘录】

《黄帝内经明堂类成》："水出井，流而动也，脉出指，流而上行，大指本节后象彼鱼形，故以鱼名之。赤白肉畔，故曰鱼际也。"

《医经理解》："掌上白肉，其隆起者形有如鱼。脉行其际，故谓鱼际。"

《经穴解》："大指本节后白肉，通为鱼腹，此穴在其际，际者，界也，乃赤白肉之界也，故曰鱼际。"

《经穴释义汇解》："本穴在掌骨之前，大指本节之后，其处肥肉隆起，如鱼腹；凡两合皆曰际，穴当赤白肉相合之处，脉行其际，故名鱼际。"

11 少商（井穴）

【**出处**】《灵枢·本输》。

【**别名**】鬼信。

【**穴义**】少，小；商，五音之一，肺属金，其音商。本穴为手少阴肺经井穴，所出为井，比喻其脉气始发，似浅小水流，故名"少商"。

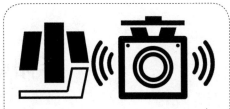

肺属金，其音"商"。"少"者小也，穴为井穴，形容脉气始发。

【**定位**】手拇指末节桡侧，指甲根角侧上方 0.1 寸。

【**主治**】①咽喉肿痛，鼻衄，咳嗽，气喘；②小儿惊狂；③手指挛痛。

【**释义摘录**】

《医经理解》："商者，金音也。言少者，以别于阳也。"

《经穴解》："穴名少商者，商者，金也。肺为阴金，大肠为阳金，阳大而阴小，故为少商。"

《古法新解会元针灸学》："少商者，阴中生阳，从少。五音六律，分宫商角徵羽，从商，属肺，肺金音商，肺经之根，故名少商。"

《经穴释义汇解》："穴为手太阴肺脉之井穴，肺音为商，位在手大指端内侧，去爪甲如韭叶。韭叶者，言少许也，以别于阳，故名少商。"

第三章
手阳明大肠经穴

1 商阳（井穴）

【出处】《灵枢·本输》。

【别名】绝阳，而明。

【穴义】商，五音之一。大肠与肺相表里，同属金，金音商。本穴为手阳明之井穴，上承肺金清肃之气，阴金在此转化为阳金，故名"商阳"。

【定位】在手指食指末节桡侧，指甲根角侧上方0.1寸。

穴属金，在时为秋，在音为商。

【主治】①咽喉肿痛，齿痛，颊肿，耳鸣，耳聋，青盲；②热病无汗、神昏；③手指麻木、肿痛。

【释义摘录】

《医经理解》："大肠则阳金矣，故其脉之起于次指端者，谓之商阳。"

《经穴解》："商者，金也。手阳明为金之表，故曰商阳。"

《经穴释义汇解》："穴为手阳明大肠脉之始穴，受手太阴脉之交，行于阳分。大肠与肺相合，肺音商。又穴属金，金音商，故名商阳。"

2 二间（荥穴）

【出处】《灵枢·本输》。

【别名】间谷。

【穴义】间，隙也，意指空陷处。穴在手大指次指本节前内侧凹陷处，是本经第二个穴位，故名"二间"。

【定位】第2掌指关节桡侧远端赤白肉际处。

【主治】①咽喉肿痛，齿痛，视物不明，鼻衄，口眼㖞斜；②热病。

【释义摘录】

《医经理解》："指凡三节，指屈数之，本节前为二间。"

《经穴解》："间者，穴也，气脉流通之称也，以前有三间，故此曰二间。"

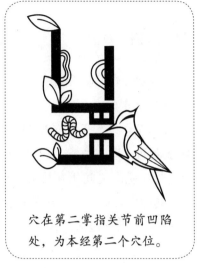

穴在第二掌指关节前凹陷处，为本经第二个穴位。

《经穴释义汇解》："间，隙也，意指空陷处。穴在手大指次指本节前内侧凹陷处，位当本经第二个穴位，故曰二间。"

《针灸穴名解》："本穴一名'间谷'。穴在次指内侧，爪后第二节后，故名'二间'。间，隔也。治症略同合谷穴。"

3 三间（输穴）

【出处】《灵枢·本输》。

【别名】少谷。

【穴义】间，间隙，指骨间空隙处。本穴位于第二掌指关节后凹陷处，为本经第三个穴位，故曰"三间"。

【定位】在手指，第2掌指关节桡侧近端凹陷处。

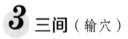

穴为本经第三个穴位。

【主治】①咽喉肿痛，齿痛，目痛；②胸满，身热而喘；③肠鸣；④手背、手指肿痛。

【释义摘录】

《医经理解》："指凡三节，指屈数之……本节后为三间也。"

《古法新解会元针灸学》："三间者，手阳明之第三空处，即名三间。又名小谷者，小骨空窍而能传达深远，医隐藏之疾邪也。"

《针灸穴名解》："本穴一名'小谷'。穴在次指内侧，爪后第三节后，故名'三间'。二间、三间，均与合谷穴交会，故二穴治病，均与合谷穴略同。"

4 合谷（原穴）

【出处】《灵枢·本输》。

【别名】虎口。

【穴义】合，开合；谷，"肉之大会为谷……肉分之间，溪谷之会"（《素问·气穴论》），指筋骨、肌肉之间相互接触的缝隙或凹陷部位，其中大者称谷。穴在第一、二掌骨之间，两骨开合如谷，故名"合谷"。

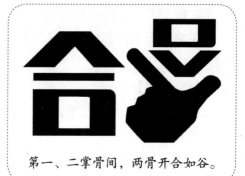

第一、二掌骨间，两骨开合如谷。

【定位】在手背，第2掌骨桡侧的中点处。取穴时可以一手的拇指指间关节横纹，放在另一手拇、食指之间的指蹼缘上，当拇指尖下是穴。

【主治】①咽喉肿痛，齿痛，头痛，目赤肿痛，鼻衄，耳聋，口眼㖞斜，口噤；②恶寒发热，无汗，多汗；③滞产，经闭，痛经；④中风失语，上肢不遂。

【释义摘录】

《医经理解》："合谷，在大指次指歧骨间，言两骨相合如谷也。"

《经穴解》："合谷者，言肺之经，由此而下行及于商阳，大肠之经，又由此而上臂也，故曰合谷。"

《古法新解会元针灸学》："合谷者，手大指次指开合之处，两手歧骨谷空，故名合谷。又名虎口者，手张之状，其形大之如虎口之状也。"

《针灸穴名释义》："合，开合、结合与合拢之意。谷，山洼无水之地，又肌肉之结合处，即古之所谓'肉之大会'，亦称为谷。合谷，山名。穴在太阴与阳明结合处。开则如谷，合则如山也。"

5 阳溪（经穴）

【出处】《灵枢·本输》。

【别名】中魁，河口。

【穴义】阳，阳位，指手背；溪，《内经》谓"肉之小会为溪……肉分之间，溪谷之会"，指筋骨、肌肉之间相互接触的缝隙或凹陷部位，其中小的称溪。穴位于拇短伸肌腱

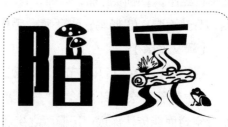

穴在手背，属阳；位于两肌腱之间的凹陷中，似处泽溪。

与拇长伸肌腱之间的凹陷处，似处泽溪，故名"阳溪"。

【定位】在腕区，腕背侧远端横纹桡侧，桡骨茎突远端，解剖学"鼻咽窝"凹陷中。

【主治】①目赤肿痛，齿痛，咽喉肿痛，头痛；②手腕肿痛、无力。

【释义摘录】

《医经理解》："阳溪，在手腕上侧两筋间陷中。溪为水所行，此则阳脉所经之溪也。"

《经穴解》："腕之中横直有三穴，小肠经有阳谷，三焦经有阳池，大肠经为阳溪，此取乎水行之义，以三穴皆自手腕而上行于臂之所也。气血遇关节之所，必稍聚而后行，故以谷、池、溪名之。阳者，以阳明经也。三穴皆以阳称，总为阳经也。"

《古法新解会元针灸学》："阳者，阳经之阳。溪者，水也。小水沟而伏阳气，故曰阳溪。又名中魁者，水火藏其中，金性相杀，魁首之属，又系腕中。"

《经穴释义汇解》："阳溪，手阳明脉之所行也，为经。在腕中上侧两旁间凹陷处，穴当阳位，其处类似山溪，故名阳溪。"

6 偏历（络穴）

【出处】《灵枢·根结》。

【别名】无。

【穴义】偏，偏斜；历，经历，通行。本穴为手阳明大肠经之络穴，其络脉由此别走，联络手太阴肺经，故名"偏历"，也因此可以同时治疗大肠经和肺经两经病变。

【定位】在前臂，腕背侧远端横纹上3寸处，阳溪与曲池连线上。

【主治】①齿痛，鼻衄，咽喉肿痛，耳鸣，耳聋；②水肿，小便不利；③手臂酸痛无力。

【释义摘录】

《黄帝内经太素》："手阳明经上，偏出此络，经历手臂，别走太阴，故曰偏历也。"

《医经理解》："偏历，为手阳明之别走太阴者。在手腕后三寸，言由此而偏斜走太阴也。"

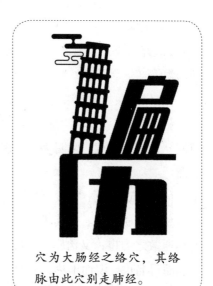

穴为大肠经之络穴，其络脉由此穴别走肺经。

《经穴解》："手阳明之别偏历，去腕三寸，别入太阴。其别者，上循臂，乘肩髃，上曲颊偏齿。以穴在臂外侧之上廉，故曰偏；而交于手太阴，亦在臂内之上廉，亦当曰偏，故曰偏历，言此络历于二经也。"

《经穴释义汇解》："偏历，手阳明络脉，在腕后三寸。手阳明脉在本穴偏行而出，此络经历手臂走向手太阴之脉，故名偏历。"

7 温溜（郄穴）

【出处】《黄帝明堂经》。

【别名】逆注，蛇头。

【穴义】温，温暖；溜，流动。本穴主治肘臂寒痛、寒厥头痛等寒湿濡滞之症；又可治疗腹痛肠鸣，有决滞通畅之力。以"温溜"命名，形容经气至此如温水流过，喻其温经散寒、温热通畅之功。

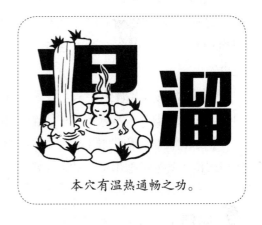

本穴有温热通畅之功。

【定位】腕背侧远端腕横纹上 5 寸，阳溪与曲池连线上。

【主治】①头痛，面肿，咽喉肿痛；②腹痛，肠鸣；③热病；④肩背酸痛，疔疮。

【释义摘录】

《医经理解》："温溜，手阳明之郄也。在手腕后五六寸间。温为阳气，阳气所注，故曰温溜。"

《经穴解》："穴名温溜者，以其出经火之后，故为温溜。温溜者，脉之细流也。"

《经穴释义汇解》："温溜为手阳明之郄，郄是人体之间隙，乃气血汇聚之处。溜与留同，含停留之意。阳明为多气多血、阳气钟聚之经，阳气温热，穴为阳气所注，故名温溜。"

《针灸穴名解》："温，和暖也。溜，顺逝也。本穴之气不弛不亢。由偏历安顺行来，具有和畅温通之意。观其所治各症，为肘臂寒痛、寒厥头痛及寒湿濡滞之症，则知其有温热通散之力也；又治肠鸣、哕、噫，则知其有决溜疏导之力也，故称'温溜'。以其功能而得名也。温而不热、通而不湍之功，昭然如见矣。"

8 下廉

【出处】《黄帝明堂经》。

【别名】手下廉。

【穴义】上、下，指高低、前后；廉，指侧边、边缘。古称堂屋之侧边为"廉"。上廉、下廉二穴位于前臂桡侧的外缘。在下端者为"下廉"，在上端者为"上廉"，以其所在部位而得名。

【定位】肘横纹下 4 寸，阳溪与曲池连线上。

【主治】①眩晕，目痛；②肘臂肿痛、挛急。

【释义摘录】

《医经理解》："廉，隅也。下廉，在辅骨下隅……肘下臂肉高起者，谓之辅兑肉也。下廉去上廉一寸。"

《经穴解》："廉者，棱隅之称。穴在臂廉隅之下，故曰下廉。"

《古法新解会元针灸学》："下廉者，廉是分肉侧，内外两片，下居者上廉之下，故名下廉。"

《经穴释义汇解》："侧边曰廉，穴为手阳明脉之腧穴。手阳明之脉沿循前臂上方至肘外侧，穴当臂之侧边，上廉穴下一寸，故曰下廉。"

《针灸穴名解》："廉，侧也，又隅也，又棱也。其穴在前膊外侧，肉棱凸起处。在此侧棱下端者，，为'下廉'，在此侧棱上端者为'上廉'。以其所在部位而得名也。"

9 上廉

【出处】《黄帝明堂经》。

【别名】手上廉。

【穴义】上、下，指高低、前后；廉，指侧边、边缘。古称堂屋之侧边为"廉"。上廉、下廉二穴位于前臂桡侧的外缘。在下端者为"下廉"，在上端者为"上廉"，以其所在部位而得名。

【定位】肘横纹下 3 寸，阳溪与曲池连线上。

【主治】①头痛；②腹痛，肠鸣；③肩臂酸痛、麻木。

【释义摘录】

《医经理解》："廉，隅也……上廉，在辅骨上隅，肘下臂肉高起者，谓之辅兑肉也……

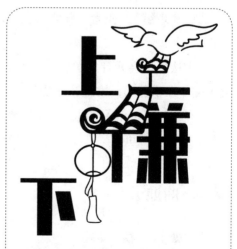

屋之边为"廉"，引申为边缘。二穴位于前臂桡侧的外缘。在下者为"下廉"，在上者为"上廉"。

上廉去三里一寸。"

《经穴解》："此穴在廉内之最高处，故曰独抵阳明之会，以在廉之上，故曰上廉。"

《古法新解会元针灸学》："上廉者，廉是洁也，内廉外廉之间，阳明清阳之气所会也。上廉郄于肺，居上而通大肠。下廉郄于心包经络，居上廉之下，而通小肠，利小便。居下廉之上，故名上廉。"

《经穴释义汇解》："侧边曰廉。穴为手阳明脉之腧穴，手阳明之脉沿循前臂上方至肘外侧，穴当臂之侧边，下廉穴之上，故曰上廉。"

10 手三里

【出处】《黄帝明堂经》作"三里"，宋代以后《针灸甲乙经》作"手三里"。

【别名】三里。

【穴义】一里，指一寸。当人屈肘时，本穴距手臂肘尖三寸，故名"三里"。因位于上肢，为与"足三里"区别，故名"手三里"。

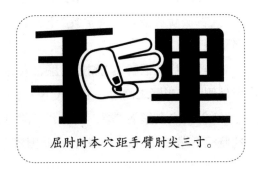
屈肘时本穴距手臂肘尖三寸。

【定位】在前臂，肘横纹下 2 寸处，阳溪与曲池连线上。

【主治】①齿痛，颊肿；②肘臂疼痛、不遂，肩背痛，腰痛。

【释义摘录】

《医经理解》："里者，脉之道也。三、五，皆阳数也。三里者，言自下廉至此凡三寸也。"

《古法新解会元针灸学》："三里者，针治逐邪远，去三里之外；又去肘端三寸，臂之上侧，在手臂部，故名手三里。"

《经穴释义汇解》："里，可作居解。穴为大肠手阳明脉之腧穴。因距手臂肘端三寸而居，故名手三里。"

11 曲池（合穴）

【出处】《灵枢·本输》。

【别名】无。

【穴义】曲，屈曲；池，水池。屈肘时，穴在肘横纹外侧端凹陷中，形似浅池，且本穴为手阳明大肠经之合穴，脉气流注此穴时，似水注入池中，故名"曲池"。

【定位】在肘横纹外侧端，尺泽与肱骨外上髁连线的中点处。

【主治】①咽喉肿痛，齿痛，目疾；②瘾疹，湿疹，瘰疬；③热病，惊痫；④手臂肿痛，上肢不遂。

【释义摘录】

《医经理解》："曲池，屈肘曲骨之中也。"

《经穴解》："此穴在肘臂屈伸之际，而本经气脉过之，故名曲池。"

《古法新解会元针灸学》："曲者，曲肘之处也；池者，阳经有阴气所聚，阴阳通化，治气分亦能养阴，故名曲池。"

《针灸穴名解》："穴在曲肘横纹外侧端，肘骨曲角内缘陷中，因名'曲池'。曲肘覆手取之，立名与'曲泽'意同。"

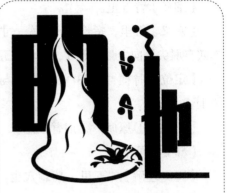

穴为合穴，脉气流注此穴时，似水注入池中。

12 肘髎

【出处】《黄帝明堂经》。

【别名】无。

【穴义】髎，骨节的空隙处。本穴位于肘关节凹陷处，故名"肘髎"。

【定位】屈肘，曲池外上方1寸，当肱骨边缘处。

【主治】肘臂酸痛、麻木、挛急。

【释义摘录】

髎，骨节的空隙处。穴位于肘关节外上方凹陷处。

《医经理解》："肘髎，在肘骨外廉陷中也。"

《经穴解》："以本经脉气之初上肘也，而穴在其上，故名肘髎以志之。"

《古法新解会元针灸学》："肘髎者，是两臂弯曲之处；髎者，骨之边髎，故名肘髎。"

13 手五里

【出处】《黄帝明堂经》。

【别名】臂五里。

【穴义】五里，指长度。古说一寸为一里，本穴自肘尖处向上量为五寸，故名"五里"。

【定位】肘横纹上 3 寸，曲池与肩髃连线上。

【主治】①瘰疬；②肘臂挛急。

【释义摘录】

《医经理解》："五里，禁刺穴也。经曰迎之五里，中道而止。五往而脏之气尽矣。故以五里名也。"

《古法新解会元针灸学》："五里者，五是五脏之阴而朝阳，里是数学之理，故名五里。"

《经穴释义汇解》："里，可作居解。五，喻中数。因穴在肘上三寸，行向里大脉中央，喻穴居手部大筋（肱二头肌）中央处，故名手五里。"

《针灸穴名解》："《内经》云：'地有五里。'里与理、裹俱通。即理其内，俾使达于外也。《针灸大成》谓主治风痨、惊恐、吐血、咳嗽、肾不纳气、心下胀满、身黄等症之有关五脏者。因名'五里'。又臂痛、嗜卧、四肢不欲动、瘰疬、疟疾、目眈眈等症，其由于内因已甚，而未现于外者，本穴亦能治之，以其病在里也。他如外因直中者，多不取此。苟辨证未明，不可莽用。故《铜人》可灸，《素问》禁针，以其关系五内，示人勿轻用也。又以其所在地位，在曲池穴上三寸处，若自肘尖向上量之，适得五寸。以古说一寸为一里计之，故名'五里'。此又一说，言其体也。"

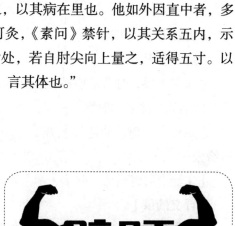

肘尖到本穴为五寸。

14 臂臑

【出处】《黄帝明堂经》。

【别名】头冲，颈冲。

【穴义】臑，指上臂部靠近腋部隆起的肌肉。本穴在曲池上七寸，臂膊肉不着骨之处，故名"臂臑"。

【定位】在臂外侧，曲池上 7 寸，三角肌前缘处。

【主治】①瘰疬；②目疾；③肩臂疼痛、不举。

【释义摘录】

《医经理解》："臑，臂上嫩白肉也。臂臑，在肘上七寸、臑肉之端也。"

穴在上臂肉不着骨处。

《经穴解》："肘之里肉曰臑，此穴在肘臑相交之处，故曰臂臑。"

《古法新解会元针灸学》："臂臑者，肩髆前廉臑肉之处，下交于臂，故名臂臑。"

《针灸穴名解》："凡肉不着骨之处，可由肉下通透者，曰臑。本穴在上膊肉不着骨之处，故名'臂臑'。举臂取之。"

15 肩髃

【出处】《黄帝明堂经》。

【别名】髃骨，中肩井，扁骨。

【穴义】肩，肩部；髃，指两边夹一角、角落，"骨"与"禺"联合起来表示骨间陷隙。本穴位于肩峰与肱骨大结节之间，举臂肩峰前凹陷中，故名"肩髃"。

【定位】在肩带部，肩峰外侧缘前端与肱骨大结节两骨间凹陷中。

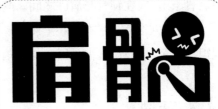

举臂时穴在肩峰前凹陷中。主治肩臂诸症。

【主治】①风疹；②上肢不遂，肩臂疼痛。

【释义摘录】

《医经理解》："骨髃，肩骨端也。"

《古法新解会元针灸学》："肩髃者，肩是肩部，髃是髃骨部。肩端髃骨与髀骨，举肩如鱼嘴开张之状也。肩端骨又名鱼骨，故名肩髃。又名中肩者，穴居肩中。又名偏骨者，偏三阳之上，肩端之下也。"

《针灸穴名解》："髃，肩骨合缝陷隙处也。又同'腢'，肩头也。穴在肩端，举臂两骨间陷者中，故名'肩髃'。"

《经穴释义汇解》："髃，指髃骨，为肩端之骨，即肩胛骨曰端，穴在肩端两骨间，故名肩髃。"

16 巨骨（手阳明经、阳跷脉交会穴）

【出处】《素问·气府论》。

【别名】无。

【穴义】巨骨，古代解剖名词，指锁骨。穴在锁骨与肩胛骨相接之处，故名。

【定位】锁骨肩峰端与肩胛冈之间凹

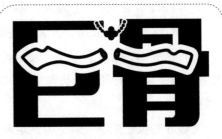

巨骨，即锁骨。穴在锁骨与肩胛骨相接之处。

陷中。

【主治】肩痛不举。

【释义摘录】

《医经理解》："巨，大也。巨骨，在肩尖上两叉骨陷中也。"

《古法新解会元针灸学》："巨骨者，巨者长而大也，大骨叉间，故名巨骨。"

《针灸穴名释义》："巨，大也。巨骨，即大骨之意。巨骨，又为古解剖名。穴与肩部之大骨相邻，故名。古之巨骨，即今之锁骨（《千金》俞府、气户、云门诸穴，均云在巨骨下）。穴在锁骨与肩胛之间。既属骨穴同名，亦为泛指肩部之大骨而言。"

《针灸穴名解》："本穴在上膊骨、肩胛骨与锁骨三骨之会，构成三角形凹隙，如循规矩，故名'巨骨'。古'巨'与'矩'通。"

17 天鼎

【出处】《黄帝明堂经》。

【别名】天顶，天盖。

【穴义】天，穴位于颈部，居天位；鼎，炉灶。本穴名有形、用两解。鼎，以三足两耳为形状特点。本穴位于缺盆上，因喻锁骨内侧端头与喉头突起部似三足鼎立，加人之两耳亦恰像其形，故名"天鼎"。按"鼎"字之义，功在水火，主治暴暗、咽肿、喉痹等火邪有碍于喉咽者，故称"天鼎"。

【定位】横平环状软骨，胸锁乳突肌后缘。

【主治】①咽喉肿痛，暴暗，呃逆；②瘰疬，瘿气。

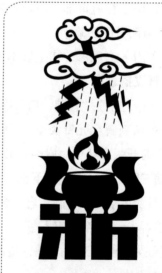

穴在缺盆上，锁骨内侧端头与喉头突起部似三足鼎立，主治火邪有碍于喉咽者。

【释义摘录】

《医经理解》："头以上为天。阳明脉出于天柱骨上，穴值其处，谓之天鼎。言天以是为鼎峙也。"

《古法新解会元针灸学》："天鼎者，肩之上谓之天部，两手阳明至肩上托头矗立，如鼎之状，故名天鼎。"

《经穴释义汇解》："鼎，为三足两耳和五味之宝器。穴在颈缺盆上，直扶突、气舍后一寸五分。因喻缺盆处两巨骨内侧端头与喉头突起部似三足鼎立，而人之两耳亦恰象其形，穴居天位，故名天鼎。"

《针灸穴名释义》:"天,见天府条。鼎,三足两耳,是古代的宝器和烹调的炊具。象人之头颈,并喻为吸入天气的贵重门户。人之头大颈细,耳在两旁,有鼎之象,乃人身之宝器也。又鼎门,城门名。《水经》榖水注:'东都城门,名曰鼎门,盖九鼎之所从入也。'穴当侧颈,自为吸入天气之重要门户。"

《针灸穴名解》:"本穴主治暴喑、气梗、咽肿、喉痹、不得息、饮食不下、喉中鸣,诸般火症之有碍于喉咽者。取此穴以通畅之。更以本穴在颈,接近于头,故能治喉咽颈项之疾。因名'天鼎'。与任脉之天突穴和协,且与挨邻也。兹以炊事喻之,鼎为炉灶,突则烟囱也。均以其有关水火,而义则调和也。故喉咽颈项有疾多用之。"

18 扶突

【出处】《灵枢·本输》。

【别名】水穴,水泉。

【穴义】扶,铺四指为扶,即一扶法。除拇指外四指并拢,四横指宽度约当同身寸3寸。突,突出、高耸,形容突起之处。本穴在喉结突起旁开三寸(一扶)处,故名"扶突"。

【定位】横平喉结,胸锁乳突肌前、后缘中间。

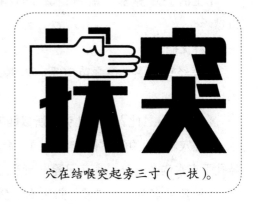

穴在结喉突起旁三寸(一扶)。

【主治】①咽喉肿痛,暴喑,呃逆;②咳嗽,气喘;③瘿气。

【释义摘录】

《医经理解》:"扶突,在曲颊下一寸。言头面突起于上,以此为扶也。"

《经穴解》:"突者,通气之名,在任经之在喉者有天突,在胃经之在于其旁者有水突,以咽水谷而有名也。"

《古法新解会元针灸学》:"扶突者,扶者扶也,突者卒跳也,故名扶突。胃水满则扶突跳动不休。又因金能生水助肾、通金津玉液,故又名水泉也。"

《针灸穴名解》:"'突',泉名,又跳跃也,又冲撞也。抚本穴则突突应手,如皮下有水泉涌突之状,因名'扶突'。又烟囱曰'突'。其所治症与天鼎穴略同。针灸者常比天鼎如炉灶,本穴犹烟囱也。借此通畅之力,泻除幽郁之火。如治暴喑、气梗、喘息等症。与任脉之天突穴所治略同。凡穴下扪之有跳突者,须以指甲深掐,然后下针,防伤动脉也。"

19 口禾髎

【出处】《黄帝明堂经》。

【别名】禾髎，长频。

【穴义】髎，空穴。本穴在口鼻之间，鼻下人中旁，鼻孔状如空穴，且此处胡须如禾，故名"口禾髎"。

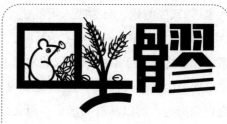

穴在鼻孔外缘下、口唇之上，口食谷。

【定位】横平人中沟上 1/3 与下 2/3 交点，鼻孔外缘直下。

【主治】① 鼻塞、鼽衄；② 口眼㖞斜，口噤。

【释义摘录】

《医经理解》："谷之苗曰禾。禾髎，在直鼻孔下夹人中旁五分，言其间髭出如禾也。"

《经穴解》："此穴近鼻孔旁，所以闻五谷之香气者，此穴近之，故曰禾髎。"

《经穴释义汇解》："髎，与窌同。窌，空穴也。穴为大肠手阳明脉之空穴，位在直鼻孔下夹水沟旁五分，言其间髭出如禾，又因穴近口处，故名口禾髎。"

《针灸穴名释义》："禾，曲头木。髎，见肘髎条。指穴在形如曲头木的鼻唇沟之下方而言。禾髎，早已误作'禾髎'，《说文》：'禾，木之曲头止不能上也。'禾，读鸡（jī）音，是典型的象形字。髎，是近骨的孔隙。'禾髎'之名最为形象。以'禾'为'禾'，传抄之误也。"

20 迎香

【出处】《黄帝明堂经》。

【别名】冲阳。

【穴义】迎，迎面，当面；香，香味，泛指气味。鼻为嗅觉器官，本穴在鼻翼旁五分，可治鼻塞不闻香臭，人性喜香恶臭，故名"迎香"。

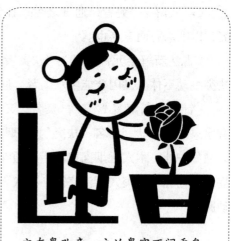

穴在鼻孔旁，主治鼻塞不闻香臭。

【定位】在面部，在鼻翼外缘中点旁，鼻唇沟中。

【**主治**】鼻渊，鼻衄，口眼㖞斜，面痒，面肿。

【**释义摘录**】

《医经理解》："迎香，在鼻孔旁五分，言鼻从此迎香而入也。"

《经穴解》："迎香以鼻闻香臭而得名也。本经于此穴而上交于足阳明也。"

《古法新解会元针灸学》："迎香者，迎者应遇；香者芳香之味。香气近鼻无知觉，刺之即知。又因足阳明宗气所和，开窍于口，脾味香，故名迎香。"

《经穴释义汇解》："本穴在鼻孔旁五分，言鼻从此迎香而入，又穴属于手阳明大肠经，与肺为表里，肺开窍于鼻，本穴可治鼻塞不闻香臭，因名迎香。"

第四章

足阳明胃经穴

1 承泣（足阳明、阳跷脉、任脉交会穴）

【出处】《黄帝明堂经》。

【别名】鼸穴，面髎，溪穴。

【穴义】承，承接；泣，无声流泪而哭。哭泣时，泪水直流而下，本穴位于瞳孔直下，眶下缘处，恰好承载眼泪，故名"承泣"。

【定位】在面部，眼球与眶下缘之间，瞳孔直下。

【主治】①目赤肿痛，迎风流泪，夜盲，近视，眼睑眴动；②口眼㖞斜。

【释义摘录】

《医经理解》："在目下陷中，上直瞳子。言泣下则此相承也。"

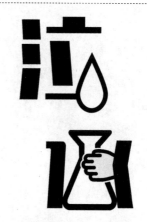

穴在瞳孔直下眶下缘，恰好承载眼泪。

《经穴解》："穴在目下为泣之所至，故曰承泣。"

《古法新解会元针灸学》："承者，承目之纲；泣者，目之酸处泪出也，故名承泣。"

《针灸穴名解》："穴在目下七分，正目直瞳子，为阳跷脉与任脉及足阳明之会。治诸般目疾。穴处俗称泪窝，因名'承泣'。口㖞泪冷者，取之效。"

2 四白

【出处】《黄帝明堂经》。

【别名】无。

【穴义】四,四方;白,明亮,光明。穴在目下一寸,主治目疾,针刺本穴能使目明四方,故名"四白"。

【定位】在面部眶下孔处。

【主治】①目赤肿痛,目翳,迎风流泪,眼睑瞤动,面痛,面肌抽搐,口眼㖞斜;②头痛,晕眩。

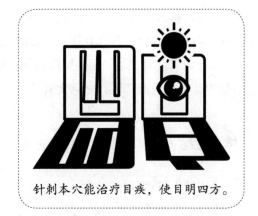

针刺本穴能治疗目疾,使目明四方。

【释义摘录】

《医经理解》:"在目下一寸,向烦骨颧空,正视取之。言四面皆白肉也,故曰四白。"

《经穴解》:"四面皆白,此穴在中,故曰四白。"

《古法新解会元针灸学》:"四白者,四是面之四方易见之处,白者目下明白也。又与目之白轮相近,肝开窍于目,至期门化气,由足阳明直通目中,化光色白,故名四白。"

《经穴释义汇解》:"白,明也。穴在目下一寸,针四分,主目疾,使目明四方而光明,故曰四白。"

3 巨髎（足阳明经、阳跷脉交会穴）

【出处】《黄帝明堂经》。

【别名】无。

【穴义】巨,大也;髎,空穴也。本穴位于鼻旁颧骨下缘,穴处凹陷甚大,故名"巨髎"。

【定位】横平鼻翼下缘,瞳孔直下。

【主治】青盲,目视不明,目翳,眼睑瞤动,口眼㖞斜,唇颊顿肿。

穴在鼻旁颧骨下缘,穴处凹陷甚大。

【释义摘录】

《医经理解》:"亦直瞳子,夹鼻孔旁八分,言其骨空最寥阔也。"

《经穴解》:"巨者,大也;髎者,穴之称也。此穴正在颧下空软处最宽,故曰巨髎。然必细按有小动脉应手,方是穴处。"

《古法新解会元针灸学》:"在颧大骨下之边髎,故名巨髎也。"

《经穴释义汇解》："巨，大也。髎，与窌同。窌，空穴也。穴为胃足阳明脉之空穴，位在夹鼻孔旁八分，其穴处骨空最寥阔，故名巨髎或巨窌。"

《针灸穴名释义》："巨，见巨骨条。髎，见肘髎条。穴在上颚骨与颧骨交接之巨大空隙中，泛指为面部髎孔之巨大者。"

4 地仓《足阳明经、阳跷脉交会穴》

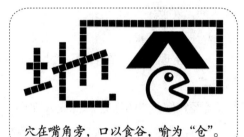

穴在嘴角旁，口以食谷，喻为"仓"。

【出处】《黄帝明堂经》。

【别名】会维，胃维。

【穴义】地，指地格。古人面分三庭，鼻以上为上庭，鼻为中庭，鼻以下为下庭，合为天人地三格。本穴在鼻下嘴角旁，属地格。仓，藏谷之处。口以食谷，食物常积储腮齿之间，故喻其处为仓。故名"地仓"。

【定位】口角旁开0.4寸。

【主治】口眼㖞斜，语言謇涩，流涎。

【释义摘录】

《医经理解》："夹口吻旁四分，外如近下，微有动脉，口以入谷，故谓之仓。唇在面之下部，故谓地也。"

《经穴解》："此穴在面最下，故有地之称。以本经为仓廪之官，乃饮食所入，故曰地仓。"

《古法新解会元针灸学》："地仓者，地是地格，因面分三庭，鼻以上为上庭，鼻为中庭，鼻以下为下庭，合而为天人地，三格局也。仓者仓廪也，五谷之精气上华面兮，冲旋面至此而上，故名地仓。"

《针灸穴名解》："穴在口角旁四分，为手足阳明、阳跷三经之会穴。人含食物常积储腮齿之间，因喻其处为仓。又以其位于口旁颐侧，故名'地仓'。口通地气也。"

5 大迎

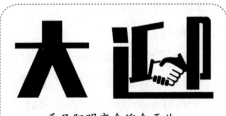

手足阳明交会迎合于此。

【出处】《素问·气穴论》《素问·气府论》。

【别名】髓孔。

【穴义】迎，相逢，交会。本穴名有两解。

其一，下颌骨古称"大迎骨"，穴当其处，故名。其二，手阳明经和足阳明经交会迎合于此，故名"大迎"。

【定位】下颌角前方，咬肌附着部的前缘凹陷中，面动脉搏动处。

【主治】口眼㖞斜，面肌抽搐，口噤，颊肿，齿痛。

【释义摘录】

《医经理解》："大迎在曲颔前一寸三分骨陷中动脉。迎，交会也。大迎为手足阳明之会。又本经自大迎循颊车上耳前，其支者自大迎前下人迎，故谓之大迎也。"

《经穴解》："此穴在颊车之前，有迎物而嚼之之象。在颈为人迎，乃迎物而吞之象。颈为人迎，此为大迎以别之。"

《古法新解会元针灸学》："大迎者，大是大冲脉也，迎者迎气血精液之来也，故名大迎。"

《经穴释义汇解》："下颌角前方之骨称'大迎骨'，穴当其处，故名。又因手阳明大肠经，上入颧骨下方遍络于齿根，而足阳明胃经下行的一支，即由此大迎穴的前面，向下经过人迎……两经交会迎合，故名大迎。"

6 颊车

【出处】《黄帝明堂经》。

【别名】曲牙，机关。

【穴义】颊，面颊，面部左右两侧；车，车轮，有运输、运转之意。古称牙床骨为牙车，且本穴位于下颌关节可以转动之处，掌管诸齿开合，故名"颊车"。穴近下齿，下齿痛宜取之。

【定位】下颌角前上方约一横指（中指）。

【主治】口眼㖞斜，齿痛，颊肿，口噤。

【释义摘录】

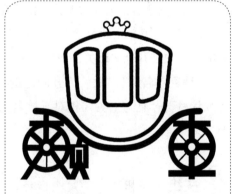

穴在下颌关节处，关节开合犹如车轮可以转动。

《医经理解》："在耳下曲颊端近前陷中。一名机关，一名曲牙，盖颊之机轴转动处也。"

《采艾编》："言齿颊转关开合，此上下牙之运纽也。"

《经穴解》："上下齿之动有车象，以在颊之侧，故曰颊车。"

《古法新解会元针灸学》："颊车者，颊是耳下牙骨也，两颊如车之有辖，即名颊车。机关者，是口开合之机关也。曲牙者，耳下八分牙尽处有曲也。"

《经穴释义汇解》："穴在耳下曲颊端牙车骨处，故名颊车。又穴位于颊之机轴转动处，故又名机关。"

《针灸穴名释义》："颊，面颊，此处指上颌骨。车，车轮，指下颌骨。颊车，即下颌关节可以转动之处。"

7 下关（足阳明经、足少阳经交会穴）

【出处】《素问·气穴论》《灵枢·本输》。

【别名】无。

【穴义】下，指颧骨弓下方，与上关相对；关，为开阖的枢机。本穴位于颧骨弓下方牙关处，司牙关之开阖，故名为"下关"。

【定位】颧弓下缘中央与下颌切迹间的凹陷中。

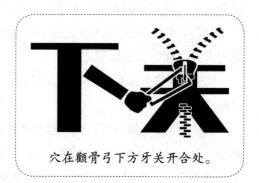

穴在颧骨弓下方牙关开合处。

【主治】①齿痛，颊肿，口眼㖞斜，下颌关节脱位；②耳聋，耳鸣。

【释义摘录】

《医经理解》："下关，在耳前动脉下廉。谓头以此为下关也。"

《经穴解》："客主人为上关，此穴正直在其下，故曰下关。"

《古法新解会元针灸学》："下关者，因牙关分上下二处，上关即客主人，下者下片部也，牙关是开合之机关，属下故名下关，手足阳明脉会此。"

《针灸穴名解》："关，为开阖之枢机。本穴有关牙齿开阖，故称之以'关'。又以其在颧骨弓下，且与上关穴相对，故名为'下关'。以治牙齿、眼、耳、偏风诸症，取意于'关'也。"

8 头维（足阳明经、足少阳经、阳维脉交会穴）

【出处】《黄帝明堂经》。

【别名】无。

【穴义】维，维护。穴在头部额角入发际处，其功用主要为抵御外感侵袭，以维护头部，有如抵角的防御作用，故名"头维"。

【定位】额角发际直上0.5寸，头正中线旁开4.5寸。

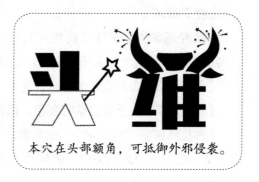

本穴在头部额角，可抵御外邪侵袭。

【主治】头痛，目痛，流泪，目视不明，眼睑眴动。

【释义摘录】

《医经理解》："在额角入发际，谓头以此为两维也。"

《经穴解》："此乃本经之脉上行，由大迎而上，所行皆手、足少阳面侧部分，而上维于额角后，横折至督经之神庭而终。此穴乃本经曲折环维之所，故曰头维。"

《古法新解会元针灸学》："头维者，手足阳明主司事治化有维之用，至头维而终致无维，动极思静，静极思动，头部维护手足阳明之会，故名头维。"

《针灸穴名解》："维，护持也。穴在额角，犹抵角之作防御也，故名'头维'。治风热头痛、目眴、泪出等病。所治以外感侵袭为主，内伤诸症次之，亦抵御外侮之意也。"

9 人迎（足阳明经、足少阳经交会穴）

【出处】《素问·气府论》《灵枢·本输》。

【别名】天五会。

【穴义】本穴居于颈部结喉旁两侧颈总动脉搏动处，即切诊部位的"人迎脉"，故名"人迎"。之所以称此动脉为"人迎脉"，可能是因为古人认为这一区域是迎候五脏六腑之气来滋养人体的地方。

【定位】横平喉结，胸锁乳突肌的前缘，颈总动脉搏动处。

【主治】①头痛，眩晕；②气喘；③咽喉肿痛，瘰疬，瘿气。

【释义摘录】

《医经理解》："一名天五会。天五，土也，胃土之会于上者也。穴在头下夹颈结喉旁一寸五分，有大动脉应手，古者从此候三阳之气。故谓是人气所迎会也。"

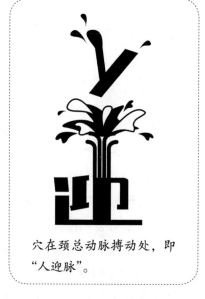

穴在颈总动脉搏动处，即"人迎脉"。

《经穴解》："穴在颈，大动脉应手，夹结喉两旁一寸五分，仰而取之，以候五脏气。足阳明、少阳之会。"

《古法新解会元针灸学》："人者，人之宗气合谷精以养先天造物之机能，五脏之气冲来所会，而收谷精，以养五脏之原，使清阳之气混合氧气冲来，走少阳养筋，还胃以安宗筋。古人以左为人迎，紧盛者伤寒；右为气口，紧盛者伤食。今以左右手寸口分之，正所谓其善思也。伤寒系天外之邪，伤食系阴积之邪，胃之经络又系行腹之正，在腹两旁、面之侧。以伤寒论之，正所谓司半阴半阳也。从阳入阴，从阴走阳，故此名人迎，又名五会之说也。"

《经穴释义汇解》："穴属阳明胃经，居颈部结喉旁两侧颈总动脉搏动处，因正值切诊部位的人迎脉，故以为名。"

10 水突

【出处】《黄帝明堂经》。

【别名】水门。

【穴义】水，指水谷之气；突，高耸、突起，此处指喉结。本穴在颈部胸锁乳突肌前，喉结突起之旁，人当饮食下咽时，穴处气向上冲，水气同源；并且针刺该穴可治疗水饮上呛、咳逆上气等症，故名"水突"。

【定位】胸锁乳突肌前缘，当人迎与气舍连线的中点。

【主治】①咳嗽，气喘；②咽喉肿痛，瘰疬，瘿气。

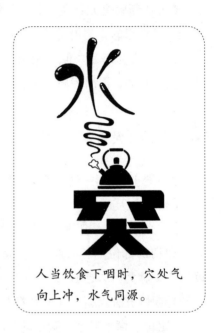

人当饮食下咽时，穴处气向上冲，水气同源。

【释义摘录】

《医经理解》："一名水门。直人迎下，夹喉咙，谓是水谷所冲突之门也。"

《经穴解》："突者，通气处也。此穴在颈之前，乃水之所由入，故曰水突。"

《古法新解会元针灸学》："水突者，水是水也；突，是仓卒而来。夫人饮水下咽，此穴必突而上也。胃伏寒水，此穴必跳动不休，故名水突。此通胃津液之官，司水津之出入，故又名水门也。"

《经穴释义汇解》："穴在颈大筋前，直人迎下，气舍上，即在颈部胸锁乳突肌前，结喉突起之旁；穴处掌握水津之出入，故名水突。"

11 气舍

【出处】《黄帝明堂经》。

【别名】无。

【穴义】气，此处指胃气；舍，指居所。本穴是足阳明胃经脉气注留之所，因名之为"气舍"。

【定位】锁骨上窝，锁骨胸骨端上缘，胸锁乳突肌胸骨头与锁骨头中间的凹陷中。

【主治】① 咳嗽，气喘；② 咽喉肿痛，瘰疬，瘿气，颈项强痛。

【释义摘录】

《医经理解》："直人迎下，夹天突陷中，气所传息之外舍也。"

《经穴解》："此穴为气上下往来之所，故曰气舍。"

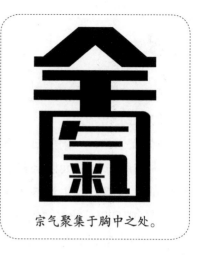

宗气聚集于胸中之处。

《古法新解会元针灸学》："气舍者，气是胃气，舍此而上经络也，故名气舍。"

《经穴释义汇解》："舍，有居留之意。穴在颈部，直人迎下，在天突穴的两旁凹陷中，为足阳明胃经脉气注留处所，故名气舍。"

12 缺盆

【出处】《素问·刺热》。

【别名】天盖。

【穴义】缺盆，缺盆骨，即锁骨。本穴在乳头直上锁骨上缘凹陷正中，故名。

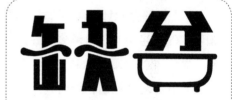

穴在锁骨上缘，凹陷如盆。

【定位】锁骨上大窝，锁骨上缘凹陷中，前正中线旁开 4 寸。

【主治】① 咳嗽，气喘；② 咽喉肿痛，瘰疬，缺盆中痛。

【释义摘录】

《医经理解》："缺盆，在肩上横骨陷中。骨形如缺盆。"

《经穴解》："此穴之名，以形有缺盆之状而名之也。然此穴乃各经上下往来入腹之处，关系甚重，断不可深刺。此处如肿，外溃则生，内溃则死，不溃亦死。"

《古法新解会元针灸学》："缺盆者，盆骨下缺处，故名缺盆。又名天盖者，肩盘象天之盖下，经气冲至而盖开，故又名天盖。"

《针灸穴名释义》："缺，空缺。盆，阔口盛器。缺盆，古代解剖名。指其位于缺盆处也。缺乃空缺与空虚之处，与残缺之意有别。故缺盆可以理解为有如无盖之盆。锁骨上窝正如盆之无盖，空虚如缺。《金针梅花诗钞》缺盆条：'肩下有窝如盆缺，横骨中央缺盆穴。'对'盆缺'和'缺盆'已经作了分别和说明。"

13 气户

【出处】《黄帝明堂经》。

【别名】无。

【穴义】户，一扇门曰"户"。"气户"在胸，内应肺，与手太阴肺经"云门"相平，均指纳气之门户，主治咳逆上气、胸背痛、胸胁满、喘息等，故名"气户"。

【定位】锁骨下缘，前正中线旁开4寸。

【主治】①咳嗽，气喘；②胸痛，胸胁胀痛。

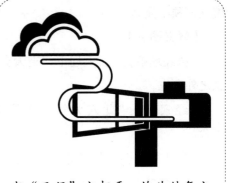

与"云门"穴相平，均为纳气之门户。

【释义摘录】

《医经理解》："气户，在巨骨下，去中行四寸，谓气之内户也。"

《经穴解》："凡各经之穴，在胸者无不主气，而胃经之下胸，此穴为首，故曰气户。"

《古法新解会元针灸学》："气户者，针巨骨，手阳明之气下降气户，而下脘痞。因手阳明主气，足阳明气血俱多。气户者，交经气出入之户口，降逆振肝之腧。又系肺之上部，肺主气，手阳明为肺之府，气逆过气户，即冲巨骨，故有气在肩背则肩背刺疼。此穴实与五脏之气相通，故名气户。"

《经穴释义汇解》："穴在巨骨下输（俞）府两旁各二寸凹陷处，按俞府乃肾足少阴经脉气会聚之处，本穴又属足阳明脉气所发之处，似可谓气之内户，即受纳气之门户，故名气户。"

14 库房

【出处】《黄帝明堂经》。

【别名】无。

【穴义】库房，指储物之仓。胸似库，藏心肺，本穴位于胸膺处，主治胸胁支满、咳逆上气等实满之证，故名"库房"。

【定位】第1肋间隙，前正中线旁开4寸。

【主治】①咳嗽，气喘，咳唾脓血；②胸

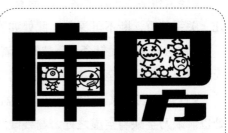

本穴主治胸肺实满之证，如储物之库。

胁胀痛。

【释义摘录】

《医经理解》:"库房,在气户下一寸六分。屋翳,在库房下一寸六分。库以藏物,翳为隐处,库之房,屋之翳,皆自户而言其深也。"

《经穴解》:"凡藏物之所,则名曰库。胸之所藏,心肺也。主气与血之本。一身之所以生者,气与血而已,而胸中藏其本,故曰库房。"

《古法新解会元针灸学》:"库房者,库是血津液之储库,房者近乳房也。妇人生子无经血,其原阴冲至膻中化气,而津液注库房,过屋翳,走膺窗,而通乳汁,故名库房也。"

《经穴释义汇解》:"库,兵车藏也,胸似库,藏心肺,穴居胸膺,又谓穴在气户之后,而喻穴居深处入库,故名库房。"

《针灸穴名解》:"本穴治症,多关肺脏,喻犹胸之储藏室也。其所治症,为胸胁满、咳逆上气、气不归根,及吐脓血浊沫诸病,均属气分上越之症,乃气逆,非气虚也。所治均属实证,有如宿积者,故曰'库房'。可治年久陈滞之病,可会意库藏之义也。"

15 屋翳

【出处】《黄帝明堂经》。

【别名】无。

【穴义】翳,用羽毛做的华盖,引申为起遮蔽作用的东西。本穴上有库房之房,下有膺窗之窗,本穴居中,犹如屋檐之遮翳,为胸部提供卫外屏障,主治咳嗽、气喘等局部病症,故名"屋翳"。

【定位】第2肋间隙,前正中线旁开4寸。

【主治】①咳嗽,气喘;②胸满,乳痈。

【释义摘录】

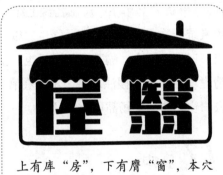

上有库"房",下有膺"窗",本穴居中,犹如屋檐之遮翳。

《经穴解》:"此穴与任脉中行紫宫平直,宫之旁则为屋之所。翳者,蔽也,故曰屋翳。"

《古法新解会元针灸学》:"屋翳者,因乳房隆起如屋,翳者如屋之顶盖,故名屋翳。"

《经穴释义汇解》:"屋,车盖也。翳,华盖也。肺者,五脏六腑之盖也。肺为华盖,穴主肺疾,又因穴在气户、库房之后而喻其深而隐曲,故名屋翳。"

16 膺窗

【出处】《黄帝明堂经》。

【别名】无。

【穴义】膺，胸膺；窗，窗牖，房屋通风透气之处。穴在胸部，性善疏利，能泄胸中郁气，犹如开窗通气，故名"膺窗"。

【定位】第3肋间隙，前正中线旁开4寸。

【主治】胸满，气喘，乳痈。

【释义摘录】

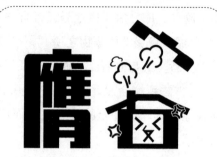

本穴性善疏利，能泄胸中郁气，如同胸膺开窗通气之处。

《医经理解》："膺窗，在屋翳下一寸六分，是胸膺所通气处也。"

《经穴解》："有屋必有窗，此穴在屋翳之下，如屋之有窗，然穴正在膺，故曰膺窗。"

《古法新解会元针灸学》："膺窗者，膺是肩臂连胸之膺，窗是孔窗窍也。足三阴由胸走手之经孔，又系妇人通乳之孔窍，故名膺窗。"

《针灸穴名解》："穴在乳盘上缘，性善疏利，能泄胸中郁气。凡属胸中积闷之症，本穴统能治之，喻犹开窗通气也。以上诸穴，曰库、曰房、曰屋、曰舍，喻其容纳储积也。曰窗、曰户，喻其开阖通畅也。窗之通，多属清；门之通，多属浊。人身以胸膺为清虚境界，腹为秽浊之域。本穴在膺，故名'膺窗'。以其所通者，为轻清之气也。本穴曰窗，非门关畅豁可比也。"

17 乳中

【出处】《黄帝明堂经》。

【别名】乳首。

【穴义】乳，乳房。穴在乳头正中，故名"乳中"。

【定位】乳头中央。

【主治】①癫狂痫；②滞产；③乳痈。

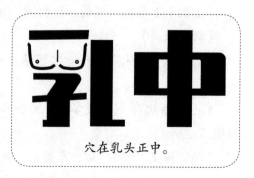

穴在乳头正中。

【释义摘录】

《医经理解》:"乳中,当乳之中。"

《经穴解》:"穴在当乳中。"

18 乳根

【出处】《黄帝明堂经》。

【别名】薛息。

【穴义】穴在乳下,乳房之根部,故名"乳根"。

【定位】第 5 肋间隙,前正中线旁开 4 寸。

【主治】①咳嗽,气喘,胸满,胸痛;②乳痈,乳癖,乳汁少。

【释义摘录】

《古法新解会元针灸学》:"乳根者,乳房下之根结也,故名乳根。"

《针灸穴名解》:"穴在乳房下缘,故名'乳根'。"

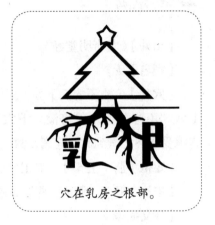

穴在乳房之根部。

19 不容

【出处】《黄帝明堂经》。

【别名】无。

【穴义】容,指容纳。穴处脐上 6 寸,对应胃上口,"不容"比喻水谷至此已满,不能再容纳,故以为名。

【定位】脐中上 6 寸,前正中线旁开 2 寸。

【主治】①腹满呕吐,食欲不振;②腹痛引背。

【释义摘录】

《医经理解》:"不容,在第四肋端,夹幽门,去中行二寸,言水谷至此,已满而不能容也。"

《经穴解》:"此穴初离胸而入腹,正在膈膜之外,环胃而生,遮隔上下之所,与肾经幽门穴平直,与中行巨阙平直。饮食之入胃者,正由上脘而下,胃脘之四外,皆为膈所环生,何一物之能容哉,故曰不容。"

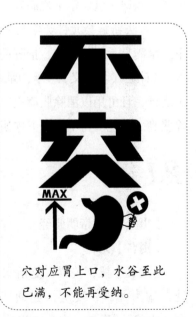

穴对应胃上口,水谷至此已满,不能再受纳。

《古法新解会元针灸学》："不容者，在膈微下，证胃之气满，不容浊气熏蒸五脏也，故名不容。"

《针灸穴名释义》："不，不能，不可。容，容纳，包容。谓其可治胃不能容诸病也。胃为水谷之海，虚而能容。用于呕吐反胃、腹满疢癖诸病，则不容者又将能容矣。"

20 承满

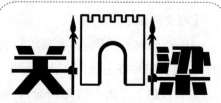

【出处】《黄帝明堂经》。

【别名】无。

【穴义】穴在不容穴下方，对应胃之上部。上穴"不容"似水谷将溢，下穴"承满"则言承受水谷之量到此已充满，故名"承满"。

胃腑承受水谷之量到此已满。

【定位】脐中上5寸，前正中线旁开2寸。

【主治】肠鸣，腹痛，腹胀，噎膈，吐血。

【释义摘录】

《医经理解》："承满，在不容下一寸，对上脘。言承者已满也。"

《经穴解》："此穴紧在中行上脘穴、二行肾经通谷穴旁，乃胃入饮食之所。承者，上之所入也；满者，下之所得也。胃之口曰贲门，饮食之精气，从此上输于脾，宣播于诸脉，故曰承满。承下之满者，而上输于脾也。"

《古法新解会元针灸学》："承满者，胃食而气至肠部，食满后而气复满于胃，食即下。承满是承胃气之满，推陈而至新，故名承满。"

《针灸穴名释义》："承，承担，承受。满，饱满，充满。承满者，上腹可以承受饱满之处，且可用以消除胀满也。上腹本可承受饱满，但过满又将不能承担，且有承担消除胀满之责也。与不容上下连属，可以互参。"

21 梁门

【出处】《黄帝明堂经》。

【别名】无。

【穴义】梁，关梁，泛指水陆交通必经之处，喻为关键、要会；亦通"梁"，泛指粮食、水谷。"胃者，水谷之海也"（《灵枢·海论》），该穴与关门对应胃脘，为胃气出入的

梁门为胃气出入的重要门户，犹如古代设防戍守的关卡。关门穴处胃腑之关卡，水谷入肠之要塞。

重要门户，故名"梁门"。

【定位】脐中上4寸，前正中线旁开2寸。

【主治】脘腹痞胀，腹痛，泄泻，食欲不振。

【释义摘录】

《经穴解》："此穴横直与中行中脘平，次行肾经阴都平，盛受饮食而化之，不宜复出，有门之象焉。梁者，所由以通于门，上下之界也。"

《古法新解会元针灸学》："梁门者，心下痞闷如伏梁，即梁门横结阴气，心火降而不下，水火未能既济，又因胃之中部瘢肉结处，故名梁门。"

《经穴释义汇解》："穴在承满下一寸。与中脘穴相对，系胃之津梁关要，为胃气出入之重要门户，故名梁门。"

22 关门

【出处】《黄帝明堂经》。

【别名】无。

【穴义】关，指关藏，关闭；门，出入之处。穴处为胃腑之关卡，水谷入肠之要塞，故名"关门"。

【定位】脐中上3寸，前正中线旁开2寸。

【主治】①腹痛，鼓胀，肠鸣，泄泻；②水肿，遗尿。

【释义摘录】

《医经理解》："关门，在梁门下一寸，对建里。盖胃之津梁关要也。"

《经穴解》："此穴与中行建里、次行石关平，正在胃中脘之下，饮食之入此者，断不可复出，如关之不可轻过也，故曰关门。"

《古法新解会元针灸学》："关门者，胃气出入食下之关，胆汁入胃助消化而润肠之门，故名关门。"

《针灸穴名释义》："关，指关藏，关闭。门，见云门条。指其为纳谷与收藏水谷之门户。穴居胃底，为胃之关。又可治完谷不化、大肠滑泄诸病。关门之名具双重意义。"

23 太乙

【出处】《黄帝明堂经》。

【别名】太一。

【穴义】太，同"大"；乙，"鱼肠谓之乙"（《尔雅》）。穴在脐上2寸，内应横结肠，肠曲似乙形，主治肠鸣、腹胀等肠疾，故名"太乙"。

【定位】脐中上2寸，前正中线旁开2寸。

【主治】①癫痫，吐舌；②腹痛，腹胀，呕吐。

【释义摘录】

《医经理解》："太乙者，东方之木，生气之神也，正对下脘。胃留水谷。是生气所从始也。"

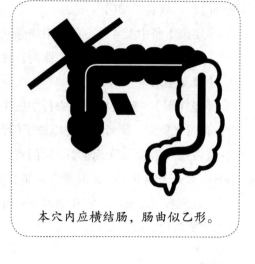

本穴内应横结肠，肠曲似乙形。

《经穴解》："太乙者，火神。此穴与中行下脘平，次行商曲平，正胃中腐化水谷之所。无火焉以主之，则水谷焉能腐化乎，故名曰太乙。"

《经穴释义汇解》："太，作通解；鱼肠谓之乙。穴在关门下一寸，肠屈曲似乙形。穴主肠疾，有通肠之意，故曰太乙；又释：太乙，星名，北辰神名。穴在腹，坤为腹，坤居正北，应古星象太乙，故名太乙。"

《针灸穴名释义》："太乙，象天地混沌之气；又神名，星名，地名。此处以穴位之所在，及其功能与大肠之形象而言。"

24 滑肉门

【出处】《黄帝明堂经》。

【别名】无。

【穴义】滑，利。穴位处皮松肉软，内应腹膜油脂，且穴属足阳明胃经，善治脾胃之疾，为通利脾胃、祛除痰湿之要穴，故名"滑肉门"，是临床常用的"减肥穴"。

【定位】脐中上1寸，前正中线旁开2寸。

【主治】①癫痫，吐舌；②腹痛，腹胀，呕吐。

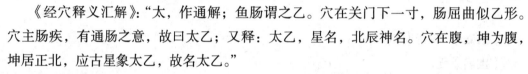

穴处皮松肉软，内应腹膜油脂。

【释义摘录】

《医经理解》："滑肉门，在太乙下一寸。穴在腹之滑肉处。"

《经穴解》："此穴与中行水分穴平直，胃中所腐之水谷，将由此而转入小肠，小肠为受盛之官，如胃中腐之不化，则下入小肠，必不能使糟粕入大肠，汁水入膀胱，如无门以阻之，而俟其腐化，则入胃即入小肠，入小肠即入大肠，为洞泄矣。滑肉者，言不可滞也；门者，又言不可速也，即拦之义也。"

《古法新解会元针灸学》："滑肉门者，滑是光滑，肉是肌肉，门是门户也。胃下附肠部有软肉生质，而滑润胃肠口门，故名滑肉门。"

《经穴释义汇解》："滑，利也。脾生肉，阳明者，胃肠也……阳明主肉，脾与胃相表里，穴为足阳明脉气所发，善治脾胃之疾，为利脾胃之门，位在太乙下一寸，腹之滑肉处，故曰滑肉门。"

25 天枢（大肠募穴）

【出处】《黄帝明堂经》。

【别名】长溪，谷门，循际。

【穴义】枢，枢纽。天枢，星名，北斗七星第一星，主持天际各星运行，为天象运行之枢纽。穴居人身上下枢要之处，为中、下二焦之气升降出入的枢纽，故名"天枢"。

【定位】横平脐中，前正中线旁开2寸。

【主治】①腹痛，腹胀，肠鸣，泄泻，便秘；②月经不调，痛经。

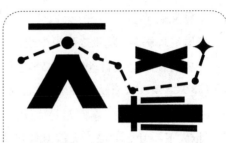

穴居腹部，为中下二焦之气升降出入的枢纽，应天枢之星象。

【释义摘录】

《医经理解》："夹脐旁二寸，为天枢。人以手指天、以足踹地，此正当人身之中，故为天之枢纽。"

《经穴解》："枢者，所以司起闭，分司上下之称也。此穴在脐之旁，而上下既分，身之前后俯仰者，此穴亦主之，故曰天枢。又曰大肠之募。"

《古法新解会元针灸学》："天枢者，天是上部之气，枢是枢纽，司转输，清气连胃府，上通肺金转浊气出肠部，故名之枢。长者，是胃肠相通；溪者，肠部金汁常注于此，似长溪之状也。谷门者，是水谷消化津液出入之门，大肠与胃化阴通脏之募也。"

《针灸穴名释义》："天，天地，此指人之上下半身而言。枢，枢机，枢纽。喻穴居人身上下枢要之处也。《素问·至真要大论》：'身半以上，天之分也，天气主之；身半以下，地之分也，地气主之。半，所谓天枢也。'《六微旨大论》：'天枢之上，天气主之；天枢之下，地气主之。'天枢，本为北斗第一星，此借喻为天地之枢机。与其外侧之大横，可以互观。"

26 外陵

【出处】《黄帝明堂经》。

【别名】无。

【穴义】外，与"内"相对；陵，大土山。腹部用力时，腹直肌隆起，外形如山陵，穴当其处，故名"外陵"。

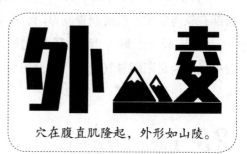

穴在腹直肌隆起，外形如山陵。

【定位】脐中下 1 寸，前正中线旁开 2 寸。

【主治】腹痛，腹胀。

【释义摘录】

《医经理解》："陵土之高阜处也。外陵在天枢下一寸。"

《古法新解会元针灸学》："外陵者，外是如地之外也，陵者高也。地外藏土募，有阴气陵天之象，穴有达高临下之功，故名外陵。"

《针灸穴名解》："本穴与足太阴之腹结穴挨近。腹结穴在大横穴下一寸三分，本穴在天枢穴下一寸。大横、天枢俱与脐平。本穴与腹结穴横距约寸半至二寸许。诸书记载不一，相差无几。又'结'字有凝滞积聚之意，即内有所结，外现棱起也。又如人在努力时，则脐腹之气，显然内结，而外表则出现硬棱，棱下是穴。因名'外陵'。本穴治绕脐腹痛，凡腹气之绕脐者，多属寒热气结。凡内有所结，则外现隆起。腹结与外陵两穴，有内外相关之象。"

27 大巨

【出处】《黄帝明堂经》。

【别名】腋门，液门，掖门。

【穴义】巨，大。本穴在腹壁肌肉方大处，故名"大巨"。

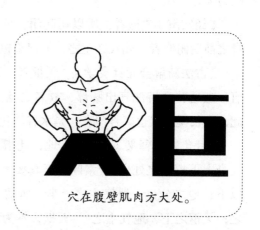

穴在腹壁肌肉方大处。

【定位】脐中下 2 寸，前正中线旁开 2 寸。

【主治】①腹胀，腹痛；②小便不利，疝气，遗精。

【释义摘录】

《医经理解》："巨，方大也。大巨，在外陵下一寸。言此为腹之方大处也。"

《针灸穴名解》："本穴内应小肠及膀胱部位，小肠属手太阳经，膀胱属足太阳经，两太阳俱称巨阳。又'太'与'大'通，故本穴命名'大巨'二字，以其功用在两太阳经也。其主治为小腹胀满，及小便不利，有关小肠及膀胱用事，故名'大巨'。即太阳与巨阳之意也。"

《针灸穴名释义》："大，饱满充实之意。巨，同钜，富也。大巨者，象腹壁之丰满光泽，而内容又复钜富也。"

28 水道

【出处】《黄帝明堂经》。

【别名】无。

【穴义】水，水液；道，通道。本穴内应膀胱，主治肾、膀胱、三焦之疾，如小便不利等，能够通调水道，使水液渗注于膀胱，功在治水，故名"水道"。

【定位】脐中下3寸，前正中线旁开2寸。

【主治】① 小便不利，小腹胀满，阴中痛，疝气；②痛经，不孕。

【释义摘录】

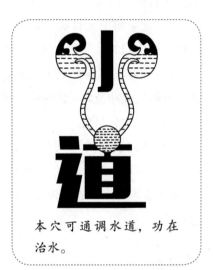

本穴可通调水道，功在治水。

《医经理解》："水道，在大巨下三寸，正当膀胱，故为出水之道。"

《经穴解》："凡经虽有各经之所治，而又以所至之部分，遂治其部分之病，而名亦命焉。如此穴实在膀胱之侧，则便之通塞，亦其所司，故曰水道，乃小肠渗水下入膀胱之道也。"

《古法新解会元针灸学》："水道者，水是水也，道是道路也，自水分化气入肺，走膈膜滤下入冲围，其胃之水化管双圈膀胱，赖肾气蒸化水湿，湛入膀胱。水常行于此，故名水道。"

《经穴释义汇解》："道，通也。肾主水，膀胱属水，三焦者水道出焉，穴主肾、膀胱、三焦之疾，通调水道，又位在大巨下一寸，正当膀胱出水之道，故名水道。"

29 归来

【出处】《黄帝明堂经》。

【别名】溪穴，肠遗，遗道。

【穴义】还者为归，返者为来。"归"和"来"均有恢复和复原之意。针灸本穴可使下垂之疾复原而愈，故名"归来"。

【定位】脐中下 4 寸，前正中线旁开 2 寸。

【主治】① 少腹疼痛，疝气；② 妇人阴冷，肿痛，月经不调。

【释义摘录】

《经穴解》："胃中所受之水谷，至此无复上逆之理，只有下行之势，故命此穴曰归来。如人之自远来归也。"

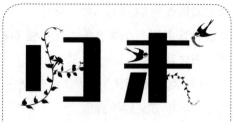

本穴主治月经不调、子宫脱垂、疝气等，可使其复原而愈。

《古法新解会元针灸学》："归者，轨道；来，去而复来。男子妇人胃气归原，谷化阴精，精化阳气，气和化质，质和精血，如归去而又复来，故名归来也。"

《经穴释义汇解》："归，还也。来，还也。穴在水道下二寸，凡因肾脏阴寒之气上逆或肝经气火冲逆而见之咳逆、骨痿、少气以及卵上入腹痛引茎等症，针灸此穴，即可还复而愈，故名归来。"

《针灸穴名释义》："归来，是返回的意思。对卵缩和阴下脱诸病，有促使恢复的作用。穴主少腹奔豚、卵上入腹引茎中痛、七疝、阴挺诸病。《金针梅花诗钞》归来条：'丸塞入腹唤归来，疝气奔豚亦妙哉。'归来者，能使不归之气、移位之丸，返回本位之意也。"

30 气冲

【出处】《黄帝明堂经》。

【别名】气街。

【穴义】其义有二。其一，冲，指冲脉。"冲脉者，起于气街，并少阴之经，夹脐上行，至胸中而散。"（《素问·骨空论》）气街为腹股沟动脉搏动处，即为气冲穴处。本穴既是足阳明之气街，又是奇经八脉之冲脉之气冲行之处，故名"气冲"，又名"气街"。其二，因功用而得名。本穴主治疝气、奔豚、妊娠子气上冲攻心等气机上冲之症。

【定位】在腹股沟，耻骨联合上缘，前正中线旁开 2 寸，动脉搏动处。

【主治】疝气，月经不调，不孕。

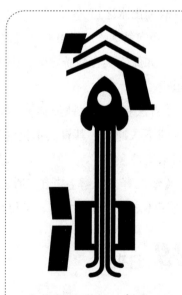

本穴主治疝气、奔豚、妊娠子气上冲攻心等气机上冲之症。

【释义摘录】

《医经理解》："气冲，又名气街。在归来下鼠蹊上一寸动脉处。气所冲行之街也。为胃脉所入，胆脉所出，冲脉所起。"

《经穴解》："此穴乃阳明直行支别内外两会之所，亦冲脉上下分行之处也。冲为血海，不曰血冲，而曰气冲，乃血之行也，非气不行，血之生也，非气不生。乃本经之要穴，亦冲脉之要穴也。"

《古法新解会元针灸学》："气冲者，三阳之气冲出，三阴之精冲来，故名气冲，气血之精道，所生大动脉，故又名气街之说也。"

《针灸穴名解》："人当呼气时，腹气下降曰归根；吸气时，腹气由本穴内部上冲，与归来穴成橐龠作用。归来穴居本穴之上，其作用为镇坠下降。本穴居归来穴之下，其作用为擎举上冲，故名气冲。"

31 髀关

【出处】《黄帝明堂经》。

【别名】无。

【穴义】髀，大腿；关，关节，此指髋关节。穴在大腿前上方，靠近髋关节处，故名"髀关"。

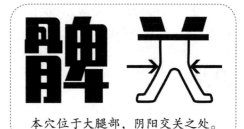

本穴位于大腿部，阴阳交关之处。

【定位】当髂前上棘与髌底外侧端的连线上，屈股时，平会阴，居缝匠肌外侧凹陷处。

【主治】下肢痿痹，屈伸不利。

【释义摘录】

《医经理解》："髀，足股骨也。髀关者，髀之机关，在膝上一尺二寸伏兔后交纹中。"

《经穴解》："胃经离腹而下行，初入于髀，有关象焉，故曰髀关。"

《古法新解会元针灸学》："髀关者，髀股骨之关节也，故名髀关也。"

《针灸穴名解》："穴在髀股外前方，膝上一尺二寸处。其经气由小腹斜走髀外侧。乃于小腹之阴达于股前之阳也。凡属经络之气，当阴侧与阳侧互通之处，不论横通斜通，多称'关'，称'门'，即阴阳交关之意。故称本穴为'髀关'。"

32 伏兔

【出处】《黄帝明堂经》。

【别名】外勾。

【穴义】伏，潜伏，伏卧。本穴在膝上六寸，大腿前隆起的股直肌处，蹲起时肌肉隆起，形似一兔伏卧，穴当其处，故名"伏兔"。

【定位】当髂前上棘与髌底外侧端的连线上，髌底上 6 寸。

【主治】下肢痿痹，膝冷，脚气。

穴在股直肌隆起处，形似卧伏之兔。

【释义摘录】

《医经理解》："伏兔，在膝上六寸起肉。其上有肉起如兔伏状也。"

《经穴解》："此以形命名者也。痈疽生此者，九死一生。"

《古法新解会元针灸学》："伏兔者，伏是潜伏，大腿肉肥如兔，跪时肉起如兔之潜而不伏也，故名伏兔。"

33 阴市

【出处】《黄帝明堂经》。

【别名】阴鼎。

【穴义】市，市集。本穴虽属阳经，但其所治多属阴寒之证，如腰膝如注水、寒疝、痿痹、阴湿、月事不调等，犹阴气之所聚，故名"阴市"。

【定位】当髂前上棘与髌底外侧端的连线上，t髌底上 3 寸。

【主治】寒疝痛引膝，下肢痿痹、屈伸不利。

本穴能消散阴翳，犹如治疗阴寒疾患之市集。

【释义摘录】

《医经理解》："阴市在膝上三寸伏兔下陷中。足为阴，此为阴之市肆也。"

《经穴解》："人之股上、膝下最寒者，皆过于此处，乃阴气之所聚也，故曰阴市。"

《针灸穴名释义》："阴，指人体的前阴部。市，遮蔽阴部的短裳。穴约当市的下缘，故名。"

《针灸穴名解》："盖谓本穴虽居阳经，而所治则多属阴症。犹与足太阴经之血海穴交易互市。故名'阴市'。本穴治腰膝如注水、寒疝痿痹、风湿、阴湿等症。凡诸阴寒疾患，皆可取此。犹治诸阴病之市集也，亦'阴市'命名之一义也。"

34 梁丘（郄穴）

【出处】《黄帝明堂经》。

【别名】无。

【穴义】梁，指物体中间高起的部分；丘，小土山，亦有突起之意。本穴在膝上二寸筋肉间隙间，穴处肌肉丰厚，隆起犹如在高地之上，故名"梁丘"。

【定位】当髂前上棘与髌底外侧端的连线上，髌底上 2 寸。

【主治】①胃痛；②乳痈，乳痛；③膝肿痛，下肢不遂。

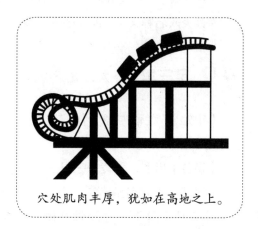

穴处肌肉丰厚，犹如在高地之上。

【释义摘录】

《医经理解》："梁丘在膝上二寸两筋间，为足阳明郄。故谓是关梁之处、丘聚之区也。"

《经穴解》："此穴在膝之后，膝之骨在其前，而股之骨又屹其两旁，有丘之象焉，故曰梁丘。"

《古法新解会元针灸学》："梁丘者，是膝梁上起肉如丘，故名梁丘。"

《针灸穴名解》："本穴在膝上筋肉隙中，阴市穴下一寸许，两筋间。曲膝取之。骨亘如梁，筋犹小丘，穴在髌上，因名'梁丘'。"

35 犊鼻

【出处】《素问·气府论》《灵枢·本输》。

【别名】无。

【穴义】犊，指小牛。穴在髌韧带外侧凹陷中，俗称"外膝眼"，膝盖骨为卵圆形，内、外膝眼在膝盖下缘，形同牛犊鼻孔，故

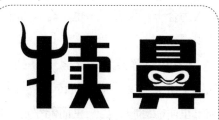

穴在外膝眼，内、外膝眼在膝盖下缘，形同牛犊鼻孔。

名"犊鼻"。足阳明胃经属土，八卦中"坤"亦属土，《易经》曰"坤为牛"，故不名猪鼻、羊鼻，而称犊鼻。

【定位】髌韧带外侧凹陷中。

【主治】膝肿痛、屈伸不利，脚气。

【释义摘录】

《医经理解》："犊鼻，在膝膑下骨解大陷中。形如牛鼻。"

《经穴解》："穴在膝膑下，胻骨上，夹解大筋陷中，形如牛鼻，故名犊鼻。"

《针灸穴名释义》："犊，小牛。鼻，口鼻。膝盖形如牛鼻，穴在膝眼中，故名。"

36 足三里（合穴，胃下合穴）

【出处】《黄帝内经》作"三里"，《太平圣惠方》始作"足三里"。

【别名】鬼邪，下陵，三里。

【穴义】本穴名解有二。其一，三里为三寸，本穴位于膝下三寸胫骨外侧，以其定位而命名。其二，里，通"理"，"三里"指本穴可统治腹部上中下三部诸症，胃痛呕吐、腹胀泄泻等均能主之，从而顾护后天之本，为强壮保健之要穴。穴在下肢，故名"足三里"，以别于"手三里"。

本穴为强壮保健要穴，故有云"常按足三里，胜吃老母鸡"。

【定位】犊鼻下3寸，距胫骨前缘一横指（中指）。

【主治】①胃痛，呕吐，呃逆，腹胀，腹痛，肠鸣，泄泻，便秘；②热病，癫狂；③乳痈；④虚劳羸瘦；⑤膝足肿痛。

【释义摘录】

《经穴解》："此穴乃胃经至要之穴，穴名三里者，言胃之经，自厉兑而上行，至其所入为合土。胃者，土也，合穴亦土也，里所以记土之远近者也，以其离井至远，故曰三里。"

《古法新解会元针灸学》："三里者，逐邪于四末，出三里之外，因其经从头至胸一气，至脐又一变，至里而转下，与太阴少阳邻里相通，所以针阳陵泉，而运胆汁入胃，补三里而能健脾，泻三里而能平肝，降逆通肠，穴在膝盖边际下三寸，故名三里。"

《针灸穴名释义》："足，指下肢，相对于手而言。三里，指长度及人身上中下三部之里。以其与外膝眼的距离长度及通乎三焦之里而言。"

《针灸穴名解》："本穴名释义有二。《灵枢·九针十二原》曰：'阳有阴疾者，取之下陵三里。'犹言陵下三寸处也。《太素·五节刺》杨上善注：'一里一寸也。'此以地位而论，言其体也。《素问·六微旨大论》云：'天枢以上，天气主之；天枢以下，地气主之；气交之分，人气从之，万物由之。'本穴统治腹部上中下三部诸症，古'理'与'里'通，是以谓之'三里'。本穴在下肢，故名'足三里'，示别于'手三里'也。"

37 上巨虚（大肠下合穴）

【出处】《黄帝内经》作"巨虚上廉"，《铜人腧穴针灸图经·足阳明胃之经左右凡三十穴》始作"上巨虚"。

【别名】巨虚上廉，上廉，巨虚，足上廉。

【穴义】巨虚，大空隙。在小腿外侧胫骨和腓骨间的大空隙中，上端和下端分别有两个穴位，本穴位于上端，故名"上巨虚"。穴为大肠下合穴，善治肠鸣、腹泻、便秘、肠痈等大肠诸疾。

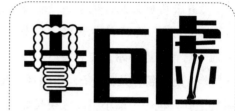

胫骨和腓骨形成的空隙上端，为巨虚上廉（上巨虚），下端为巨虚下廉（下巨虚）。

【定位】犊鼻下6寸，距胫骨前缘一横指（中指）。

【主治】①腹痛，泄泻，便秘，肠鸣，乳痈；②半身不遂，下肢痿痹，脚气。

【释义摘录】

《医经理解》："巨虚，谓胻外方大空虚处也。巨虚上廉，在三里下三寸。"

《古法新解会元针灸学》："上廉者，是腿胻筋骨肉，内外廉之上部，故名上廉。又曰膝胻骨屈曲如钜，骨与筋肉之内外分间，其虚空如巨长之状，故又名上巨虚。"

《针灸穴名解》："本穴原名'巨虚上廉'。按'巨虚'二字之义，即大空隙也；廉，侧也，隅也。本穴位于下腿外侧，大空隙之上端，故简称'上巨虚'。"

38 条口

【出处】《黄帝明堂经》。

【别名】无。

【穴义】条，形容狭长；口，缝隙。本穴与上、下巨虚同在一条狭长的缝隙中，上巨虚在缝隙上端，下巨虚在缝隙下端，本穴位于两穴之间，故名"条口"。

【定位】犊鼻下8寸，距胫骨前缘一横指（中指）。

【主治】下肢痿痹。

【释义摘录】

《医经理解》："条口，在上廉下二寸，下廉上一寸，其地按之虚大有口，又直上而下，故谓条口。"

《经穴解》："以本经之脉下行膝胻骨之外，筋之裹，直下行，有条之象，而此穴在其中，有口之象焉，故曰条口。"

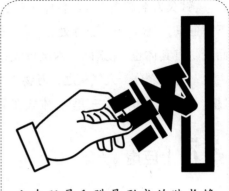

穴在胫骨和腓骨形成的狭长缝隙中。

《古法新解会元针灸学》："条口者，胫肉与筋骨分间，两筋间中有筋，白如板一条，上通于胃，下连足跗，故名条口。"

《针灸穴名释义》："条，指条风，即东北风。口，同孔，空也。条口，乃治疗下肢风病之孔穴也……谓小腿前缘狭长如条，形如刀口。穴在其处，因而得名，亦无不可。"

39 下巨虚（小肠下合穴）

【出处】《黄帝内经》作"巨虚上廉"，《铜人腧穴针灸图经·足阳明胃之经左右凡三十六》始作"上巨虚"。

【别名】下廉，巨虚下廉。

【穴义】巨虚，大空隙。在小腿外侧胫骨和腓骨之间的大空隙中，上端和下端分别有两个穴位，本穴位于下端，故名"下巨虚"。穴为小肠下合穴，故主要治疗小腹疼痛、泄泻等小肠疾患和下肢痿痹等。

【定位】犊鼻下9寸，距胫骨前缘一横指（中指）。

【主治】①小腹疼痛，泄泻，腰脊痛引睾丸；②乳痈；③半身不遂，下肢痿痹。

【释义摘录】

《医经理解》："巨虚，谓胫外方大空虚处也。巨虚下廉，在上廉下三寸。"

《经穴解》："小肠在胃之下，大肠在小肠之下，则治大肠之上廉者应在下，治小肠之下廉者应在上，然脊上大肠俞亦在上，小肠俞亦在下。乃以肺在上，心在下之位次为上下，而不以大小肠之上下为上下也。"

《古法新解会元针灸学》："胻骨跗筋分内、中、下部，故名下廉，下巨虚是一空长之下部也，故又名下巨虚。"

40 丰隆（络穴）

【出处】《灵枢·经脉》。

【别名】无。

【穴义】本穴名解有二。其一，丰，丰满；隆，隆起。穴在胫骨前肌与趾长伸肌之间，该处肌肉丰满而隆起，又处多气多血之胃经上，故名"丰隆"。其二，"丰隆"，雷神名，假借该词拟"轰隆"之声。本穴在人体下肢，祛痰利湿效果非常明显，治疗胸膈痰

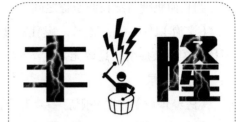

穴可祛痰利湿，治疗阴气弥漫之症，犹如雷起地下。

滞、沉昏头痛等阴气弥漫之症，犹如雷起地下，地气升为乌云，天气降为大雨，雨过天晴，乌云消散，故名"丰隆"，寓有云雷之意。

【定位】外踝尖上8寸，条口外，距胫骨前缘二横指（中指）。

【主治】①腹痛，腹胀，便秘；②咳嗽，哮喘，痰多，咽喉肿痛，胸痛；③头痛眩晕，癫狂；④下肢不遂，痿痹。

【释义摘录】

《医经理解》："丰隆，在外踝八寸，言肌肉至此而丰隆也。"

《经穴解》："血气俱盛者，胃经也，而有络焉以通于足太阴，则必盛之极者，而始溢焉络而入于他经。曰丰隆者，言盛之极也。

《古法新解会元针灸学》："丰隆者，阳血聚之而隆起，化阴络，交太阴，有丰满之象，故名丰隆。"

《针灸穴名解》："丰隆，雷神名也。《离骚》屈原吟'召丰隆使先导兮''吾令丰隆乘云兮'。《淮南子》'季春三月，丰隆乃出'，注曰'雷神也'。本穴在人体下肢，犹雷起地下也。于《易》在卦，则为'复''豫'之象，'顺动来复也'。本穴司气分之升降，于体则豫，于用则复。犹地气升为云，天气降为雨。《广雅·释天》曰：'云师，谓之丰隆。'"

41 解溪（经穴）

【出处】《灵枢·本输》。

【别名】鞋带。

【穴义】本穴在足踝部，当系解鞋带之处，故名以"解"；穴位于足背横纹正中凹

陷处，姆长伸肌腱与趾长伸肌腱之间，如溪谷之状，故名以"溪"。

【定位】在踝前侧，踝关节前面中央凹陷处，姆长伸肌腱与趾长伸肌腱之间。

【主治】①头痛，眩晕，癫狂；②腹胀，便秘；③下肢痿痹，足踝无力。

【释义摘录】

《医经理解》："在冲阳后一寸五分，足腕上系鞋带处，骨解陷中也。"

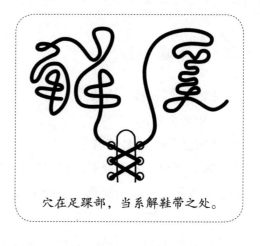

穴在足踝部，当系解鞋带之处。

《经穴解》："此穴乃古人系鞋带处。胃之别者、直行者，由膝而下行者，至此统入于足跗上，有溪之象焉。解者，膝之旁曰解，此乃解之最下之处，其脉则自解而来者，故曰解溪。"

《古法新解会元针灸学》："解溪者，是足腕陷上系带之处，解之而开，故名解溪。"

42 冲阳（原穴）

【出处】《灵枢·本输》《灵枢·根结》。

【别名】会原，跗阳。

【穴义】冲，冲击；阳，此处指足背面。穴在足背动脉处（即"跗阳脉"），以手切脉有搏动感，故名"冲阳"。

【定位】在足背最高处，足背动脉搏动处，当姆长伸肌腱与趾长伸肌腱之间。

【主治】①胃痛，腹胀；②口眼㖞斜，齿痛，面肿；③癫狂；④足痿无力、肿痛。

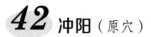

穴在足背动脉"跗阳脉"处，以手切脉有搏动感。

【释义摘录】

《医经理解》："冲阳，阳之冲，故动脉独大，在足跗上五寸高骨间动脉，去陷谷二寸。"

《经穴解》："穴名冲阳者，以冲脉下行之别者并于少阴，既渗三阳，而又斜入踝，伏行出属跗，上循跗入大趾之间，渗诸络而温足胫内……此穴虽为足阳明胃经之穴，乃亦冲、阳二脉之处，故曰冲阳。又此脉可决死生，别谷气之有无。"

《经穴释义汇解》："穴在足跗上五寸，骨间动脉上，解溪下二寸。冲，通道也。阳明多气多血，喻穴处为本经阳气之通道，故名冲阳。"

《针灸穴名释义》："冲，冲要，冲动。阳，指足背，在上。穴当定背最高处，且位于太冲之上方，故名。"

43 陷谷（输穴）

【出处】《灵枢·本输》。

【别名】无。

【穴义】陷，凹陷；谷，两山之间的夹道或者流水道。本穴位于第二、三跖骨结合部前方处，穴处凹陷如山谷，故名"陷谷"。

【定位】第2、3跖骨间，第2跖趾关节近端凹陷中。

【主治】①腹痛，肠鸣；②面肿，水肿；③足背肿痛。

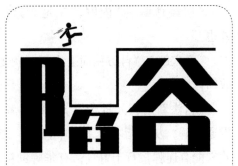

穴在第二、三跖骨结合部，凹陷如山谷。

【释义摘录】

《医经理解》："陷谷，在足大趾次趾外间本节后陷中也。"

《经穴解》："谷者，水之注也。自冲阳而至此穴部分，下于前穴，故曰陷谷。"

《针灸穴名释义》："陷，陷阱，自高而下亦谓之陷。谷，见合谷条。指经气自高而下如入于谷，及能治水病也。陷，坑也。坑，阱也，又自高而下也。《说文》：'陷，高下也。'段注：'高下者，高与下有悬殊之势也。高下之形曰陷，故自高入于下亦曰陷。凡深没其中曰陷。'经气自高处之冲阳而走向第二、三跖趾关节如阱如谷之处，陷谷之名至为恰当。"

44 内庭（荥穴）

【出处】《灵枢·本输》。

【别名】无。

【穴义】内，内部；庭，庭堂，居所，即通于门内部之庭堂。胃之经气经内庭出厉兑交隐白，厉兑在本穴之后，八卦中"兑"为门（《易经》），故此穴名为"内庭"。本穴为足阳明胃经之荥穴，荥主身热，故本穴最善退胃火，主治胃火导致的齿痛，咽喉肿病，

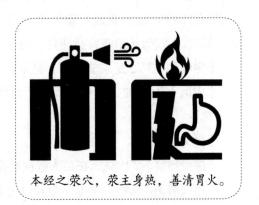

本经之荥穴，荥主身热，善清胃火。

鼻衄，便秘等。

【定位】足第2、3趾间，趾蹼缘后方赤白肉际处。

【主治】①齿痛，咽喉肿痛，鼻衄，口眼㖞斜；②腹胀，泄泻，食欲不振；③热病；④足背肿痛。

【释义摘录】

《医经理解》："内庭，在足大趾次趾外间两歧骨后三分陷中，言此犹内而未及外也。"

《经穴解》："自厉兑而上入于足跗上，在二指之间，有庭之象焉。以其在二指之内，故曰内庭。"

《古法新解会元针灸学》："内庭者，是通于内部之庭堂。因胃之精气下连于厉兑，贯通于脾，从次指本节下横串直上，交经于隐白。由外可连内，脾为黄庭，胃为使臣，此穴能直连脾，行于胃气，有华脾助精之功，故名内庭。"

《针灸穴名解》："门内曰'庭'，主屋正室亦曰'庭'。本穴之下为厉兑穴。'兑'于《易·说卦》为口，为门。本穴犹在门庭之内也。又其所治证，多不在穴位近处，而在头脑腹心者居多，是其功用有关于内也。于体则庭，于用则内，故名内庭。"

45 厉兑（井穴）

【出处】《灵枢·本输》《灵枢·根结》。

【别名】无。

【穴义】本穴名解有二。其一，厉，岸危处曰厉，本穴位于第二脚趾爪甲后方一分许，犹如身处岸边，故以"厉"名。兑，为门（《易经》）。本穴为足阳明胃经之井穴，乃胃经经气出入之门，故名"厉兑"。其二，厉，"砺"的本字，意为质地粗硬的磨刀石。兑，

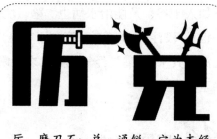

厉，磨刀石；兑，通锐。穴为本经之井穴，五行属金。

通"锐"。本穴为足阳明胃经井穴，位于足趾尖锐处，且五行属金，故名。

【定位】足第2趾末节外侧，趾甲根角侧后方0.1寸。

【主治】①鼻衄，齿痛，面肿，口眼㖞斜，咽喉肿痛；②热病，癫狂，多梦，善惊，神昏。

【释义摘录】

《医经理解》："厉兑，在足大趾次趾端，正足趾坚锐处也。"

《经穴解》："兑者，悦也，为开口之象。又曰：为口、为饮食之象，皆合于胃之义，

故曰厉兑。"

《古法新解会元针灸学》："厉兑者，厉者天地间之厉气也；兑者实现也。由胃之阳得吸脾土之阴，同化而分阴阳，实为厉气充现于络，以御天地时行之疫厉也，故名厉兑。"

《经穴释义汇解》："岸危处曰厉；兑，穴也。穴在足大趾次趾之端，去爪甲角如韭叶，即第二趾外侧爪甲后方一分许，喻穴居临岸危处；又穴与脾脉相通，兑为口，主口疾，故名厉兑。"

第五章

足太阴脾经穴

1 隐白（井穴）

【出处】《灵枢·本输》。

【别名】无。

【穴义】隐，有潜藏孕育之义；白，五行对应金，指手太阴肺经。本穴为足太阴脾经之井穴，经气出于此，然后上走胸部，与手太阴肺金之脉相接于中府。隐白者，金色白，金隐于土，有脾母孕育肺子之义，所以本穴不仅可以治疗腹胀、便血、崩漏等脾胃病和

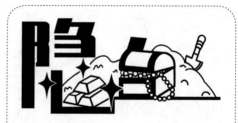

白，五行属金，金隐于土，有脾母孕育肺子之义。

脾不统血之证，亦可治疗喘满不得安卧等肺气逆乱之证，故名"隐白"。

【定位】在大趾末节内侧，趾甲根角侧后方 0.1 寸。

【主治】①腹胀，泄泻，呕吐；②月经过多；③便血，尿血，鼻衄；④昏厥。

【释义摘录】

《医经理解》："隐白，土者金之母，白者金之色。足太阴坤土，上接手太阴乾金，故谓足大趾端所起之脉为金气所隐也。"

《经穴解》："穴名隐白者，以脾经为土，而土生金，金之色白。土生金，金隐于土中，故曰隐白。"

《古法新解会元针灸学》："隐白者，隐，是逸藏也；白者，无色也，金属也。隐白穴属土，有生金荣肺之象。中隐木，有酸甘化阴之功。又在足大趾内侧白肉际，故名隐白。"

《针灸穴名解》："本经承厉兑之金，由足阳明之阳传交足太阴之阴。金，色白，坚

刚，为阳。本穴居阴经之下，在足大趾之端，独潜龙之隐，故名'隐白'。太阴根于隐白，喻金气之藏也。"

2 大都（荥穴）

【**出处**】《灵枢·本输》。

【**别名**】无。

【**穴义**】大，盛大；都，都城，引申为汇聚。穴处为足太阴脾经经气丰盛与聚集之处，故名"大都"。

【**定位**】在足内侧缘，当第一跖趾关节前下方赤白肉际凹陷处。

【**主治**】① 腹胀，胃痛，泄泻，便秘；②发热。

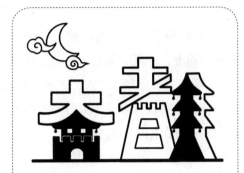

脾土为四象之母，如一国之都，故名"都"。

【**释义摘录**】

《医经理解》："都者，土之会。大都，在大趾本节后内侧骨缝陷中。"

《经穴解》："凡气血交汇聚之地，则以都名之。穴名大都者，以此穴在足大趾之本节，故曰大都。"

《古法新解会元针灸学》："大都者，大都会也，乘其妻助之润下，秉燥火而旺于四时。此穴司脾土之阳，而生运会，故名大都也。"

《针灸穴名释义》："大，盛大，丰富。都，都会，储积，又是池的意思。指穴为土气丰富与储积之处，如水入于池也。"

《针灸穴名解》："大，广泛也；都，丰盈也，又汇聚也。二字连用，喻犹诸病汇聚一大都市也……又以穴在足下，承前穴之潜隐，犹阳气下踵，得时而出，挈发其蕴蓄之性能也。其力无限，故名'大都'。"

3 太白（输穴、原穴）

【**出处**】《灵枢·九针十二原》《灵枢·本输》。

【**别名**】无。

【**穴义**】太，大也，穴在足大趾内侧后方

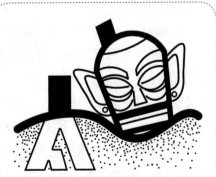

白，金之色。此穴为本经土穴，有全土生金之功。

赤白肉际处。白，金之色，此穴为本经土穴，有全土生金之功，故名"太白"。

【定位】第一跖趾关节近端赤白肉际凹陷中。

【主治】①胃痛，腹胀，肠鸣，泄泻，便秘；②身重节痛。

【释义摘录】

《医经理解》："太，大也，始也。太白为土，为金气所始，在大趾后内侧核骨下陷中。"

《经穴解》："穴名太白者，本经为土，土所生者为金，井名隐白，已含金之义矣，至此为输土，土所生者金，故名太白。"

《经穴释义汇解》："太，大也。穴在足大趾后，内侧核骨下，赤白肉际中，故名太白。又释：察日行以处位太白，太白者，西方金之精。穴为土穴，土生金。西方金，其色白。西方白色……其应四时，上为太白星，穴应太白之星名，故名太白。"

4 公孙（络穴；八脉交会穴，通冲脉）

【出处】《灵枢·经脉》。

【别名】无。

【穴义】公，众，支属之总汇；孙，支脉、旁系。本穴为足太阴脾经之络穴，足太阴之脉为正经如公，阳明之别络如孙，故曰"公孙"。

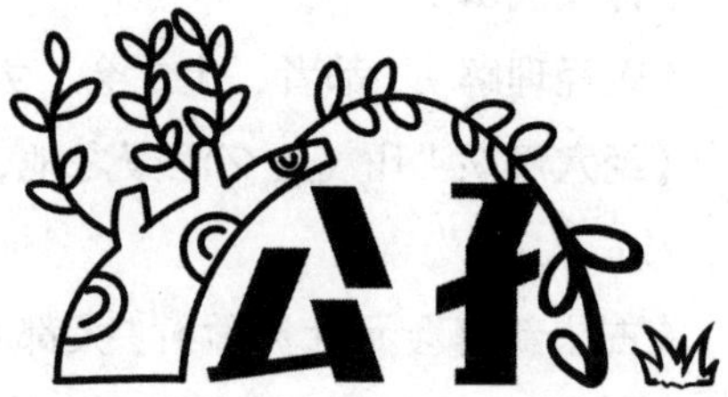

【定位】第一跖骨底的前下缘赤白肉际处。

【主治】①胃痛，呕吐，腹痛，腹胀，泄泻；②心烦。

本穴为络穴，足太阴之脉为正经如公，阳明之别络如孙。

【释义摘录】

《医经理解》："公孙，在大趾本节后内侧一寸，足太阴络别走阳明者。又合冲脉，会阴维。凡同支之脉，自孙而分之。自组而分之，分于斯合于斯，故谓其穴为公孙也。"

《经穴解》："穴名公孙者，万物生于土，而土又以火为父，以金为子。脾经自井隐白木生大都火，以及太白上又将生商丘金，有祖孙父子之义，故曰公孙。"

《古法新解会元针灸学》："公孙者，公者象也、贵也；孙者细也，传代也。脾主运血而络于阳，传脾之络，主化气。又脾之大络出于脾之大包，运通五脏六腑，公孙运通十二经络，是以有经络、细络、孙络之名称。公孙亦经络之一也。由经之络可连孙络，取穴公正，端坐贵如王孙，四通八连，周行脏腑络脉，化气通经，换五脏六腑之气，出于四肢，故名公孙。"

《经穴释义汇解》："肝木为公，心火为子，脾土为孙，穴在公孙之脉，因名公孙也。又释：古史以火德旺者曰炎帝，以土德旺者曰黄帝。黄帝姓公孙，名轩辕。公孙穴，乃脾土别络，人体五脏，脾居中央，中央黄色，入通于脾，以土德旺。此别络穴，别于太阴土位，络于阳明燥金之位，土以生金，亦犹以土德旺之后裔，由流溯源，赐其姓也，故名。"

5 商丘（经穴）

【出处】《灵枢·本输》。

【别名】无。

【穴义】商，五音之一，属金；丘，山丘。穴为足太阴脾经之经穴，五行属金，且本穴位于足内踝前方凹陷中，其处内踝隆起似小丘，故名"商丘"。

【定位】在足内踝前下方凹陷中，当舟骨结节与内踝尖连线的中点处。于内踝前缘直线与内踝下缘横线的交点处取穴。

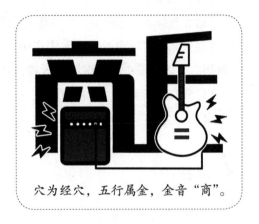

穴为经穴，五行属金，金音"商"。

【主治】①腹胀，泄泻，便秘，痔疾；②足踝痛，疝气痛引膝股。

【释义摘录】

《医经理解》："商丘，在内踝下微前陷中。商，金也。太阴所行，谓是金气之所聚也。"

《经穴解》："穴名商丘者，金为商，土为丘，脾土而生经金，故曰商丘。"

《古法新解会元针灸学》："商丘者，商者肺音也，丘者土丘也。土丘有宝土聚而生金之象，肺曜于此，故名商丘。"

《经穴释义汇解》："丘，喻土之高处。商丘者，金也。穴为太阴所行，金气之所聚。位在足内踝下微前凹陷中，其处骨隆起似小丘，故名商丘。"

6 三阴交（足太阴经、足少阴经、足厥阴经交会穴）

【出处】《千金翼方·针灸》。

【别名】三交。

【穴义】三阴为足之三阴经；交，交会。本穴为足太阴、足少阴、足厥阴三经之交会穴，统治三阴经所主治的病症，特别是经带胎产①、子宫精室等泌尿生殖系统疾病，此穴为首选，故名"三阴交"。

【定位】内踝尖上 3 寸，胫骨内侧缘后际。

【主治】① 月经不调，崩漏，带下，阴挺，不孕，滞产；② 遗精，阳痿，遗尿，小便不利，疝气；③ 腹胀，肠鸣，泄泻；④ 下肢痿痹。

经带胎产首选穴。孕妇禁针；与合谷同用有催产作用。

【释义摘录】

《医经理解》："三阴交，在内踝上除踝三寸骨下陷中，是三阴脉之交会也。"

《经穴解》："三阴者，足太阴在中，厥阴在前，少阴在后，三阴所生者皆经血。如经血闭，泄之立通；经脉虚耗不行者，补之则亦通。"

《经穴释义汇解》："穴在内踝上三寸骨下凹陷处，足太阴厥阴少阴之会。穴为足三阴之交会，故名三阴交。"

7 漏谷

【出处】《黄帝明堂经》。

【别名】太阴络。

【穴义】本穴名解有二。其一，漏，指渗漏；谷，指凹陷。本穴为足太阴络②，比喻本经络脉由此漏而别走分出，故名"漏"，且位于胫骨内侧缘后方凹陷处，故名"谷"。其二，"漏谷"亦有谷子漏出之意，比喻本穴可治疗消化不良导致的完谷不化、腹胀肠鸣，故有"消化不良失营养，地机漏谷公孙强"之说。

【定位】在小腿内侧，当内踝尖与阴陵泉的连线上，距内踝尖 6 寸，胫骨内侧缘后方。

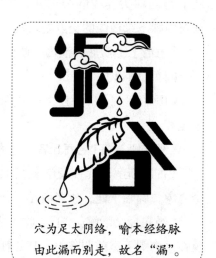

穴为足太阴络，喻本经络脉由此漏而别走，故名"漏"。

---

① 孕妇禁针。《铜人腧穴针灸图经》记载医案："昔有宋太子性善医术，出苑逢一怀娠妇人，太子诊曰：是一女也。令徐文伯亦诊之，此一男一女也。太子性急欲剖视之，臣请针之，泻足三阴交，补手阳明合谷，应针而落，果如文伯之言，故妊娠不可刺也。"因本穴与合谷可促进宫缩，故有文献报道应用电针三阴交、合谷的方法促分娩。

② 《针灸穴名解》："本穴又名'太阴络'。盖以本穴外表部位，与足阳明络穴'丰隆'部位相对，当与足阳明经有所沟通，故别名'太阴络'也。"

【主治】①腹胀，肠鸣；②小便不利，遗精，疝气；③下肢痿痹。

【释义摘录】

《医经理解》："漏谷，在内踝上六寸骨下陷中，是太阴之络也。谓有漏而别走者也。"

《经穴解》："穴名漏谷者，盖以此穴正在内踝上六寸之所，又为太阴络在下之公孙，所以交足阳明之在足跗者。此穴之络，乃在膝之下，上行而交于膝之阳明，有交必有隙，故曰漏谷。"

《经穴释义汇解》："穴在内踝上六寸骨下凹陷处，为足太阴络，因喻本经络脉由此漏而别走分出，穴似谷孔，故名漏谷。"

《针灸穴名释义》："漏，是渗泄和穴洞的意思；谷，见合谷条，又同穀。水湿与水谷漏出不止诸病，用之为有效也……功能渗湿止淋、固肠止利，因其功用而得名。"

8 地机（郄穴）

【出处】《黄帝明堂经》。

【别名】脾舍。

【穴义】地，土为地之体，脾属土，此处指足太阴脾经；机，机要，关键。本穴为足太阴脾经之郄穴，是足太阴经气血深聚之要穴，故名"地机"。

【定位】阴陵泉下3寸，胫骨内侧缘后际。

【主治】①腹胀，泄泻；②月经不调，疝气。

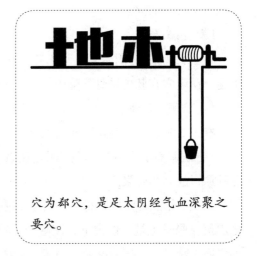

穴为郄穴，是足太阴经气血深聚之要穴。

【释义摘录】

《医经理解》："地机者地之机杼，太阴郄也。在膝下五寸，内侧辅骨下陷中。"

《经穴解》："穴名地机者，地者，脾之为言属土也；机者，比近膝，为上下转动之关，故曰机。又名脾舍。"

《古法新解会元针灸学》："地机者，是所居地部之中也。一身分上中下三部，自足至脐为下部，属于地部；机者，本能也，地机穴居地之中部，运膝之机关，故名地机。又名脾舍者，是脾之膏泽舍此，润活肌络，荣筋以利关节，故名脾舍也。"

《针灸穴名解》："机者，灵运之动能也。本穴治历节风，麻木，风湿，鹤膝风。凡属不良于行之症均可取之，俾以复其灵运机动之能也。穴在下肢，故名地机。本穴兼治水肿、腹坚、胁胀、不欲食，诸症之关于脾者，故又名'脾舍'，亦含有'地'字之义，脾属土也。"

9 阴陵泉（合穴）

【出处】《灵枢》作"阴之陵泉"，《黄帝明堂经》始作"阴陵泉"。

【别名】阴之陵泉。

【穴义】穴位于胫骨内侧髁后下方凹陷中，比喻本穴犹如阴侧山陵下的深泉，故名"阴陵泉"。

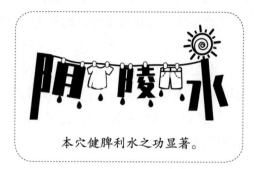

本穴健脾利水之功显著。

【定位】胫骨内侧髁下缘与胫骨内侧缘之间的凹陷中。

【主治】①腹痛，腹胀，泄泻；②妇人阴中痛，痛经，小便不利，遗尿，遗精；③水肿；④腰膝酸痛。

【释义摘录】

《医经理解》："阴陵泉，与阳陵泉相对，泉出于下，陵起于上，谓其当膝骨高起之下也。阴陵穴在膝内辅骨下陷中。"

《经穴解》："地之高者曰陵，脾经自足上行至膝之下，可谓高矣，故曰陵。脉过其处，有泉之象，以其与阳陵相对而处，此在内，彼在外，故曰阴陵泉。"

《古法新解会元针灸学》："阴陵泉者，是阴筋陵结甘泉，升润宗筋，上连胸膈，以养肺原，故名阴陵泉。"

《针灸穴名解》："《灵枢·九针十二原》云：'疾高而内者，取阴之陵泉。'本穴在膝之内侧，胫骨上端，髁突下，凹隙中。喻犹阴侧陵下之深泉也，简称'阴陵泉'。所治为腹坚，喘逆，疝气，癥瘕，遗精，遗尿，暴泻，飧泄，俱阴象症也。"

10 血海

【出处】《黄帝明堂经》。

【别名】百虫窠，血郄。

【穴义】海，百川归聚之处。本穴主要治疗崩漏、月经不调、闭经等血分诸病，以及血不归经者，有引血归经之功，犹如导洪流入江海，故名"血海"。

【定位】髌底内侧端上2寸，股内侧肌隆起处。

【主治】①月经不调，经闭，崩漏；②湿疹，风疹。

【释义摘录】

《医经理解》："血海，在膝髌上一寸内廉白肉际陷中。脾统血，故谓是血海也。"

《经穴解》："穴名血海者，脾生血，此穴离而上，血渐生旺，而腹中饮食所生之血，亦能于此所上下，血生于此地，故曰血海。"

《针灸穴名释义》："血，指气血；海，百川皆归之处。血海者，言其可以统血摄血也。太阴为多血少气之脏，又与多气多血之阳明为表里，故可以治血症见长。"

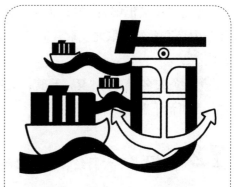

此穴有引血归经之功，犹如导洪流入江海。

《古法新解会元针灸学》："血海者，是心生血，肝藏血，肾助血。足三阴，肾之阴谷，肝之曲泉，脾之阴陵泉，皆生潮之处。三阴并行，通血之要路。若刺委中大筋，亦赖脾运之血而涌出，故能止少腹胀与水泻绞痛，是其验也，故名血海。"

11 箕门

【出处】《黄帝明堂经》。

【别名】无。

【穴义】箕，指簸箕。穴在大腿内侧，因取穴时需两腿分张，前大后小，形如簸箕，故名"箕门"。

【定位】当血海与冲门连线上，血海上6寸。

【主治】①小便不通，遗尿；②鼠蹊肿痛。

【释义摘录】

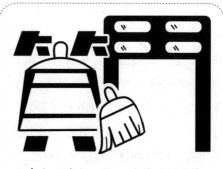

穴在大腿内侧，取穴时需两腿分张，形如簸箕。

《医经理解》："箕门，在血海上六寸，在鱼腹上越两筋间动脉应手，谓箕坐则此穴两张如门也。"

《经穴解》："穴名箕门者，以足之两股在此，其形并列如箕，经脉之动脉皆以门称，故曰箕门。"

《古法新解会元针灸学》："箕门者，言其两筋间穴列如箕星。又曰箕等于簸箕，因两筋间之槽前大后小，如簸箕之状，是箕之前口，故名箕门。"

《经穴释义汇解》："箕，为扬米去糠之具。穴在鱼腹上越两筋间阴股内廉，即于膝盖内缘直上八寸取之。取穴时，需两展其足，状如箕舌，又为脾气所出之门，故名箕门。"

《针灸穴名释义》："箕，簸箕，又星座名，风名。门，见云门条。以其必须箕踞取穴，及可治下肢之风病也。"

12 冲门 （足太阴经、足厥阴经、阴维脉交会穴）

【出处】《黄帝明堂经》。

【别名】慈宫，上慈宫，前章门。

【穴义】本穴位于腹股沟髂外动脉外侧，与"气冲"相平，为足太阴脾经上冲入腹之门，故名"冲门"。

【定位】在腹股沟外侧，距耻骨联合上缘中点3.5寸，当髂外动脉搏动处的外侧。

【主治】①腹满，积聚疼痛；②疝气，癃闭；③滞产。

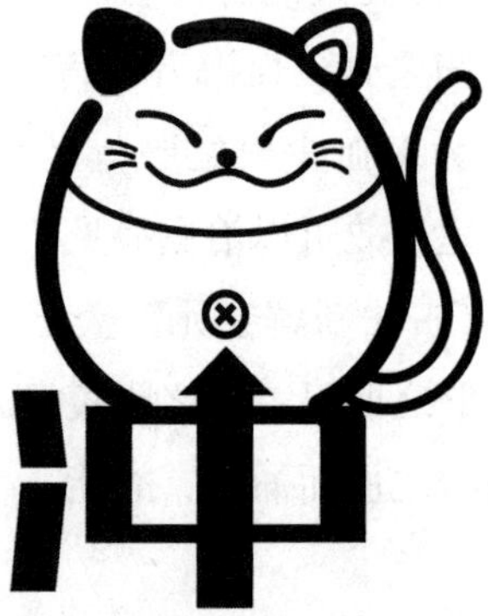

【释义摘录】

《医经理解》："冲门，一名慈宫。太阴，母道也，故有慈称。太阴之气由此而上冲于腹，故谓之

穴在股动脉外侧，与"气冲"相平，为脾经上冲入腹之门。

冲门，上去大横五寸，在府舍下横骨两端约纹中动脉应手。"

《经穴解》："此穴乃脾经入腹之始，足三阴经并足阳明自股入腹者，横列数之。足少阴在里，其入腹之始穴为横骨穴，去中行各一寸。次则阳明经，入腹为气冲穴，去中行各二寸。次则足厥阴肝经，入腹为阴廉穴，去气冲穴二寸。次则足太阴脾经，入腹为冲穴。以气冲已在中，去中行二寸之际，而此穴乃在去中行四寸半之际，反在气冲之外，以其近于胃经入腹穴之气冲也，故曰冲门。"

《古法新解会元针灸学》："冲门者，由脏气交经通冲之门，胞中化冲气不得循经，肝胃气冲来害血，留于腹中而发奔豚、瘕聚、狐疝，上有腹舍肠结止之，大横阻之。若脾虚失守，冲气上冲，必发狂疯、中风、厥闭之急症，故名冲门。"

13 府舍 （足太阴经、足厥阴经、阴维脉交会穴）

【出处】《黄帝明堂经》。

【**别名**】无。

【**穴义**】本穴在少腹之下，犹如储藏内府元气的舍宅，故名"府舍"。

【**定位**】当脐中下 4 寸，冲门上方 0.7 寸，距前正中线 4 寸。

【**主治**】①妇人疝气；②腹痛，腹满，积聚，呕吐，泄泻。

【**释义摘录**】

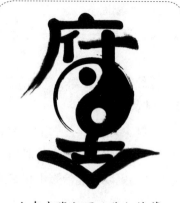

穴在少腹之下，犹如储藏内府元气的舍宅。

《医经理解》："府舍，在腹结下五寸，上直两乳。此脉上下入腹络胸结心肺，从胁上至肩，为太阴郄，三阴阳明支别，故谓是诸脏腑之舍也。"

《经穴解》："穴名府舍者，以入门则为舍，舍之所藏，乃六腑也，故名府舍。"

《古法新解会元针灸学》："府舍者，府是六腑之腹部，五脏三阴之气舍此，而应府之营养，故名府舍。"

《经穴释义汇解》："府，指脏腑。舍，言其所居。穴位足太阴脾脉之腧穴，足太阴、阴维、厥阴之会，位在腹结下三寸。足太阴脉贯胃，属脾络嗌。三阴脉上下一一入腹，络肝脾，结心肺。穴如诸脏腑聚集所居之处，并主其症，故名府舍。"

《针灸穴名解》："本穴在少腹之下，犹内府元气储藏之舍宅也，故曰'府舍'……在腹部呼吸，有府舍、腹结之收，而佐以冲门、气冲之放，亦即往复升沉之道也。其所治为疝、痹、积聚等症。由此观之，针穴命名，乃养生静坐调气，体验有得，而定之也。"

14 腹结

【**出处**】《黄帝明堂经》。

【**别名**】腹屈，肠屈，肠结。

【**穴义**】当小腹用力时，穴处肌肉硬结处，且本穴善治腹中积聚诸症，如腹痛、便秘、疝气，故名"腹结"。

【**定位**】大横下 1.3 寸，距前正中线 4 寸。

【**主治**】绕脐腹痛，泄泻。

【**释义摘录**】

《医经理解》："在大横下一寸三分，谓腹

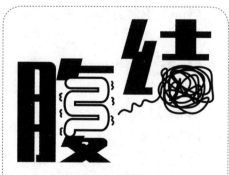

本穴善治腹中积聚诸症。

气之所结聚也。"

《经穴解》："此穴一名肠屈，盖大肠盘曲折叠之所，曰结、曰屈，可以会其命名之义。"

《经穴释义汇解》："穴在腹部大横下一寸三分，为腹气之所结聚，主腹内诸疾，故名腹结。"

《针灸穴名解》："结，凝聚也。本穴与足阳明经之外陵穴挨近。人当小腹努力时，则外陵穴处肌肉与本穴处肌肉，同时硬结。腹结穴在阴经，结于内；外陵穴在阳经，结于外也。更以其能治腹中积聚诸症，而名以'腹结'。"

15 大横（足太阴经、阴维脉交会穴）

【出处】《黄帝明堂经》。

【别名】无。

【穴义】横，齐平。穴位于脐旁4寸，与肚脐齐平，故名"大横"。

【定位】脐中旁开4寸。

【主治】腹痛，泄泻，便秘。

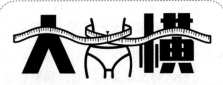

穴在脐旁4寸，与肚脐相平，主治大肠诸疾。

【释义摘录】

《医经理解》："大横，上直两乳，横直脐旁，故谓之大横也。"

《经穴解》："穴名大横者，以此穴在肝经期门之下五寸半，而期门乃在巨阙之旁四寸五分，而巨阙为任脉之经穴，在脐上六寸半，此穴在其下五寸半，正当离脐之上一寸许，乃腹中至广至横之所，故曰大横。"

《古法新解会元针灸学》："大横者，是腹部肠膜横结，足太阴之膏泽，横贯肠胃以助消化，对人体健康有伟大之功效，故名大横。"

《针灸穴名解》："本穴平脐，内应横行结肠，故名'大横'。能治肠腹气分之痛。"

16 腹哀（足太阴经、阴维脉交会穴）

【出处】《黄帝明堂经》。

【别名】无。

【穴义】哀，哀鸣，指肠鸣声。穴居上腹部，本穴主治消化不良、腹痛肠鸣，犹如腹部发出哀鸣之状，故名"腹哀"。

【定位】当脐中上3寸，距前正中线4寸。

【主治】下痢脓血，腹痛，便秘，食不化。

【释义摘录】

《医经理解》："腹哀，在胆日月下一寸五分，上直两乳，谓腹常于此哀鸣也。"

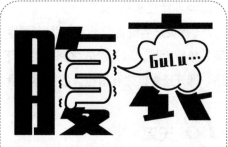

哀，肠鸣声。穴居上腹部，此处常有肠鸣之声。

《经穴解》："哀者，衰也。脾之气至此将衰，故曰衰。正当胁下空隙，腹之上左右两空内缩之地，故其名如是也。"

《古法新解会元针灸学》："腹哀者，穴居腹部，哀是乞求也，因足太阴磨胃助消化之工作，腹求胃之精气、谷气养脾润五脏，以助四肢之行动。语云，足得血能行，手得血能舞，此之谓也。故名腹哀。"

《针灸穴名释义》："腹，腹腔，也是重复和富有之意；哀，哀痛，也是爱护之意。指腹裹肠胃，为土气之所在，须加爱护以免腹中哀痛，而腹中哀痛用之亦有效也。"

17 食窦

【出处】《黄帝明堂经》。

【别名】命关。

【穴义】窦，有孔穴之意。脾脉由此穴上入于胸肺，食谷之精气穿透腹膈，以助肺气，故名"食窦"。本穴有宽胸利膈、通利食道之功，故"食窦"亦可理解为"食道"。

【定位】当第5肋间隙，距前正中线6寸。

【主治】胸满，胁痛。

【释义摘录】

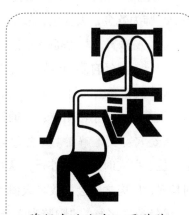

脾经由此穴上入于胸肺，食谷之精气穿透腹膈以助肺气。

《医经理解》："食窦，在天溪下一寸六分陷中，直乳旁一寸半，谓食气从此窦入也。食窦，犹胃之分至天溪、胸乡，则肺之分矣。"

《经穴解》："窦者，隙也。饮食自胸而下，入于上脘，而脾为之运化。此穴乃脾经入胸之始，而脾气受而化之，故曰食窦。"

《古法新解会元针灸学》："食窦者，饮食入胃，胃之原气出注于肠，谷精入脾养肺，使食谷之精气穿透腹膈，以助肺气，故名食窦。"

《针灸穴名释义》："食，指食物与饲养。窦，指洞穴与水道。意为穴乃婴儿食物之所出与乳汁之水道也。"

《针灸穴名解》："'食窦'即食道也。本穴与食道有关，故能治食道各症状。本穴取法，须先单臂上举，以开经穴之路，然后下针，乃有疗效。有此经孔道之开，乃通传导谷气之路。即开通食饮之孔道也。故简称'食窦'。'窦'，孔窍也。去中庭穴五寸，五肋间。"

18 天溪

【出处】《黄帝明堂经》。

【别名】无。

【穴义】天，指天位，横膈以上的部位；溪，溪流。穴位于胸部，乳房外侧肋间隙凹陷中，因凹陷处狭长如溪流，故名"天溪"。

【定位】当第4肋间隙，距前正中线6寸。

【主治】①胸痛，咳嗽，气喘；②乳痈。

【释义摘录】

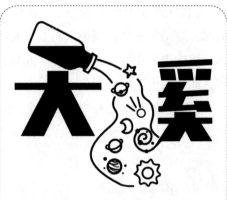

穴在乳房外侧肋间隙凹陷中，凹陷处狭长如溪流。

《医经理解》："天溪，在胸乡下一寸六分陷中。肺为乾金，天象也，故谓此为天溪。"

《经穴解》："体之高处则名曰天，脉之行处名曰溪。脾经自隐白入胸至此穴，可谓高矣，故曰天溪。"

《古法新解会元针灸学》："天溪者，天是膈之上部也，溪者水之小沟川也。肺得氧气从天下降雾露于小川溪，不通即生嗽痰，赖食窦冲和之气以通透之，故名天溪。"

《经穴释义汇解》："肉之大会为谷，肉之小会为溪。穴在胸乡下一寸六分凹陷处，居天位。取穴时，需手外开，从膻中穴旁开六寸，在第六肋间肌肉之会合处，连于筋骨间是穴，应肉之小会，故名天溪。"

《针灸穴名解》："胸腔为人身轻清境界，其象比天。本穴平于乳房外侧陷处，故名'天溪'。"

19 胸乡

【出处】《黄帝明堂经》。

【别名】无。

【穴义】乡，指处所。本穴位于胸廓外侧平坦处，因其所在之处而得名，故名"胸乡"。

【定位】当第3肋间隙，距前正中线6寸。

【主治】胸胁胀痛引背。

【释义摘录】

《医经理解》："胸乡，在周荣下一寸六分陷中，谓此为胸之乡也。"

《经穴解》："此穴在乳之上旁，正为胸之部分，以土有邑聚之象，故曰乡。"

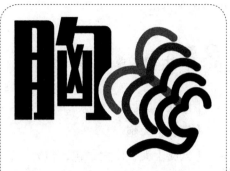

穴位于胸阔外侧平坦处，当第3肋间隙，因其所在之处而得名。

《经穴释义汇解》："乡，所在处之意。穴在周荣下一寸六分凹陷处，若卧不得转侧，本穴主之。因穴居胸侧所在处而称胸之乡，故名胸乡。"

《针灸穴名解》："乡，原野寥阔处也。即气行胸廓，得以扩张，因名'胸乡'。"

20 周荣

【出处】《黄帝明堂经》。

【别名】无。

【穴义】周，指周身；荣，同"营"，营养。穴属脾经，脾主肌肉，主统血。针灸该穴则可统血散精，周荣全身，故名"周荣"。

【定位】当第2肋间隙，距前正中线6寸。

【主治】胸胁胀满，气喘，咳唾脓血。

【释义摘录】

《医经理解》："周荣，在中府下一寸六分陷中，仰而取之。言肺气周养于一身也。"

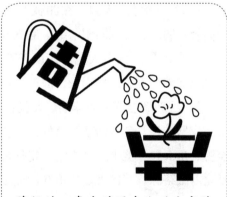

脾经的一条支脉至本穴后上交肺经，输布精气荣养周身。

《经穴解》："穴名周荣者，以土生金，而上与中府相近。土有四经，有周义焉，上生肺经之金，故曰荣。"

《古法新解会元针灸学》："周荣者，周始于身，荣行脏腑，润和肌肉，调理阴阳，交于络脉，开于肌表，故名周荣。"

《经穴释义汇解》："穴位足太阴脾脉之腧穴，位在中府下一寸六分凹陷处。脾主运化；诸湿肿满，皆属于脾。因穴主胸胁胀满，饮食不下，针灸则统血散精，周荣全身，故以为名。"

《针灸穴名释义》："周，周身，周遍。荣，荣茂，荣养。周荣者，言先后天之气可以荣敷周身也。"

21 大包（脾之大络）

【出处】《灵枢·经脉》。

【别名】大胞。

【穴义】大，广大；包，包容、容纳。因总统阴阳诸络，脾气散精灌溉五脏六腑。刺激本穴可以振奋脾气，促进运化功能，调节人体营养的摄取、代谢和水液的合理分布，故可治疗不明原因的周身困重、疼痛、无力及脾功能失调导致的肥胖和水肿，无所不包。故名"大包"，又名"脾之大络"。

【定位】第6肋间隙，当腋中线上。

【主治】胁痛，全身疼痛，四肢倦怠。

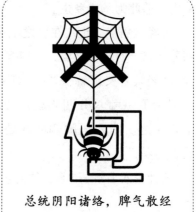

总统阴阳诸络，脾气散经灌溉五脏六腑，无所不包。

【释义摘录】

《医经理解》："大包，在渊腋下三寸，直胁下六寸。为脾之大络，布胸胁中，出九肋间及季胁端，总统阴阳诸络，灌溉五脏，故谓大包，言无所不包也。"

《经穴解》："穴名大包者，以五脏以土为主，土为坤象，无所不载，无所不容，脾以此络而灌注五脏以润周身，故曰大包。"

《古法新解会元针灸学》："大包者，大者十二经之大络，再加阴络、阳络，通体周身，安慰神经，各有治病之奇妙。大包布五脏，连细络，通心连心包络，走七系，由肺至脾，出大包，会十二经之络。走任督二脉络，安脑府而润脑膜，连系三焦之络脉，包括全身之络脉，其伟大之功不在治症多寡，而在维护各部络之门径，故名大包。"

《针灸穴名解》："'大包'，为脾之大络。其经气行经，由周荣斜抵胁肋，交贯肝胆心包各经。又与心肾肺胃经挨近。十二经中独此经与他经挨连最广，故以脾经为总统十二经络，称其最终斜行一段经线，为脾之大络，而名其大络之末穴为'大包'。寓广大包容，通连周布之意也。"

第六章

手少阴心经穴

1 极泉

【出处】《黄帝明堂经》。

【别名】无。

【穴义】极，顶端，最高点；泉，泉水，水之源。本穴位于手少阴心经的最高处，喻经气犹如水流自极高之泉而下，故名"极泉"。

【定位】腋窝中央，腋动脉搏动处。

【主治】① 心痛；② 干呕，咽干；③ 瘰疬；④ 胁痛，肩臂痛。

【释义摘录】

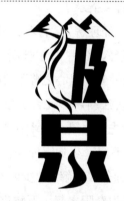

穴在心经最高点，经气由此流注，似泉水下流。

《医经理解》："心者，君主之官，神明出焉，有建极之义，有通灵之称。水之始出曰泉。维皇建极，维此出泉，心为生血之源也。"

《经穴解》："心，至尊者也，故曰极，其脉之发源第一穴，故曰泉。"

《古法新解会元针灸学》："极泉者，极者极深，泉是水泉也。心阳化液，由心系通肺出腋下，心火生脾土，而续交经之孔窍，相酬以甘液，故名极泉。"

《针灸穴名解》："少阴脉于六经为最里，而心脏居胸部之极深。本经之气，承足太阴经，循经内行。'其支者，复从胃，别上膈，注心中'之线，传交手少阴经，与旁出腋下者相接，由本穴透出，循行于臂，喻犹出于极深之泉也。故名'极泉'。"

2 青灵

【出处】《太平圣惠方·明堂》。

【别名】青灵泉。

【穴义】青，万物初生之色；灵，神灵，心藏神。本穴属手少阴心经，"心者，生之本，神之变也"（《素问·六节藏象论》），即心是生命的根本，是精神意志之所在，故名"青灵"。且本穴主治目黄、头痛、胁痛、肩臂不举、不能带衣等虚弱之症，有振奋神气之功，具有生发之象，故名。

穴属心经，有振奋神气之功，具有生发之象。

【定位】肘横纹上3寸，肱二头肌的内侧沟中。

【主治】①瘿气；②腋痛，肩臂疼痛。

【释义摘录】

《医经理解》："青者，最高之色，心为万物之灵，故谓其通于青玄之表也。"

《经穴解》："心主神明，故曰灵。曰青灵者，如青天之称，亦清净无为之象，且本穴不载针分，以心之尊不可轻刺耳。"

《古法新解会元针灸学》："青灵者，青者木之所生也，灵者灵机也。心阳过青灵，有先知先觉之灵。因木在天为玄，在地为木，在人为肝，木阳生火，补心之真阴生阳，循经主青灵，生觉感神经，有青而通灵之功，故名青灵。"

《针灸穴名解》："少阴君火之气，出于极泉，犹《易》震卦之一阳居下也。震居东方，东为春阳之起，万物借以发生。春色青青，故名'青灵'。……再考本穴主治为目黄、头痛、胁痛、肩臂不举、不能带衣，均属虚弱之症。针之助使神气振发，而促青阳兴起也。所谓青阳者，东方青气之灵也，犹云朝气也。"

《经穴释义汇解》："穴在肘上三寸，为心经之腧穴。心者，生之本，神之变，意即心是生命的根本，神露智慧变化起源之处。穴属心脉，主头部神志疾患，故以为名。"

3 少海（合穴）

【出处】《黄帝明堂经》。

【别名】无。

【穴义】少，指手少阴心经；海，为百川之汇。少海者，为手少阴心经之合水穴，本经脉气汇聚之处，故名"少海"，喻少阴之海。

【定位】横平肘横纹，肱骨内上髁前缘。

【主治】①心痛；②呕吐；③瘰疬；④胁痛，腋痛，肘臂挛痛。

【释义摘录】

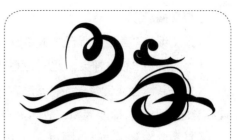

穴为手少阴心经之合穴，为脉气汇聚之处。

《经穴解》："穴名少海者，海之象，取本经所入为合水也。凡骨节过经之所，皆以池、泽、海名之者，以经至其地，必存聚蓄潴，而方能过骨节曲折之处，此乃少阴之合水穴，故曰少海。"

《古法新解会元针灸学》："少海者，少是手少阴也，海者由经达心脏之海，故名少海。曲者肘之曲也，节者两臂相交之关节也，故又名曲节也。"

《针灸穴名解》："海为诸川之汇，深阔无量。在人身六经，以少阴经为最里。又本穴治症，极为复杂，牵及多经之病，有如众症来归者。故曰'少海'。所谓'少'者，初也、始也。此则由里扩外之始也，意指少阴言也。其所治症为表里、虚实、寒热，以及七情志意等病，如癫狂、呕吐、项强、臂痛、齿痛、目眩、头风、气逆、瘰疬等等，即'海'之含意也。"

《针灸穴名释义》："少，指手少阴心经。海，见血海条。少海，古地名。喻为手少阴心经所入为合之海也。少海，地名。《韩子·外储说左》：'齐景公游少海。'注：'少海，即渤海也。'又《淮南·地形》：'东方曰少海。'注：'少海，泽名。'此为手少阴经之合穴，即以之假借命名。"

4 灵道（经穴）

【出处】《黄帝明堂经》。

【别名】无。

【穴义】灵，神灵，心藏神，故称之"灵"；道，通道。本穴为手少阴心经之经穴，"所行为经"，喻心经经气通行之道，故名"灵道"。是治疗冠心病、心绞痛之要穴。

【定位】腕掌侧远端横纹上1.5寸，尺侧腕屈肌腱的桡侧缘。

【主治】①心痛，悲恐善笑；②暴喑；③肘臂挛急。

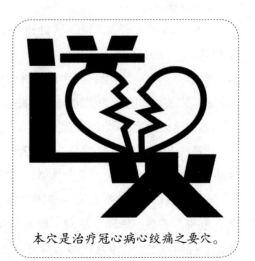

本穴是治疗冠心病心绞痛之要穴。

【释义摘录】

《采艾编》："言心灵所行之道路也。"

《经穴解》："心主神灵，此穴为心经所行，故曰灵道，走而不守也。"

《古法新解会元针灸学》："灵道者，灵为心灵之毅力。道为经穴之常道。手指相握，仗心意之灵力到，即能握物，故名灵道。"

《针灸穴名解》："道，顺也，远也，万事之通行也。本穴秉少阴之气，由少海穴直道而来，主治心痛、干呕、悲恐、瘛疭、肘挛、暴喑以及诸般郁滞之症。刺之俾使其灵通顺适也。故名'灵道'。"

5 通里（络穴）

【出处】《灵枢·经脉》。

【别名】通理。

【穴义】通，通达；里，表里。本穴是手少阴心经的络穴，其络脉由本穴分出，别而上行，循经入于心中，系舌本，属目系。其络脉还走向相应表里经，起沟通表里两经和补充经脉循行不足的作用，故名"通里"。

【定位】腕掌侧远端横纹上1寸，尺侧腕屈肌腱的桡侧缘。

【主治】①心悸，心痛；②咽喉肿痛，暴喑；③肘臂挛痛。

穴为心经络穴，沟通其表里经手太阳小肠经。

【释义摘录】

《黄帝内经太素》："里，居处也。此穴乃是手太阴脉气别通，为络居处，故曰通里也。"

《医经理解》："通里，在手内侧腕骨后一寸，谓是通灵之里道也。"

《经穴解》："前穴为灵道，道，路也。此穴为通里，里亦路也。以此穴别通于手太阳，必有路以通之，故曰通里。"

《古法新解会元针灸学》："通里者，由手少阴络通于手太阳也，与手厥阴邻里相通。手少阴心之经脉会于此，支走其络，连络厥阴太阳，故名通里。"

《针灸穴名解》："本穴为手少阴之络，可由本穴横通手太阳经。其所治症为目痛、汗闭、喉痹、心热、悸动、胀满、崩漏等症。凡此诸症，多由涩滞抑郁所生者，本穴统能治之。综而观之，是本穴以通为治也。故名'通里'，即通而理之也，亦即功通于里也。"

6 阴郄（郄穴）

【出处】《黄帝明堂经》。

【别名】手少阴郄，少阴郄。

【穴义】阴，指手少阴心经；郄，同"隙"，有孔窍、空隙之义，又指郄穴。本穴为手少阴心经的郄穴，心经气血深聚的孔隙，故名"阴郄"，有滋阴养血之功，故多用于骨蒸盗汗、心烦失眠等心阴虚诸证。

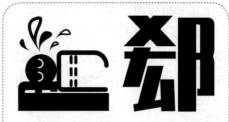

本穴多用于骨蒸盗汗、心烦失眠等心阴虚诸证。

【定位】腕掌侧远端横纹上 0.5 寸，当尺侧腕屈肌腱的桡侧缘。

【主治】①心痛，心悸；②咯血，骨蒸盗汗；③鼻衄。

【释义摘录】

《医经理解》："阴郄，少阴之郄也。在手掌后，前直小指，去腕五分动脉中。"

《经穴解》："穴名阴郄者，指少阴经而言也。郄者，空也。前有神门，后有通里，此有动脉，故以郄名。又《内经》注云：手少阴之郄穴，乃手少阴发脉之处。"

《经穴释义汇解》："穴在掌后脉中，去腕五分，手少阴郄，穴为心手少阴脉之郄穴，故名阴郄。"

7 神门（输穴、原穴）

【出处】《黄帝明堂经》。

【别名】兑冲，中都。

【穴义】神，神明、神志，心藏神；门，出入之门户。本穴为心经原穴，心气出入之处，且主治恐、悸、呆、痴、健忘、狂、痫等神志不清之症，故名"神门"。

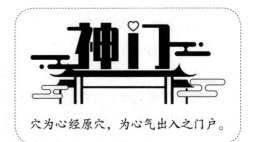

穴为心经原穴，为心气出入之门户。

【定位】腕掌侧远端横纹尺侧端，尺侧腕屈肌腱的桡侧缘。

【主治】心痛，心烦，惊悸，痴呆，健忘，失眠，癫狂，惊痫。

【释义摘录】

《医经理解》："神门，在掌后锐骨端陷中，是为神所出入之门。"

《经穴解》："心者，神明之主。心经有病，独取此穴者，以心经之输土，为心火之所生，有病则泄其子也。曰门者，以本经初离腕而入掌，在锐骨之端动脉处，有门象焉，故曰神门。"

《古法新解会元针灸学》："神门者，手腕之骨相对，其形如门。血支从郄回络归经，火生土化精和神，从经之神而安心主之神，故名神门。"

《针灸穴名解》："《内经》曰：'心藏神。'《道藏》云：'玉房之中神门户。''玉房'，心也。本穴为本经主要穴位。治恐悸、呆痴、狂痫、健忘，及神识不清等症。取本穴以开心气之郁结，故称'神门'。治以泻法开之，使神志得舒也。"

8 少府（荥穴）

【出处】《黄帝明堂经》。

【别名】兑骨。

【穴义】少，指少阴；府，聚集之意。穴为手少阴心经经气所聚之处，故名"少府"。

【定位】横平第 5 掌指关节近端，第 4、5 掌骨之间。取穴时嘱患者握拳，小指尖所指处取穴，横平劳宫。

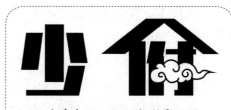

穴为手少阴心经经气所聚之处。

【主治】①心悸，烦满，胸痛；②肘臂痛，掌中热，手指拘挛。

【释义摘录】

《医经理解》："少府者，少阴之府。"

《经穴解》："少者，指少阴经而言也。府者，藏物之名。以火经而遇火穴，有藏物之象焉，故曰少府。"

《古法新解会元针灸学》："少府者，手少阴心脉，出腋走手小指，交少府而通心之府小肠也，故名少府。"

《经穴释义汇解》："穴在小指本节后凹陷处，与手厥阴经劳宫穴相平直。府，文书藏也，引申聚集之义。因喻本穴为手少阴脉气汇聚之处，故名少府。"

《针灸穴名解》："本穴与劳宫穴为邻，同在掌握之中，犹宫中、府中也。本穴通及心肾，能舒二经抑郁之气。其治为烦满、悲恐、心中痛、阴挺、阴痒、遗尿、偏坠、太息、小便不利等症。为手、足两少阴之通达内府者，故名'少府'，即犹治两少阴之内府病也。"

9 少冲（井穴）

【出处】《黄帝明堂经》。

【别名】经始。

【穴义】少，既指手少阴心经，又可指小，喻经气幼小。冲，为要冲、直冲之义，指阴阳经气通行之处。本穴为手少阴心经之井穴，"所出为井"，形容脉气幼小而未盛，且穴为手少阴和手太阳交接之处，故名"少冲"。又因井如水泉之突出者，所以"冲"寓有冲进之意，为冲气之和。所治为烦满、上气、心虚、热壅、口臭、喉痹，皆取其冲通而和之力。

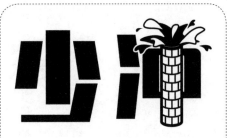

穴位心经之井穴，井如水泉之突出者。

【定位】小指末节桡侧，指甲根角侧上方 0.1 寸。

【主治】①心痛，心悸，心烦，神昏；②胁痛。

【释义摘录】

《经穴解》："少冲云者，以本经为手少阴，故曰少。以井为木，故曰冲。木有上腾之象，火有上炎之义，故以少冲名之。"

《古法新解会元针灸学》："少冲者，因肝之母为肾，心之母为肝，肾肝相生而化冲气，合于任脉，而通心脏。肝性味酸同木，木生火化养气，赖冲气之根原，而通经筋，合肾真阴所主，而交手小指。心生血入肝以填之，气血实满冲变，经脏交换，故名少冲。又名经始者，心经终始于此，而交手太阳之经，以御外邪也，故又名经始。"

《针灸穴名解》："冲，通行而直进也。又幼也，和也。冲气以为和也。本经之气，由其络穴通里，传接手太阳经。为由阴转阳，化阴沉之气为阳春之和。运行手太阳之径路。而本经络穴以下各穴，则本经行气之余也。犹行驶虽停，贯力仍在也。故名之以'冲'，而曰'少冲'。"

《经穴释义汇解》："本穴在手小指内侧之端，若去指甲角如韭叶之处，属本经井穴，犹如井泉之发，脉气正深，为手少阴心脉冲出之所在；又少也可喻小，韭叶者，也作少许解，故以为名。"

第七章
手太阳小肠经穴

1 少泽（井穴）

【出处】《灵枢·本输》。

【别名】小吉，少吉。

【穴义】少，小；泽，光泽、润泽。本穴为手太阳小肠经之井穴，位于手小指之端，为本经脉气之所出，其气微小，故名"少泽"。其所治症，为口热、心烦、喉痹、目翳、舌强等，多取其泽润之力。

【定位】小指末节尺侧，指甲根角侧上方 0.1 寸。

【主治】①乳痈，乳汁少；②目翳，咽喉肿痛；③热病，昏迷；④头痛，颈项强痛。

【释义摘录】

《医经理解》："少泽，在手小指外侧端，手太阳所发端也，故谓之少。"

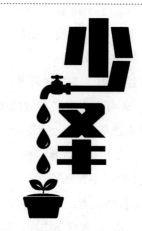

穴有泽润之力；穴为井穴，脉气微小。

《采艾编》："自少阴心而络通于此，彼以少冲名，此以少泽名，泽取井养，少从少冲也。"

《经穴解》："泽者，水之所聚也。以其在小指之端，而又为小肠之井，故名少泽。"

《经穴释义汇解》："少，小也。穴在手小指之端，去爪甲一分凹陷处，手太阳脉井穴，心脉交于本穴，心与小肠相合，似山泽通气，故名少泽。"

《针灸穴名释义》："少，指小指及幼小。泽，指光泽，滑润。泽门，古代城门名。少泽，为小指末节经气门户之光泽处。"

《针灸穴名解》："本经承少阴君火之气。君火具阳刚之性。故少阴末穴，名之以

'冲'。迨至本经，则为太阳寒水之气，火从胜己，而化成阴柔之水性，故本经首穴名之以'泽'。此阴阳互济、相辅相成之义也。泽，在卦属兑，兑为少女，女具柔顺之阴象。又兑为口，口外柔而内刚，此为阴阳互济也。人能体'泽'字之义，以调阴阳则和乐而无病。泽而曰少者，承冲气之和也。本经由少阴君火之气之络穴通里，转注而来。火气为阳，犹天日之热照彻下土，冲和之气，蒸蒸而生，化为膏雨甘霖，泽及万物。本穴为本经受泽之初，故称'少泽'。"

2 前谷（荥穴）

【出处】《灵枢·本输》。

【别名】无。

【穴义】谷，山谷，两山之间。本穴在手小指掌指关节前，其所在处凹陷如谷，故名"前谷"。

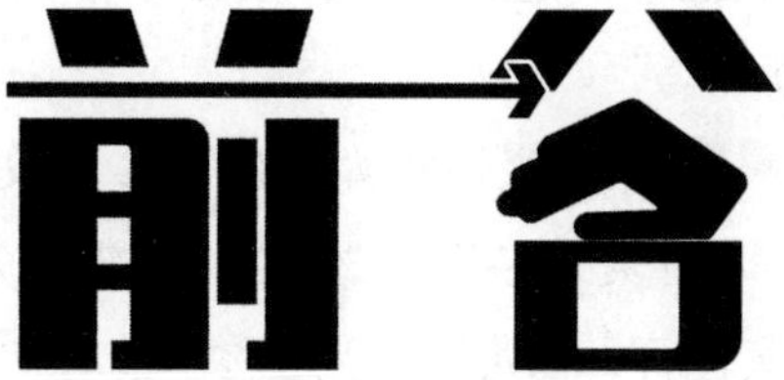

【定位】第5掌指关节尺侧远端赤白肉际凹陷中。

前谷

穴在手小指掌指关节前，所在处凹陷如谷。

【主治】①目痛，耳鸣，咽喉肿痛；②乳痛，乳少；③热病，癫狂；④头痛，颈项强痛；⑤手指肿痛。

【释义摘录】

《经穴解》："谷者，水之所行也。以本穴在指本节前，故为前谷。"

《古法新解会元针灸学》："前谷者，前是手小指本节之前也。谷者，谷之空洞也。手小指本节前，骨之空处，通于经孔，与分泌之孔窍，故名前谷。"

《经穴释义汇解》："穴当手小指外侧本节凹陷处，其所在处骨肉相会凹陷如谷，故名前谷。"

3 后溪（输穴；八脉交会穴，通督脉）

【出处】《灵枢·本输》。

【别名】无。

【穴义】后，方位词，指手小指本节后；溪，小水沟、沟渠。本穴位于手小指掌指关节后的横纹头处。握拳时手小指掌指关节外侧肉起如山峰，按之似小溪之处，故名"后溪"。

【定位】第5掌指关节尺侧近端赤白肉际凹陷中。

【主治】①耳聋，目赤，鼻衄；②癫狂病；③疟疾；④头痛，颈项强痛，肘臂痛。

【释义摘录】

《经穴解》："谷溪皆水过之称，以本节前为前谷，所以本节后为后溪，与奇经督脉相通。盖足太阳在督脉之两旁，而此经自肩上与督横交，故与督脉相通。"

《古法新解会元针灸学》："后溪者，后是手小指本节后也；溪者，小水沟也。手小指外侧握拳肉起如山峰，按之似小豁之曲，故名后溪。"

《经穴释义汇解》："握拳时，穴处肉起如山峰，按之似小溪之曲处，故名后溪。"

《针灸穴名解》："前谷、后溪两穴，俱承少泽穴之'泽'，犹雨露充沛，沟渠盈溢，经气流行，如走溪谷，故称'前谷''后溪'。"

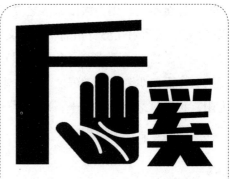

小指掌指关节后横纹头，握拳时，穴处横纹犹如沟溪。

4 腕骨（原穴）

【出处】《灵枢·本输》。

【别名】无。

【穴义】本穴在手腕前凹陷处，靠近腕骨（今之豌豆骨），骨穴同门，故名"腕骨"。

【定位】第5掌骨底与三角骨之间的赤白肉际凹陷中。

【主治】①耳鸣，目翳；②黄疸；③热病，惊风，抽搐；④疟疾；⑤头痛，颈项强痛，肩臂腕指痛。

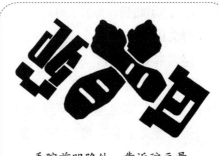

手腕前凹陷处，靠近豌豆骨。

【释义摘录】

《经穴解》："穴在腕骨之前，故曰腕骨。"

《古法新解会元针灸学》："腕骨者，是臂骨与腕骨相交接之处。骨者，腕前之骨曰起骨，腕后之骨曰手髁骨。手腕前之起手下陷处，故名腕骨。"

《针灸穴名释义》："腕骨，古解剖名。手外侧腕前起骨名腕骨，骨穴同名。杨上善引《明堂》曰：'腕骨在手外侧腕前起骨下陷中，即此起骨为腕骨，此经名腕骨。'古之腕骨，即今之豌豆骨，穴在其前方陷中，故名。"

5 阳谷（经穴）

【出处】《灵枢·本输》。

【别名】无。

【穴义】阳，指手臂外侧；谷，山谷，两山之间。本穴位于手外侧腕中，尺骨茎突和三角骨之间的凹陷处，且其处不如"阳溪""阳池"之宽深，形似小山谷，故名"阳谷"。

【定位】尺骨茎突与三角骨之间的凹陷中。

【主治】①头痛，眩晕，耳鸣，耳聋；②热病，癫狂痫；③颈肿，颊肿，腕臂疼痛。

穴在手腕外侧尺骨茎突前凹陷中，形似小山谷。

【释义摘录】

《经穴解》："阳指太阳经而言也，谷指本经离腕而上臂，至锐骨之前，经脉过之有空，似水从谷出之象也，故曰阳谷。"

《古法新解会元针灸学》："阳谷者，手太阳经，锐骨下空处如洞，故名阳谷。"

《经穴释义汇解》："本穴为手太阳脉之经穴，位在手外侧腕中，兑骨下凹陷处，其处不如阳溪、阳池之宽深，形似小谷，故名阳谷。"

《针灸穴名释义》："以其属于阳经阳穴，且有兴阳之效也。"

6 养老（郄穴）

【出处】《黄帝明堂经》。

【别名】无。

【穴义】本穴常用于治疗目视不明、耳闭不闻、肩臂疼痛等老年病，针此穴有益于老人的健康长寿，为调治老年病的要穴，故名"养老"。

【定位】腕背横纹上1寸，尺骨头桡侧凹陷中。

【主治】①目视不明；②肩臂疼痛不举。

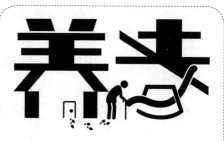

本穴主治目视不明、耳闭不闻等老年病。

【释义摘录】

《医经理解》："太阳故谓之老，此则其气所养也。"

《古法新解会元针灸学》："养老者，元老之称也，因此有折冲经络之能，故名养老。"

《经穴释义汇解》："考小肠之功能为吸收水谷所化之精微，以供养全身；又因本穴可治由外因侵犯本经脉气所发生的病变，以及本经主液体所发生的病变，如耳聋、目视不明、肩臂疼痛等老年病，故名养老。"

《针灸穴名释义》："养，奉养。老，年老，老迈。以其功能明目舒筋，治老年阳气不足诸病也。"

7 支正（络穴）

【出处】《灵枢·经脉》。

【别名】无。

【穴义】支，分支，支离；正，正经。本穴为络穴，手太阳络脉自此别走其表里经手少阴心经，故名"支正"。也因此既能治疗颈痛之手太阳病症，亦能安神志，治疗癫狂、健忘等心经病症。

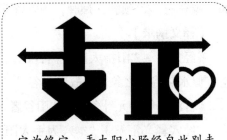

穴为络穴，手太阳小肠经自此别走其表里经手少阴心经。

【定位】腕背侧远端横纹上5寸，尺骨尺侧与尺侧腕屈肌之间。

【主治】①热病，癫狂；②疣；③头痛，颈项强痛，肘臂酸痛。

【释义摘录】

《黄帝内经太素》："正，正经也。支，络脉也。太阳正经之上，支别此络，走向少阴，故曰支正也。"

《医经理解》："支正，在手腕后五寸，手太阳络别走少阴者，走手少阴者为支，此则其正也。"

《经穴解》："此络之别者，上走肘，络肩髃，经之别行者曰支，以通于心经，故曰正。"

《针灸穴名解》："手太阳经气，行至前膊，偏走外侧。本穴无显著标示。取穴时以手托颐，指尖于本侧向外旁竖，本经转成当前直线，穴位适当腕肘折中之处，因名'支正'。盖以取穴姿式而得名也。"

8 小海（合穴）

【出处】《灵枢·本输》。

【别名】无。

【穴义】小，指小肠经；海，百川之汇。本穴为手太阳小肠经的合穴，喻小肠经脉气至此犹如江河之水入海，故名"小海"。

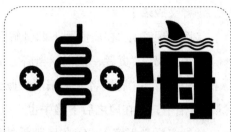

穴为合穴，脉气至此犹如江河之水入海。

【定位】尺骨鹰嘴与肱骨内上髁之间凹陷中。取穴时令患者微屈肘，在尺骨鹰嘴与肱骨内上髁之间的尺神经沟中取穴，用手指弹敲此处时有触电麻感直达小指。

【主治】①癫痫；②头痛，颈项强痛，肘臂疼痛。

【释义摘录】

《医经理解》："小海，在肘内大骨外大筋内，去肘端五分陷中，盖小肠经之海也。"

《经穴解》："此穴为小肠脉所聚，故曰小海。"

《古法新解会元针灸学》："小海者，小是手太阳小肠经，海者得金水木火相之气，合土会肘而通脾脏，正合火生土，土和脾，主运四末。五脏之海合于经络之海，司运五脏之气。手太阳经，曲肘处，乃小肠经脉之海，经脏出入之朝会，故名小海。"

《经穴释义汇解》："小肠与胃相连，胃为水谷之海，又六经为川，肠胃为海，穴为小肠经脉气汇合之处，喻为小肠经之海，故名小海。"

《针灸穴名释义》："小，指手太阳小肠经。海，见血海条。为手太阳经所入为合之海也，与少海可以互参。"

《针灸穴名解》："本穴与少海穴虽不同经，而穴底极为接近，故名'小海'。其治症亦甚复杂，亦有汇治诸经各病意势，犹江海之汇百川也。

9 肩贞

【出处】《素问·气穴论》。

【别名】无。

【穴义】肩，肩部；贞，正。一指正中，本穴位于肩关节正中直下；二指正气，针此穴可扶正气，驱邪气，主治风痹不举、肩中

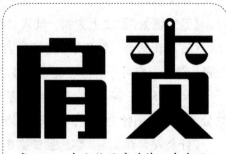

贞，正。本穴位于肩关节正中直下。

热痛等一切肩部不适，故名"肩贞"。

【定位】肩关节后下方，腋后纹头直上1寸。

【主治】①瘰疬；②肩痛，上肢不遂。

【释义摘录】

《医经理解》："在肩曲胛下两骨解间，肩髃后陷中，是肩之正处也。"

《采艾编》："贞者，正也。当肩之正也。"

《经穴解》："肩髃者，手阳明大肠经穴，在肩端臑上陷中，斜举臂取之。此穴在肩髃之后陷中，当在肩之后下陷中也，以其将离肩也，故曰肩贞。"

《经穴释义汇解》："穴在肩胛骨外缘弯曲处之下，两骨（指肩胛骨与肱骨）分解之间，肩髃穴后之凹陷处，即是肩之正处，故名肩贞。"

《针灸穴名释义》："肩，肩部。贞，指正气，精气。穴为肩部正气所居之处，不容外邪干犯也。贞，正也。《书·太甲》：'万邦以贞。'《释名·释言语》：'贞，定也，精气不动惑也。正者不正，邪所干也；不定者定，精气复也。'肩贞之名具有双重涵义。"

10 臑俞

【出处】《黄帝明堂经》。

【别名】无。

【穴义】臑，上臂；俞，同"腧"，腧穴。本穴靠近腋部，位于腋后纹头直上肩胛冈下，且主治臂酸无力、肩胛痛等局部病症。故名"臑俞"。

【定位】腋后纹头直上，肩胛冈下缘凹陷中。

【主治】肩臂疼痛。

【释义摘录】

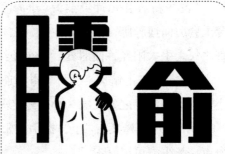

臑指肱骨上端靠近腋部的肌肉，穴在局部。

《经穴解》："肘之上为臑，此穴紧在臑尽处，故曰臑俞。"

《古法新解会元针灸学》："臑俞者，臑者骨之起处，前伏胸后通胁，中有空，如龟之前胸骨，有空可穿。俞者经气所过之穴道，在臑骨空穴，故名臑俞。"

《经穴释义汇解》："穴在肩髎穴后内下方肩胛骨上廉凹陷处，即当上肢的上节内侧之处，为手太阳脉之腧穴，因膊下对腋为臑，穴当其处，故名臑俞。"

《针灸穴名释义》："臑，见臂臑条。俞，同腧，同输，又通枢。指其为臂部臑肉之枢纽与臂臑经气之所注输也。"

《针灸穴名解》："臑，其处肉不着骨。穴在肩胛突下缘，其处肉下有通隙，可由肩胛下透过。故名之以'臑'。'俞'为腧之简，即通透内外之腧穴也。因名'臑俞'。"

11 天宗

【出处】《黄帝明堂经》。

【别名】无。

【穴义】天，天空、天部，此指身体上部；宗，有尊崇之意，指日、月、星。此穴与臑俞、曲垣、秉风等数穴分列如星座，故名天宗。

【定位】肩胛冈中点与肩胛骨下角连线上1/3 与下 2/3 交点凹陷中。

【主治】肩臂疼痛不举。

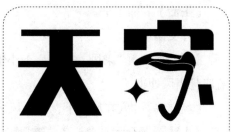

本穴与秉风、曲垣等穴排列如星座，故仿星名以名之。

【释义摘录】

《医经理解》："天宗，在秉风后大骨下陷中，言从此上而之天部也。"

《经穴解》："自少泽而至此穴，可谓高矣，故曰天宗。"

《古法新解会元针灸学》："天宗者，天是上部肩盘骨之边际；宗者根宗于天部，合覆宗气，故名天宗也。"

《针灸穴名释义》："天，天空，此指人身之上部。宗，宗仰之意。天宗，星名；又统指天象、天神，或如帝王之宗室，乃众所瞻仰之处也。天宗为天上之星辰。《礼记·月令》：'天子乃祈来年于天宗。'注：'天宗，谓日月星辰也。'《书·尧典》：'禋于六宗。'疏：'六宗者，天宗三，日月星也；地宗三，江河岱也。'《汉书·天文志》：'太岁在子曰困敦，十一月出。石氏曰：名天宗。'又《淮南·时则》天宗注：'凡属天上神，日月星辰，皆为天宗。'《晋书·天文志》谓宗星是象征帝王宗室之星。穴当肩胛骨中部，与曲垣、秉风诸穴彼此相望，有天宗之象焉。"

《针灸穴名解》："本穴与曲垣、秉风等穴，排列如星象，故皆仿取星名以名之……又以本穴在肩胛冈下，受曲垣、秉风外绕，本穴居中如枢，故称之为'天宗'。"

12 秉风

【出处】《黄帝明堂经》。

【别名】肩解，景风。

【穴义】秉，执掌之意；风，气动为风，引申为"风邪"。本穴主治风邪入侵导致的肩臂疼痛不举、上肢酸麻、咳嗽等病症，如同掌管风邪者，故名"秉风"。

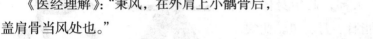

本穴主治风邪入侵导致的疾病，如"秉风政之官"。

【定位】肩胛冈中点上方冈上窝中。

【主治】肩痛不举。

【释义摘录】

《医经理解》："秉风，在外肩上小髃骨后，盖肩骨当风处也。"

《经穴解》："穴在肩之下，正为风之自外来者所中，故曰秉风。"

《古法新解会元针灸学》："秉风者，从风之所行也。肩夹后肉筋起如围瓶之状，风从背来，秉风迎之，顺风而高起天空，以防外邪所入，故名秉风。"

《针灸穴名解》："气动为风，即今之所谓气流也。人体气息周行，同于大气运转，故名之以'风'。本穴主治风痛、风痹、气逆作喘等症之有关于风者，如司风者之掌理诸风也，故名'秉风'。"

13 曲垣

【出处】《黄帝明堂经》。

【别名】无。

【穴义】垣，矮墙。穴在肩胛骨中央曲陷处，其四旁骨起如垣，故名"曲垣"。

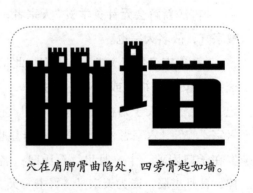

穴在肩胛骨曲陷处，四旁骨起如墙。

【定位】肩胛冈内侧端上缘凹陷中。

【主治】肩痛不举。

【释义摘录】

《医经理解》："曲垣，在肩中央曲胛陷中，其四旁骨起如垣也。"

《经穴解》："以其骨形如垣而曲，故曰曲垣。"

《古法新解会元针灸学》："曲垣者，肩中央骨之曲处，四面如坚壁之围，曲如天之北斗星，周似紫衡星之垣，故名曲垣。"

《经穴释义汇解》："卑曰垣，墙也。穴在肩中央胛骨曲陷处。胛似墙，其穴比秉风低卑，故名曲垣。"

《针灸穴名释义》："曲，见曲池条。垣，短墙，又是天体划分的范围。指穴在肩胛骨弯曲高起处之内方也。"

《针灸穴名解》："本穴在肩胛冈上窝凹曲处。肩背各穴，列如星象，环绕如垣，故名'曲垣'。"

14 肩外俞

【出处】《黄帝明堂经》。

【别名】无。

【穴义】本穴位于肩胛内侧，因其位于肩中俞外侧，故称之"肩外俞"。

【定位】第一胸椎棘突下，后正中线旁开3寸。

【主治】肩背痛引项臂。

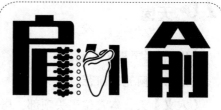

本穴虽在后正中线旁开三寸处，但不属于膀胱经。

【释义摘录】

《医经理解》："肩外俞，在肩胛上外廉，去脊三寸陷中。"

《经穴解》："以穴在肩之外也，故名之。"

《古法新解会元针灸学》："肩胛上肩中偏外，小肠脉所过之腧穴，故名肩外俞。"

《经穴释义汇解》："穴在肩胛上廉，去脊三寸陷中，因其位于肩中俞之外侧，故名肩外俞。"

15 肩中俞

【出处】《黄帝明堂经》。

【别名】无。

【穴义】本穴在肩胛内侧，位于大椎与肩井中间，故名"肩中俞"。

【定位】第7颈椎棘突下，后正中线旁开2寸。

【主治】①恶寒发热，咳嗽，气喘；②目视不明；③肩背疼痛。

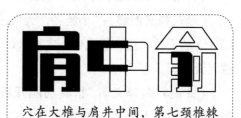

穴在大椎与肩井中间，第七颈椎棘突下，旁开2寸处。

【释义摘录】

《医经理解》："肩中俞，在肩胛内廉，去脊二寸陷中也。"

《经穴解》："肩之所以负重者，以骨会大杼也，此穴近大杼，故曰肩中俞。"

《古法新解会元针灸学》："肩臂胛相直于肩中，手太阳脉所过之腧，故名肩中俞。"

《经穴释义汇解》："穴在肩胛内廉，去脊二寸凹陷处，即在肩井与大椎之中间，故名肩中俞。"

《针灸穴名释义》："肩，指肩背。中与外，是互相比较之意。俞，腧穴。穴居肩背，距脊柱稍远者称为肩外俞，距脊柱较近者称为肩中俞。"

16 天窗

【出处】《灵枢·本输》。

【别名】窗笼，窗聋。

【穴义】天，本穴位于头项部，居天位；窗，为房屋通风透气之孔。本穴能治疗聋、暗、咽肿、噤口等人体头部诸孔窍疾患，犹如开窗通气，故名"天窗"。

【定位】横平喉结，胸锁乳突肌的后缘。

【主治】①耳鸣，耳聋，咽喉肿痛，②暴暗；③颈项强痛。

【释义摘录】

《医经理解》："天窗，在颈大筋前，曲颊下，扶突后，动脉应手陷中，言是天部通气处也。"

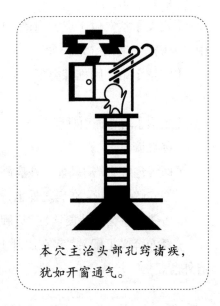

本穴主治头部孔窍诸疾，犹如开窗通气。

《经穴解》："此穴在颈之侧，如室之有窗，在室之侧也，故名天窗。"

《古法新解会元针灸学》："天窗者，项颈筋间之孔穴，在天部之上，故名天窗。"

《经穴释义汇解》："小肠者，天气之所生也。穴在曲颊下，扶突穴后，颈升动脉凹陷处，居天位。窗，通孔也。穴系天部通气之孔穴，故名天窗。"

《针灸穴名释义》："指其功能开通头面孔窍诸病，犹如人身上部之窗户也。"

17 天容

【出处】《灵枢·本输》。

【别名】无。

【穴义】肩之上为天部；容，面容、容貌。本穴位于下颌角后方，手太阳小肠经自此上面颊而入面

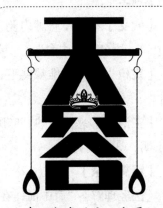

穴在下颌角后方，当耳环所垂之处。

容，且位于耳环所垂之处，故名"天容"。

【定位】下颌角后方，胸锁乳突肌的前缘凹陷中。

【主治】①胸痛，气喘；②耳聋；③咽喉肿痛，瘿气，颈项肿痛。

【释义摘录】

《医经理解》："天容，在耳下曲颊后，言其处广而有容也。"

《经穴解》："耳下曲颊后，乃颈侧最上之所，衣领所以不能蔽人之容，于此呈露之处，故曰天容。"

《经穴释义汇解》："容，盛也。穴为小肠脉之腧穴。小肠者，天气主之，其脉自此入面容。又穴在耳下曲颊后，居天位，其处广而有容，故名天容。"

《针灸穴名释义》："天，见天宗条。容，容貌，容体，防身之具亦名容。穴当扶持头容正直与防护头颈之处也。"

18 颧髎（手少阳经、手太阳经交会穴）

【出处】《黄帝明堂经》。

【别名】兑骨。

【穴义】颧，颧骨；髎，骨的空隙处。本穴以定位命名，穴在颧骨下缘凹陷中，故名"颧髎"。

【定位】颧骨下缘，目外眦直下凹陷中。

【主治】口眼㖞斜，眼睑瞤动，目赤，目黄，齿痛，颊肿。

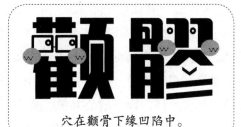

穴在颧骨下缘凹陷中。

【释义摘录】

《医经理解》："在颧骨下廉陷中。"

《经穴解》："此穴在颧骨下，故曰颧髎。"

《古法新解会元针灸学》："颧髎者，是颧衡之骨，空髎之处，故名颧髎。此穴禁灸，恐灸破伤颧部，因人之时运由此定休咎，忧其气色有变也。"

《经穴释义汇解》："髎，与窌同。窌，空穴也。穴在顊骨下廉陷中之空穴。顊，即颧，故名颧髎或颧窌。"

《针灸穴名释义》："指其为颧部之深孔也。"

19 听宫（手少阳经、手太阳经、足少阳经交会穴）

【出处】《灵枢·刺节真邪》。

【别名】多所闻。

【穴义】听，聆听，指耳的功能；宫，五音之首。本穴位居耳前，针之能使耳听五音，助恢复听力，为治耳疾要穴，故名"听宫"。

【定位】耳屏正中与下颌骨髁突之间的凹陷中。

【主治】①耳鸣，耳聋，聤耳；②癫狂病。

【释义摘录】

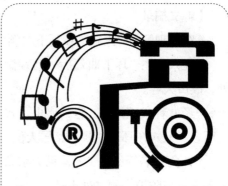

宫，五音之首。本穴为治耳疾要穴，针后能使耳听五音。

《医经理解》："听宫，又名多所闻，耳为听官，穴在耳中珠子，故名也。"

《古法新解会元针灸学》："听宫者，听是耳之所司；宫者心意通脾之返音也。心气出于太阳，行运太阳之终，二火一水而化土，其返应仍存心音。太阳通于耳窍，如管律例，心意内通，其意象徵。脾音为宫，因火能生土，意达则响应，即能知音，故名听宫。又名多所闻者，肾通于耳膜，心气通于耳窍，心肾相交，水火即济，耳即能听闻，故又名多所闻。禅家清心静欲，神安气爽，回光返照，听而不闻，视而不见，气神合一，无所出入，精神内守，只知有命而已矣。"

《经穴释义汇解》："宫，五音之首，针此穴后能听五音，可助恢复听力；又因此穴在耳屏前，深居于耳轮之内，而以宫相喻，故名听宫。"

《针灸穴名释义》："听，指耳的功能。宫，王者之所居。穴在耳前，意为此乃管理听力的高贵之处。"

《针灸穴名解》："宫，深室也，以喻耳窍。"

第八章

足太阳膀胱经穴

1 睛明（手太阳经、足太阳经、足阳明经、阴跷脉、阳跷脉交会穴）

【出处】《黄帝明堂经》。

【别名】目内眦，泪孔。

【穴义】睛，指眼睛；明，光明。本穴在目内眦处，主治目疾，有明目之功，故名"睛明"。

【定位】目内眦内上方眶内侧壁凹陷中（闭目，在目内眦内上方0.1寸的凹陷中）。

【主治】①目赤肿痛，迎风流泪，目视不明，夜盲，目翳；②眩晕。

【释义摘录】

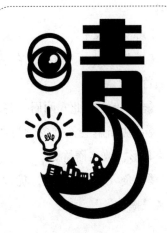

主治目疾，有明目之功，如黑夜中的灯给人带来光明。

《经穴解》："睛之所以明者在瞳仁，而何以此穴为睛明？盖目虽为五脏之所俱属，而目独为肝之窍，然心犹为目之本也，目眦乃心之部分，故以此穴为睛明。禁灸者，恐火气熏目也。此穴所治，皆治目病。"

《古法新解会元针灸学》："睛明者，诸阳气上行而达目，明者五脏六腑之精华，乘阴跷之升冲而返光，如天气之晴朗，发生日光，地气之阴精，而化月光，日月如天地之双睛。人目有二，亦可谓日月。人之双睛能明者，赖五脏六腑之精华返射，诸阳发光而能明，故名睛明。"

《针灸穴名释义》："睛，目睛。明，光明。为治目病之要穴，能使目睛光亮明白也。"

《针灸穴名解》："本穴在目内眦，红肉际。近于睛，能治风热目疾，以复其明，故曰'睛明'。本穴为督脉，手、足太阳，足阳明，阳跷，阴跷六脉之会。故治一切目疾。对郁热之证最宜，如暴赤肿痛、眦痒、翳、障，诸目疾俱效。"

2 攒竹

【出处】《黄帝明堂经》。

【别名】员柱，始光，明光，夜光，鱼头。

【穴义】攒，聚集；攒竹，簇聚之竹。本穴位于眉头凹陷处，眉毛犹如聚簇在一起的新生竹叶，故名"攒竹"。

【定位】眉头凹陷中，额切迹处。

【主治】①头痛，眉头痛；②目赤肿痛，目视不明，流泪，眼睑瞤动，眼睑下垂，口眼㖞斜。

【释义摘录】

《医经理解》："攒竹，在眉尖陷中，言聚眉如竹也。"

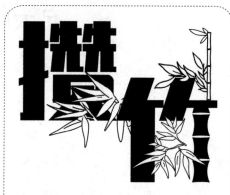

眉毛犹如聚簇在一起的竹叶，穴在眉头凹陷处。

《经穴解》："此穴两眉一蹙，有攒竹之形，故曰攒竹。"

《古法新解会元针灸学》："攒竹者，诸阳之气攒聚于眉头，如新竹之茂，又如竹字以象其形，故名攒竹。"

《针灸穴名解》："眉，犹竹叶，穴在眉内侧端，喻如新篁攒生，本穴犹竹叶之蒂柄，故名'攒竹'。"

3 眉冲

【出处】《脉经·平三关病候并治宜第三》。

【别名】小竹。

【穴义】眉，眉毛；冲，直上。本穴位于两眉头直上入发际处，故名"眉冲"。

【定位】额切迹直上入发际 0.5 寸。

【主治】①头痛，眩晕；②鼻塞；③癫痫。

【释义摘录】

《采艾编》："眉上近中之处，直冲而上也。"

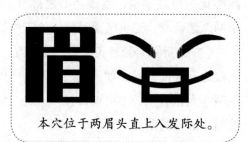

本穴位于两眉头直上入发际处。

《经穴解》："眉冲者，其穴直在眉之上也，为本经上冲至额之所，故曰眉冲。"

《古法新解会元针灸学》："眉冲者，经气从眉直冲入发际，故曰眉冲。"

《针灸穴名释义》："眉，眉头；冲，冲要与向上之意。穴在眉头直上，正当前额冲要之处。"

4 曲差

【出处】《黄帝明堂经》。

【别名】鼻冲。

【穴义】曲，曲折；差，参差不齐。本穴为眉冲旁开横行向外处，因其处经脉曲折参差，故名"曲差"。

【定位】前发际正中直上 0.5 寸，旁开 1.5 寸。

【主治】①头痛，眩晕；②目视不明；③鼻塞。

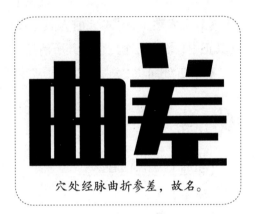

穴处经脉曲折参差，故名。

【释义摘录】

《医经理解》："言自攒竹而上，曲而向外，略有参差也。"

《经穴解》："穴名曲差者，自眉冲而上，乃直行也，自督经中行神庭平处，乃横折一寸五分，其形曲，故曰曲差。"

《古法新解会元针灸学》："曲差者，头为九阳之会，参差不齐，在眉冲穴两旁曲发之处，故名曲差。"

《针灸穴名释义》："曲，见曲池条。差（chā），差错，不齐。指穴当经脉曲折不齐之处。足太阳经自睛明直行向上，行至眉冲处即横行向外，曲而不齐也。"

5 五处

【出处】《黄帝明堂经》。

【别名】无。

【穴义】处，处所。因本穴居于足太阳膀胱经起始的第五个穴位处，故名"五处"。

【定位】前发际正中直上 1 寸，旁开 1.5 寸。

【主治】①头痛，头重，眩晕；②癫痫，

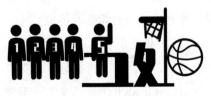

本穴为膀胱经第五个穴位。

抽搐，热病。

【释义摘录】

《医经理解》："五处，上曲差一寸五分。五者尊称也。"

《经穴解》："此穴之后有四穴，并此穴为五穴，皆直行相去一寸五分，至天柱，则夹项后发际大筋外廉陷中，而不在头矣，故名五处，以志之也。"

《针灸穴名释义》："前头部在道经中称为天庭（两眉之间也称天庭），穴居其间，正有天上诸星（五星）罗列之象，且在本经序次亦为第五，或系因此而得名。"

《针灸穴名解》："本穴前为曲差穴，后为承光穴，两旁为上星及目窗穴，加以本穴在其正中，恰为五个穴位。其所治症，均以目病为主。其通孔窍，解郁热，则小异而大同，似有五处同功之意，而本穴居四者之中，故名为'五处'。"

6 承光

【出处】《黄帝明堂经》。

【别名】无。

【穴义】承，承载；光，阳光，光照。承光，承载光照。本穴位置近头顶，主治目疾，如青盲、目翳等，使目光明，有"承受光照恩泽"之意。

【定位】前发际正中直上 2.5 寸，旁开 1.5 寸。

【主治】①头痛，眩晕；②鼻塞。

【释义摘录】

《医经理解》："承光，在五处上一寸五分，言其高将及天，可承天光也。"

《采艾编》："承光，似言上穴通天之牖，此是承光照也。"

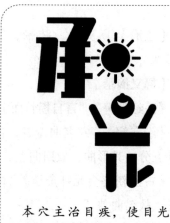

本穴主治目疾，使目光明，故名"承光"，寓意蒙受光明恩泽。

《经穴解》："承者，以下承上之象，光者，指百会穴而言也。百会在人顶上，有人君北辰之象，此穴在其左右之下，有人臣侍君之象，故曰承光。"

《古法新解会元针灸学》："承光穴，本太阳经之光，搏结如太阳之光辉，故两目能视，赖承光之力，能察万物也。"

《经穴释义汇解》："承，下载上也。穴在五处后二寸。足太阳之脉，起目内眦睛明穴，上额，循攒竹，过神庭，历曲差、五处、承光、通天，自通天斜行左右，相交于顶上百会，有下载上之意；又穴主目疾，使目光明，故名承光。"

7 通天

【**出处**】《黄帝明堂经》。

【**别名**】天臼。

【**穴义**】通，通达；天，天部。因本穴位于发际上 4 寸，所处为人体至高之地，喻脉气通于天，故名"通天"。本穴主要功能在于通彻上窍，主治头痛头重、鼻塞多涕、口喎、目盲等上窍不灵之证。

【**定位**】前发际正中直上 4 寸，旁开 1.5 寸。

【**主治**】①头痛，眩晕；②鼻塞，鼻渊，鼻衄。

【**释义摘录**】

《医经理解》："通天，在承光上一寸五分，言此为至高之地，脉气之通天者也。"

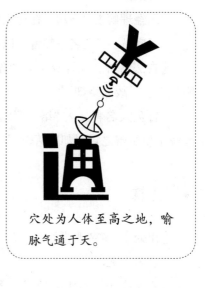

穴处为人体至高之地，喻脉气通于天。

《采艾编》："上为脑，下为鼻，言气之通于颠也。"

《经穴解》："此穴在督之百会左右，乃太阳经横络入足少阳胆经诸穴，养筋脉之所也，又为左右交督经之所，故曰通天。"

《古法新解会元针灸学》："夫天心、地心、足心、人心、顶心、囟，皆相通也。善人之清气，与天心相接，故名通天。"

《针灸穴名解》："《针灸大成·百证赋》云：'通天去鼻内无闻之苦。'鼻司呼吸，亦通天也，故名为'通天'。"

8 络却

【**出处**】《黄帝明堂经》。

【**别名**】脑盖。

【**穴义**】络，联络；却，退却，向后撤退，此处指向脑后循行。足太阳膀胱经经脉循行有云"其直者，从颠入络脑，还出别下项"，意即膀胱经从头顶处入里联络于脑，然后还出下行时转向脑后，穴当其处，故名"络却"。

【**定位**】前发际正中直上 5.5 寸，旁开

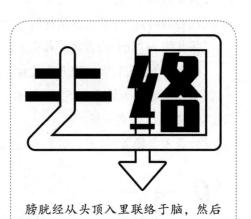

膀胱经从头顶入里联络于脑，然后还出下行时转向脑后，穴当其处。

1.5 寸。

【主治】①头痛，眩晕；②耳鸣，癫狂。

【释义摘录】

《医经理解》："络却，在通天后一寸五分。言脉络至此，始却而向后也。"

《经穴解》："穴名络却者，以本经至通天，乃在顶际，此则却行向后，故曰络却。"

《古法新解会元针灸学》："络却者，络者阴络也，却者去脑后也，脑血冲来，而生阳复去也，故名络却。"

《针灸穴名释义》："络，联络，缠绕。却，退却，脱落。穴当古人系冠之处，联络缠绕不使所戴之冠退却脱落也。"

9 玉枕

【出处】《黄帝明堂经》。

【别名】无。

【穴义】玉，石头之精华，形容贵重。脑为人体中枢系统之所在，颅骨保护脑的重要性犹如执玉，其中枕骨为仰卧位时着枕的部位，故将枕骨两旁的突起称为"玉枕骨"。穴当其处，故名"玉枕"。

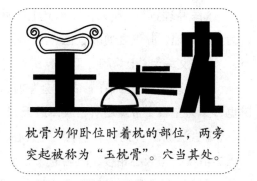

枕骨为仰卧位时着枕的部位，两旁突起被称为"玉枕骨"。穴当其处。

【定位】横平枕外隆凸上缘，后发际正中旁开 1.3 寸。

【主治】①头痛，颈项强痛；②目痛，鼻塞。

【释义摘录】

《医经理解》："玉枕，在络却后一寸五分，夹脑户一寸三分，起肉枕骨上也。"

《采艾编》："起骨为吉象，其贵如玉也。"

《经穴解》："玉枕者，以穴在枕骨上也。"

《古法新解会元针灸学》："玉枕者，玉者贵重也；枕骨也，仰卧着枕，脑后之骨要保重甚于执玉，故名玉枕。"

《针灸穴名释义》："玉，贵重之意；枕，指枕骨。穴与枕骨为邻，故名。"

10 天柱

【出处】《灵枢·本输》。

【**别名**】无。

【**穴义**】天，上部、头部；柱，支柱。人体以头为天，颈椎犹如攀天之柱，故被称为"天柱骨"。穴在项部，斜方肌起始部，天柱骨两旁，故名"天柱"。

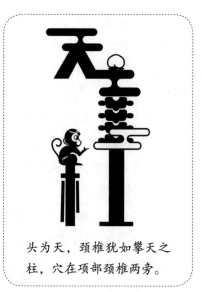

头为天，颈椎犹如攀天之柱，穴在项部颈椎两旁。

【**定位**】横平第 2 颈椎棘突上际，斜方肌外缘凹陷中（后发际正中直上 0.5 寸，斜方肌外缘凹陷中）。

【**主治**】①头痛，眩晕；②目痛；③癫狂痫，热病；④颈项强痛，肩背痛。

【**释义摘录**】

《医经理解》："天柱，夹项后大筋外廉发际陷中。是天柱骨际也。"

《经穴解》："天者，指首而言也。此穴紧在两大筋之旁，以载夫首，有柱之象，故曰天柱。"

《针灸穴名释义》："天，指头部，柱，支柱，梁柱。天柱，山名，又星名。意为穴处乃头部之支柱。天柱，星名，见《晋书·天文志》。山名，见《史记·封禅书》。星譬其高，山象其用。柱，支柱也。《国语·周语》：'天之所支，不可坏也。'《金针梅花诗钞》天柱条：'天柱将颓眩晕生。头疼项强脊难伸。'擎天有柱，则诸症自除。"

《针灸穴名解》："人体以头为天，颈项为其支柱。穴在颈上，故名'天柱'。凡患颈项痛委，不能支持头脑者，谓为天柱骨折，绝症也。小儿有患之者，刺此穴或能得救。"

11 大杼（八会穴之骨会，手、足太阳经交会穴）

【**出处**】《素问·水热穴论》《灵枢·刺节真邪》。

【**别名**】无。

【**穴义**】杼，织布机的梭子。椎骨横突形如织机上的梭子，第一胸椎横突尤大。因本穴位于第一胸椎棘突下两旁，故名"大杼"。

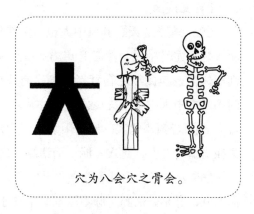

穴为八会穴之骨会。

【**定位**】第 1 胸椎棘突下，后正中线旁开 1.5 寸。

【**主治**】①咳嗽，气喘；②发热；③颈项强痛，肩背痛。

【释义摘录】

《医经理解》："大杼，在项后第一椎下，两旁相去脊中各二寸。《海论》曰：'冲脉者其输上出于大杼。'《气穴论》注曰：'督脉别络，手足太阳三脉之会，故为经脉之大机杼也。'"

《经穴解》："又杼之名义即梭也，乃经之持纬者，此下肋枝皆横列于背，而太阳经脉从此穴直行而下，次第纬之，有梭纬经之象，故名大杼。"

《古法新解会元针灸学》："大杼者，两肩骨大如杼中，形如杼箧，足太阳经形如水槽出入在其杼中。"

《经穴释义汇解》："穴为背中大腧，因在背俞穴之中，它的部位高居于五脏六腑各穴之上，又位在杼骨之端，故名大杼。"

《针灸穴名释义》："脊旁肌肉长大，经气自此下行，具有机杼与水槽之状，故名。"

12 风门（足太阳经、督脉交会穴）

【出处】《黄帝明堂经》。

【别名】热府。

【穴义】风，指代风邪，为六淫之一。本穴为风邪入侵人体的门户，可用于治疗一切因风而致的疾病，故名"风门"。

【定位】第2胸椎棘突下，后正中线旁开1.5寸。

【主治】①咳嗽，发热，头痛，鼻塞，鼻流清涕；②颈项强痛，胸背痛。

【释义摘录】

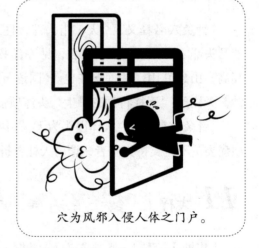

穴为风邪入侵人体之门户。

《经穴解》："天之邪风中人也，多在于上，而人之背尤易中风，然必有窍焉，以招其中。故在督之中行，于项之侧，足少阳之经，则曰风池，与此经之在背者，则又有风门焉。其入风最易，犹开门以受风者，故曰风门。风之中人，皮毛先受之，肺主皮毛，故此穴之下，而肺俞紧接焉。皆自然之理也。古人云：'若频刺此穴，泄诸阳热气，背永不发痈疽。'盖以本经为一身之巨阳，而此穴又在诸腧穴之上，此穴一泄，而诸腧穴之热俱泄，风热去则毒气解，而痈疽何由生哉。"

《古法新解会元针灸学》："风门者，风所出入之门也。此穴在肺之上部，肺属金，而振肝，肝阳鼓荡肺，肺不受邪，上冲于背，遁开风门则外邪乘虚来攻，经络大血管则闭，即发中风半身不遂之类，故名风门。又名热府者，诸热生风行于背，肺之上空，当积瘀热，故又名热府。"

《针灸穴名释义》："风，指气，又指风邪。门，见云门条。风门者，既为肺气出入与风邪犯人之门户，也为治风治气之所宜取。《广雅·释言》：'风，气也。'故风并不单指风之邪气而言。穴在肺俞之上方，为肺气出入之所必由。用治风邪外感、上气咳逆诸病，将有双重意义。"

《针灸穴名解》："本穴与督脉之陶道穴相近，'陶道'喻其旋转也。凡物体旋转，则必生风。风生则大气清凉，正合本穴能治诸般热证之义。本穴内应肺体，为气息出纳之道路，故名'风门'。如旧式风匣前后有风门也。养生家称之为橐龠。观此穴大意，治气管病，当能有效。"

13 肺俞（肺之背俞穴）

【出处】《灵枢·背腧》。

【别名】无。

【穴义】肺，肺脏；俞，同"输"，运输、输注。本穴位置近肺，为肺脏之气输注于背部之处，有宣肺平喘、化痰止咳、清热理气之功，是治疗肺部疾患的重要穴位，故名肺俞。

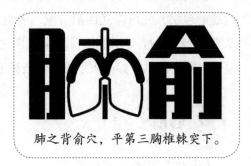

肺之背俞穴，平第三胸椎棘突下。

【定位】第 3 胸椎棘突下，后正中线旁开 1.5 寸。

【主治】①咳嗽，气喘，肺痨，咳血，潮热，盗汗；②小儿龟背。

【释义摘录】

《采艾编》："凡言俞者，本经所注也。"

《古法新解会元针灸学》："肺俞者，系在于背，足太阳经所过肺之系部，故名肺俞。"

《针灸穴名释义》："肺，指肺本脏，又为火气勃郁之意。俞，见膈俞条。内通肺脏，可治病火病气诸病。《释名·释形体》：'肺，勃也，言其气勃郁也。'"

14 厥阴俞（心包之背俞穴）

【出处】《千金要方·肺脏方·积气第五》。

【别名】心包俞，阙输，巨阙俞。

【穴义】厥阴，指手厥阴心包。本穴为心包之气输注背部之处，有宽胸理气之功，是治疗心及心包疾患的重要穴位，故名"厥阴俞"。

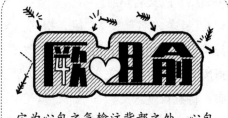

穴为心包之气输注背部之处。心包为心之宫城，代心受邪，平第四胸椎棘突下。

【定位】第4胸椎棘突下，后正中线旁开1.5寸。

【主治】①心痛，胸闷；②咳嗽；③呕吐。

【释义摘录】

《经穴解》："厥阴，心包也；俞，输也。心包之气血，输于此穴也。"

《经穴释义汇解》："厥阴俞，即心包络俞也。穴在肺俞与心俞之间，是手厥阴心包络气血输注之处。厥阴有消尽之意，本穴可治心气不固、四肢厥逆之证，故名厥阴俞。"

《针灸穴名释义》："厥阴，指心包络，又为阴气至极与厥逆之意。俞，见臑俞条。内通心包络，并可降逆回阳。厥，逆也，冷也，又极与尽也。《释名·释疾病》：'逆气从下厥起，上行入心腹也。'厥阴，阴之尽也，手厥阴出自胸中，足厥阴下起大敦上至颠顶。阴极阳生，如心阳不振、四肢厥逆及逆气上冲者，皆可选用。"

15 心俞（心之背俞穴）

【出处】《灵枢·背俞》。

【别名】背俞，伍焦之间，心之俞。

【穴义】本穴位置近心，为心气输注于背部之处，有疏通心络、调理气血、宁心安神之功，是治心脏疾患的重要穴位，故名"心俞"。

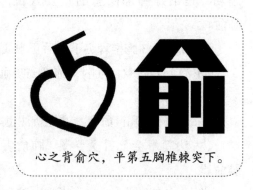

心之背俞穴，平第五胸椎棘突下。

【定位】第5胸椎棘突下，后正中线旁开1.5寸。

【主治】①心痛，惊悸，失眠，健忘，梦遗；②咳嗽，咳血，盗汗；③癫痫。

【释义摘录】

《古法新解会元针灸学》："心俞者，心脏系于背部，足太阳之所穿行，故名心俞。"

《经穴释义汇解》："心形如未敷莲花，附着于脊之第五椎。穴在第五椎下两旁各一寸五分，是心气转输、输注之穴，是治心疾之重要腧穴，故名心俞。"

《针灸穴名释义》："心，指心本脏，又是'任'与'容'的意思。俞，见臑俞条。内通心脏，可以益气行血，安神定惊。"

《针灸穴名解》："本穴与督脉之神道穴平。心藏神也，本穴为心脏之俞，故名'心俞'。其所治症为有关心脏及其近旁诸症，以及食道、气道诸病。如心风、偏瘫、狂癫、神乱、胸闷、吐衄、目䀮、健忘等症。"

16 督俞

【出处】《太平圣惠方·卷第九十九》。

【别名】高盖，督脉俞。

【穴义】督，指督脉。本穴为督脉之气输注于背部之处，可治疗督脉所过部位的疾病，如腰、脊、头脑之病，故名"督俞"。

【定位】第6胸椎棘突下，后正中线旁开1.5寸。

【主治】①心痛；②腹痛，腹胀，肠鸣，气逆。

穴为督脉之气输注于背部之处，督脉是统率全身阳气之脉。

【释义摘录】

《古法新解会元针灸学》："督起诸阳，统阳气于足太阳经之所过，通督脉之系，故名督俞。"

《经穴释义汇解》："督俞，亦称督脉俞。在六椎下两旁各寸半。言督脉之气转输、输注之腧穴，故名督俞或督脉俞。"

《针灸穴名释义》："督脉贯脊而行，为脏腑诸俞之所依附，故能督正诸俞，贯通腰脊。"

《针灸穴名解》："本穴即督脉之俞也，能治腰、骨髓及头脑诸病之有关于督者，故名'督俞'。"

17 膈俞（八会穴之血会）

【出处】《灵枢·背腧》。

【别名】无。

【穴义】膈，指横膈膜。本穴位于第七胸椎棘突下两旁，内应横膈膜，有宽胸理气、和胃降逆之功，是治疗呃逆、噎膈等膈肌疾患的要穴，故名"膈俞"。此外，本穴位于心

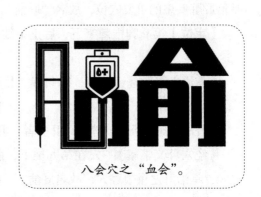
八会穴之"血会"。

俞与肝俞之间，心主血，肝藏血，有活血祛风的功效，可用于治疗咯血、衄血等血证以及荨麻疹等，故为八会穴之"血会"。

【定位】第7胸椎棘突下，后正中线旁开1.5寸。

【主治】①呕吐，呃逆，吐血；②气喘。

【释义摘录】

《古法新解会元针灸学》："膈俞即横膈之所系于背。俞者，过也，足太阳之所过，故名膈俞。"

《经穴释义汇解》："穴在第七椎下两旁各一寸五分，内应横膈，为主膈胃寒痰、噎膈等疾之腧穴，故名膈俞。"

《针灸穴名释义》："膈，指胸膈，关格。俞，见臑俞条。内通胸膈，可以开通关格。《玉篇》：'膈，胸膈。'《释名·释形体》：'膈，隔也。隔塞上下使气与谷不相乱也。'又，格拒也。膈俞者，可以开通胸膈之关格及格拒否塞诸病之处也。"

《针灸穴名解》："本穴内应横膈膜，而为之俞，故名'膈俞'。治膈肌有病，如格忒心跳之类。因动脉血管贯膈下行，静脉血管贯膈上行，全部膈肌与血液循环大有关系，故本穴又为血之会穴，而治吐衄、血晕诸病。又以食道下行，亦由膈肌穿过，故治胃脘痛、反胃、食不下、脉胀、肢肿、积气、周痹，诸有关膈肌、食管、气道之症。以及便血、肠痈、脏毒等症，凡属有关血瘀者，均可取此。因血之会穴，乃膈俞也。瘀者多凝，得热可散，故宜多灸。"

18 肝俞（肝之背俞穴）

【出处】《灵枢·背腧》。

【别名】无。

【穴义】本穴位置近肝脏，为肝脏之气输注于背部之处，有疏肝理气、凉血明目之功，是治肝脏疾患的重要穴位，故名"肝俞"。

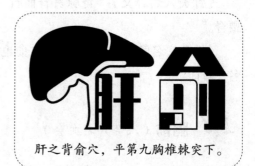

肝之背俞穴，平第九胸椎棘突下。

【定位】第9胸椎棘突下，后正中线旁开1.5寸。

【主治】①胁痛，黄疸；②目赤，目视不明，夜盲，流泪；③吐血；④癫狂病。

【释义摘录】

《古法新解会元针灸学》："肝俞者，肝之系于背，太阳脉之所过，故名肝俞。"

《经穴释义汇解》："穴在第九椎下，两旁各一寸五分，内应肝，是肝气转输、输注之穴，是治肝之重要腧穴，故名肝俞。"

《针灸穴名释义》："肝，指肝本脏，又木也，干也。俞，见膈俞条。内通肝脏，可达木气之郁滞。"

《针灸穴名解》："肝在膈下。本穴内应肝脏而为之俞，故名'肝俞'。"

19 胆俞 （胆之背俞穴）

【出处】《黄帝明堂经》。

【别名】无。

【穴义】本穴位置近胆，为胆气输注于背部之处，有疏利肝胆、清泄肝胆湿热之功，是治胆腑疾患的重要穴位，故名"胆俞"。

【定位】第 10 胸椎棘突下，后正中线旁开 1.5 寸。

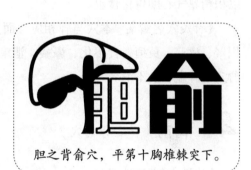

胆之背俞穴，平第十胸椎棘突下。

【主治】呕吐，口苦，黄疸，胁痛。

【释义摘录】

《古法新解会元针灸学》："胆俞者，胆在肝之下，而连系于背，足太阳脉之所过胆部，故名胆俞。"

《经穴释义汇解》："穴在第十椎下两旁各一寸五分，为胆气转输、输注之穴，是治胆之重要腧穴，故名胆俞。"

《针灸穴名释义》："胆，指胆本腑，为连肝之府。俞，见膈俞条。内通胆腑，利胆疏风。"

《针灸穴名解》："胆附于肝，本穴内应于胆，而为之俞，故名'胆俞'。"

20 脾俞 （脾之背俞穴）

【出处】《灵枢·背腧》。

【别名】无。

【穴义】本穴位置近脾，为脾气输注于背部之处，有健脾利湿之功，是治脾脏疾患的重要穴位，故名"脾俞"。

【定位】第 11 胸椎棘突下，后正中线旁开 1.5 寸。

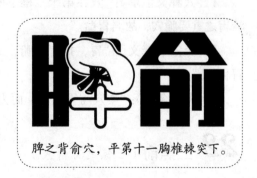

脾之背俞穴，平第十一胸椎棘突下。

【主治】①腹胀，呕吐，泄泻；②水肿，黄疸；③多食善饥，身瘦。

【释义摘录】

《古法新解会元针灸学》："脾俞者，所系背部，太阳经之所过，故名脾俞。"

《经穴释义汇解》："穴在第十一椎下两旁各一寸五分，是脾气转输、输注之穴，是治脾之重要腧穴，故名脾俞。"

《针灸穴名释义》："脾，指脾本脏；又裨也，并也。俞，见膈俞条。内通脾脏，可以积精禀气、助胃化食也。"

《针灸穴名解》："本穴与脾相应，而为之俞，故名'脾俞'。治胀满、吐逆、疹癖、积聚、痎疟、黄疸、食不化、羸瘦、泄痢等症。凡关于脾病者，以本穴治之，兼取膀胱俞穴治脾虚、食不消。"

21 胃俞（胃之背俞穴）

【出处】《黄帝明堂经》。

【别名】无。

【穴义】本穴位置近胃，为胃气输注于背部之处，有健脾和胃、消食化滞之功，是治胃腑疾患的重要穴位，故名"胃俞"。

【定位】第 12 胸椎棘突下，后正中线旁开 1.5 寸。

【主治】①胃痛，呕吐，腹胀，肠鸣；②多食善饥，身瘦。

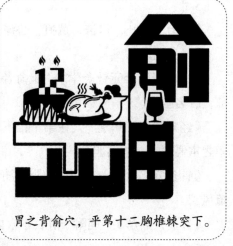

胃之背俞穴，平第十二胸椎棘突下。

【释义摘录】

《古法新解会元针灸学》："胃俞者，胃为五谷之海，胃膜连系于背，足太阳之所过，故名胃俞。"

《经穴释义汇解》："穴在第十二椎下两旁各一寸五分，是胃气转输、输注之穴，是治胃之重要腧穴，故名胃俞。"

《针灸穴名释义》："胃，指胃本腑，又围也，委也。俞，见膈俞条。内通胃腑，调胃化气。"

《针灸穴名解》："本穴与胃相应，而为之俞，故名'胃俞'。"

22 三焦俞（三焦之背俞穴）

【出处】《黄帝明堂经》。

【**别名**】无。

【**穴义**】本穴为三焦之气输注于腰部之处，有通调水道之功，是治三焦疾患之重要穴位，如水肿、小便不利等水液代谢障碍，故名"三焦俞"。

【**定位**】第1腰椎棘突下，后正中线旁开1.5寸。

【**主治**】①腹胀，呕吐，肠鸣，泄泻；②小便不利，水肿；③腰背痛。

【**释义摘录**】

《经穴解》："十三椎下为三焦俞，督之十三椎为悬枢，枢所以主开闭者在乎中，而三焦之俞即在乎旁，观此，则三焦之气化可见一斑矣。"

《经穴释义汇解》："穴在第十三椎下两旁各一寸五分，是三焦之气转输、输注之穴，是治三焦病患之重要腧穴，故名三焦俞。"

《针灸穴名释义》："三焦，指胸腹腔上中下三停之空松处。俞，见膈俞条。内应全身，升阳决渎。"

《针灸穴名解》："本穴与人体上中下各部脂膜相应，而为之俞，故名'三焦俞'。治胀满、膈塞不通、呕逆、饮食不化、肩背急、腰脊强、少腹坚硬、注泻下痢、目眩、头痛、妇人癥聚。凡病之有关脂膜者，俱应取此，以舒三焦郁滞之气。"

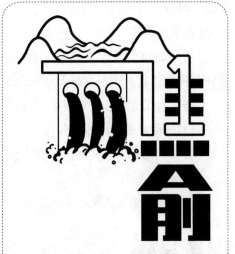

穴平第一腰椎棘突下，为三焦之气输注于腰部之处，有通调水道之功。

23 肾俞 （肾之背俞穴）

【**出处**】《灵枢·背腧》。

【**别名**】无。

【**穴义**】本穴位置近肾，为肾气输注于腰部之处，有益肾助阳、强腰利水、聪耳明目之功，是治疗肾脏疾患的重要穴位，故名"肾俞"。

【**定位**】第2腰椎棘突下，后正中线旁开1.5寸。

【**主治**】①耳鸣，耳聋；②遗尿，遗精，

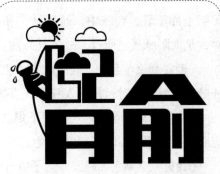

肾之背俞穴，有益肾气，强腰膝之功，平第2腰椎棘突下。

阳痿，早泄；③月经不调，带下，不孕；④多食善饥，身瘦；⑤腰痛。

【释义摘录】

《古法新解会元针灸学》："肾俞者，肾为作强之官，智巧出焉，与膀胱表里相通，带脉相连系。其系于背，足太阳脉之所过，故名肾俞。"

《经穴释义汇解》："穴在第十四椎下两旁各一寸五分，应肾，是肾气转输、输注之穴，是治肾重要腧穴，故名肾俞。"

《针灸穴名释义》："肾，指肾本脏，又藏也，写（泻）也。俞，见臑俞条。内通肾脏，引水藏精。"

《针灸穴名解》："本穴与肾脏相应，而为之俞，故名'肾俞'。"

24 气海俞

【出处】《太平圣惠方·卷第九十九》。

【别名】无。

【穴义】本穴对应任脉气海穴，是人身原气输注于腰背部之处，有助肾纳气之功，故名"气海俞"，其所治各症与气海穴略同。

【定位】第 3 腰椎棘突下，后正中线旁开 1.5 寸。

【主治】①腰痛，痛经；②痔疾。

【释义摘录】

《经穴解》："气海穴乃任经脐下第二穴也，去脐之下一寸半，乃男女生气之海也。"

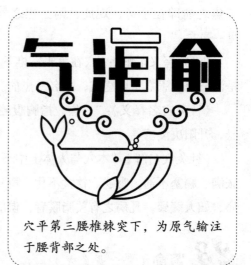

穴平第三腰椎棘突下，为原气输注于腰背部之处。

《古法新解会元针灸学》："化血之精，从阳明上冲至乳，会膻中，通任脉，和心血，归经入血海而化气，再归气海，与背俞相对，足太阳脉气之所过，故名气海俞。"

《经穴释义汇解》："气海俞在十五椎下两旁各寸半，为人之生气注输所出之处，与任脉之气海穴相对，是与人身原气直接关系之穴位，故名气海俞。"

《针灸穴名释义》："气，指下焦之原气。海，是富饶藏聚之意。俞，见臑俞条。内应脐下之肓原，吞吐下焦之原气。"

《针灸穴名解》："俗云'男子以气为主'，因男子腹呼吸，依气海处主持吐纳，故本穴所治各症，多与任脉之气海穴略同。"

25 大肠俞（大肠之背俞穴）

【出处】《黄帝明堂经》。

【别名】无。

【穴义】本穴为大肠之气输注于腰背部之处，有疏调肠腑、理气化滞之功，是治疗大肠疾患的重要穴位，故名"大肠俞"。

【定位】第4腰椎棘突下，后正中线旁开1.5寸。

【主治】①腹胀，腹痛，肠鸣，泄泻，便秘；②腰痛。

【释义摘录】

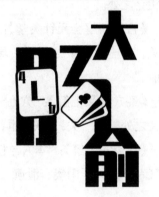

大肠之背俞穴，平第4腰椎棘突下。

《古法新解会元针灸学》："大肠俞者，在左回叠积十六曲，直肠在右（即盲肠），长七寸，系于十六椎之两旁。足太阳之所过，故名大肠俞。"

《经穴释义汇解》："穴在第十六椎下两旁各一寸五分，是大肠之气转输、输注之穴，是主大肠病之重要腧穴，故名大肠俞。"

《针灸穴名释义》："大肠，指大肠本腑，又畅也。俞，见臑俞条。内通大肠，畅胃去滓。《释名·释形体》：'肠，畅也。通畅胃气，去滓秽也。'大肠司传导，主变化，体之俞，腑之应也。"

《针灸穴名解》："本穴与大肠相应，而为之俞。治肠鸣、泻痢、绕脐切痛、腰痛、腹胀、食不化、大小便难。诸症之有关于大肠者，皆可取此以舒之，故名'大肠俞'。"

26 关元俞

【出处】《太平圣惠方·卷第九十九》。

【别名】无。

【穴义】本穴对应关元穴，为人身元气输注于腰背部之处，可培补元气，主治阳痿、遗精、带下、泄痢等，与关元穴相似，故名"关元俞"。

【定位】第5腰椎棘突下，后正中线旁开1.5寸。

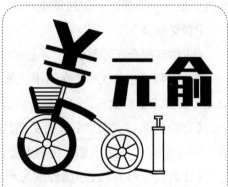

穴为人身元气输注于腰背部之处，可培补元气，故名。穴在第五腰椎棘突下旁开1.5寸。

【主治】①腹胀，泄泻；②尿频，遗尿，小便不利；③腰骶痛。

【释义摘录】

《经穴解》："关元乃任经穴，在脐下三寸，为小肠之募，乃足三阴肾、肝、脾与任脉相会之处。"

《古法新解会元针灸学》："关元即膀胱下口，司气化，卫气所出之门，小水外出之机关，亦全身重要之关窍，导阴于下，导阳于上，有系于背，足太阳之所过，故名关元俞。"

《经穴释义汇解》："穴在十七椎下两旁各寸半，与任脉之关元穴相对，为人体阳气交关之处，又'关'，联络也，也称联络元气之俞穴，故名关元俞。"

《针灸穴名解》："本穴与任脉关元穴相应，而为之俞，故名'关元俞'。凡病之关于元气者，如男子阳痿、泄遗，女子癥瘕、白带，便难、泻痢、虚胀等症，皆可取之。"

27 小肠俞（小肠之背俞穴）

【出处】《黄帝明堂经》。

【别名】无。

【穴义】本穴为小肠之气输注于腰背部之处，有通调肠腑之功，是治疗小肠疾患的重要穴位，故名"小肠俞"。

【定位】横平第1骶后孔，后正中线旁开1.5寸。

【主治】①遗精，遗尿，尿血，小便涩痛，疝气，带下；②泄泻；③腰骶痛。

穴为小肠之背俞穴，有泌别清浊之功。

【释义摘录】

《古法新解会元针灸学》："小肠俞者，系于背，足太阳之所过，故名小肠俞。"

《经穴释义汇解》："穴在第十八椎下两旁各寸五分，是小肠之气转输、输注之穴，是主小肠疾之重要腧穴，故名小肠俞。"

《针灸穴名释义》："小肠司受盛，主化物。张隐庵曰：'小肠居胃之下，胃之运化者，赖以受盛。'受盛失职，化物无能，自可于此处求之。"

《针灸穴名解》："按小肠外围为水，与三焦、膀胱均有连系，故本穴所应之症，常有选取三焦、膀胱两经之穴协助取效者。"

28 膀胱俞（膀胱之背俞穴）

【出处】《黄帝明堂经》。

【别名】无。

【穴义】本穴位置近膀胱，为膀胱之气输注于腰背部之处，是治疗膀胱疾患的重要穴位，故名"膀胱俞"。

【定位】横平第 2 骶后孔，后正中线旁开 1.5 寸。

【主治】①小便不利，遗尿；②泄泻，便秘；③腰骶痛。

【释义摘录】

《经穴解》："足太阳之正，行入腰中，循膂络肾，下属膀胱矣，而膀胱之腑气，又输于此，为膀胱俞。"

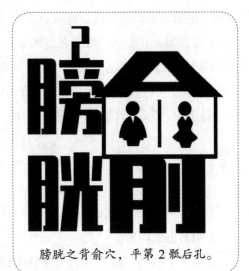

膀胱之背俞穴，平第 2 骶后孔。

《古法新解会元针灸学》："膀胱之膜系于背，其经之所过，故名膀胱俞。"

《针灸穴名释义》："膀胱，指膀胱本腑。俞，见臑俞条。内通膀胱，藏津决水。膀胱津之府，水之门，外俞内府，彼此互通。"

《针灸穴名解》："本穴与膀胱相应，而为之俞，故名'膀胱俞'。"

29 中膂俞

【出处】《黄帝明堂经》。

【别名】中膂，中膂内俞，脊内俞。

【穴义】中，中点；膂，指背脊肉，即脊柱旁背、腰、臀部的肌肉。本穴位于人体全长的折中处，且穴下为脊柱旁的臀大肌，故名"中膂俞"。

【定位】横平第 3 骶后孔，后正中线旁开 1.5 寸。

【主治】①腹胀，泄泻，痢疾；②腰骶痛。

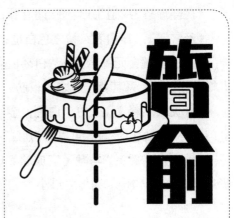

本穴位于人体全长的折中处，故名"中"。

【释义摘录】

《医经理解》："中膂俞，在第二十椎下。膂，脊中肉也，故又名脊中俞。"

《经穴解》："膂者，夹脊两旁肉也，在内则为夹脊之脂络，在外则为夹脊之膂，内以系各脏腑，外以载各穴，亦在背之至要者也，故有俞焉。"

《经穴释义汇解》："膂，背脊肉也。腧穴在第二十椎下两旁各一寸五分，夹脊胂而起，即夹脊椎两旁隆起的肌肉之中，故名中膂俞或中膂内俞，或脊内俞。"

《针灸穴名释义》："中，指人身的中部。膂，背脊。俞，见膈俞条。穴在骶部，约居人身之中，为腰膂之气所注输。"

30 白环俞

【出处】《黄帝明堂经》。

【别名】玉环俞。

【穴义】白环，指玉环，道家认为这是人体的藏精之处。本穴为玉环精华之气输注于腰部之处，主治白浊、带下、遗精、月经不调、虚劳骨蒸等精气不足之证，故名"白环俞"。

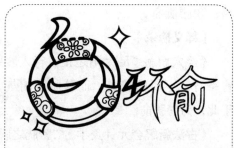

本穴为玉环精华之气输注于腰部之处。

【定位】横平第 4 骶后孔，后正中线旁开 1.5 寸（骶管裂孔旁开 1.5 寸）。

【主治】①遗尿，遗精白浊，赤白带下，月经不调；②腰骶痛。

【释义摘录】

《医经理解》："道书曰：'腰间有脉，其白如绵，其连如环。'盖指肾也。"

《经穴解》："曰白者，精之色白也；环者，督、任二脉如环之无端也。"

《古法新解会元针灸学》："白环俞者，其大板筋色白，下系于环跳，上通肾带，至九椎总连韧筋，系其背连胯之大板筋，足太阳之所过，故名白环俞。"

《针灸穴名释义》："白，白色，金气；环，圆环；俞，见膈俞条。白环，可能是指肛门或臀部，故白环俞者可以意为肛门或臀部之俞也。"

《针灸穴名解》："马融《广成颂》曰：'纳焦侥之珍羽，受王母之白环。'即人身最贵最密处也。'焦侥'喻体之最小，'王母'喻体之受生处也。"

31 上髎

【出处】《黄帝明堂经》。

【别名】无。

【穴义】髎，孔隙，此指骶骨后孔。穴在骶骨第一孔中，居上，故名"上髎"。本穴平于关元俞，有调经、益气、固脱之功，主治月经不调、带下、遗精、腰痛膝软等生殖系统和腰骶部疾患。

穴在骶骨第一孔中，居上。

【定位】正对第 1 骶后孔中。

【主治】①月经不调，带下，阴挺，阴疝；②腰骶痛。

【释义摘录】

《古法新解会元针灸学》："上髎者，腰髁下方骨空髎陷中上空，故名上髎。"

《经穴释义汇解》："髎，与窌同。窌，空穴也。人身骶骨叫髎骨。穴为足太阳脉之空穴，位在第一空腰髁下一寸，夹脊凹陷处，即在骶骨第一孔中，居上，故名上髎或上窌。"

《针灸穴名解》："荐骨左右八孔，排序次第曰上、次、中、下，名曰'八髎'。本穴居上，故名'上髎'。与关元俞穴相邻，治症同于关元俞穴。"

32 次髎

【出处】《黄帝明堂经》。

【别名】无。

【穴义】次，第二；髎，孔隙，此指骶骨后孔。穴在骶骨第二孔中，位居上髎穴之次，故名"次髎"。主治同"上髎"，是治疗痛经的首选穴位。

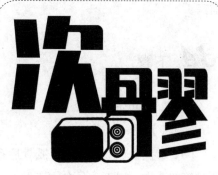

穴在骶骨第二孔中，位居上髎穴之次。

【定位】正对第 2 骶后孔中。

【主治】①月经不调，痛经，带下，遗精，小便不利，疝气；②腰痛，下肢痿痹。

【释义摘录】

《医经理解》："次髎，夹脊旁第二空。"

《经穴释义汇解》："人身骶骨叫髎骨。穴为足太阳脉之空穴，位在第二空夹脊凹陷处，即在骶骨第二孔中，居次上，故名次髎或次窌。"

《针灸穴名解》："本穴居次，故名'次髎'。相邻小肠俞穴，故其治症与小肠俞穴同。"

33 中髎

【出处】《黄帝明堂经》。

【别名】无。

【穴义】髎，孔隙，此指骶骨后孔。穴在骶骨第三孔中，居中，故名"中髎"。

【定位】正对第3骶后孔中。

【主治】①月经不调，带下，小便不利；②便秘，泄泻；③腰骶痛。

【释义摘录】

《医经理解》："中髎，夹脊旁第三空。"

《经穴解》："穴在三空夹脊陷中，足厥阴肝经、足少阳胆经所结之会。"

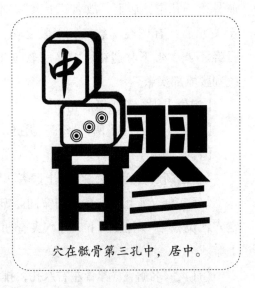

穴在骶骨第三孔中，居中。

《古法新解会元针灸学》："中髎者，在背部方骨第三空髎处，夹脊各开一寸空中，故名中髎。"

《针灸穴名解》："本穴居第三，而强名之为'中髎'。相邻膀胱俞穴，故其治症同膀胱俞穴。"

34 下髎

【出处】《黄帝明堂经》。

【别名】无。

【穴义】髎，孔隙，此指骶骨后孔。穴在骶骨第四孔中，居下，故名"下髎"。

【定位】正对第4骶后孔中。

【主治】①带下，便秘，便血，小便不利；②疝痛引小腹，腰痛。

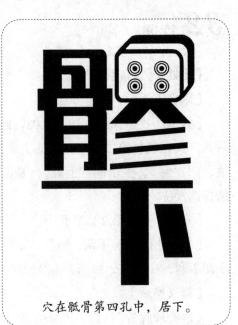

穴在骶骨第四孔中，居下。

【释义摘录】

《医经理解》:"下髎,夹脊旁第四空。"

《经穴解》:"穴在四空夹脊陷中。"

《古法新解会元针灸学》:"下髎者,八髎之中居其下,在背部方骨空髎陷中,足太阳脉所过之郄空,故名下髎。"

《针灸穴名解》:"本穴居下,故名'下髎'。与中膂俞穴相邻,故其治症同于中膂俞穴。"

35 会阳

【出处】《黄帝明堂经》。

【别名】利机。

【穴义】会,交会;阳,指阳经。本穴乃足太阳膀胱经与督脉交会之处,为阳经之会,故名"会阳"。

【定位】尾骨端旁开 0.5 寸。

【主治】①痔疾,痢疾;②阳痿,带下。

【释义摘录】

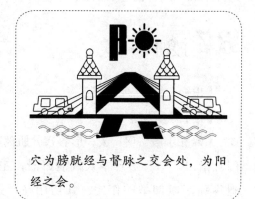

穴为膀胱经与督脉之交会处,为阳经之会。

《医经理解》:"会阳,阳脉气所会也。"

《采艾编》:"会阳者,向也,前会阴,此会阳,二行三行分为两,此则并而合会。"

《经穴解》:"穴名会阳者,乃太阳左右四行,俱会于此尾尻之两旁,而有是名也。"

《古法新解会元针灸学》:"会者,足三阳冲于背,从谷道过尾闾而从督脉自会阳双关而上,故名会阳。"

《针灸穴名释义》:"穴与会阴相邻,自有交通结合与互相对待之义。"

36 承扶

【出处】《黄帝明堂经》。

【别名】扶承,肉郄,阴关,皮部。

【穴义】承,承受;扶,扶持。穴在臀下横纹正中,臀之下,大腿之上,有承托上身而辅助下肢的作用,故名"承扶"。

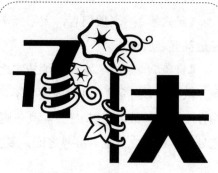

穴在臀之下,大腿之上,有承托上身而辅助下肢的作用。

【定位】臀沟的中点。

【主治】①痔疾，脱肛，便秘，小便不利；②腰、骶、臀、股痛。

【释义摘录】

《医经理解》："承扶，在尻臀下股阴上约文中，言此乃承身部而相扶也。"

《古法新解会元针灸学》："承扶者，承于上而至于下也，扶护臀下。足太阳筋夹于骨，承上而辅之下，故名承扶。"

《经穴释义汇解》："承，止也。扶作匍匐同音。穴在尻臀下股阴上陷纹中，即臀之尽止处，因穴当承受上身而辅助下肢，故名承扶。"

《针灸穴名释义》："承，见承光条。扶，扶持，扶助，又风名。谓其对扶持人体与治疗下肢风病，俱可承担也。"

37 殷门

【出处】《黄帝明堂经》。

【别名】无。

【穴义】殷，盛、大，形容穴处肌肉丰厚。门，指出入口，形容本穴宣泄瘀滞，主治腰腿疼痛难以伸举的作用，其功用在于通泻，犹如邪气的出口。故名"殷门"。

【定位】臀沟下6寸，股二头肌与半肌腱之间。

【主治】腰痛，下肢痿痹。

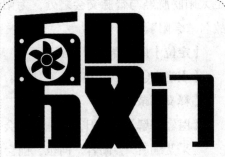

穴处肌肉殷实丰厚，其功用在于通泻，犹如邪气的出口。

【释义摘录】

《医经理解》："殷盛也，其地最广，其气最深也。"

《经穴解》："名殷门者，太阳经至此下行大盛，殷者，盛也，而此穴其门也，乃本经血甚盛之所也。"

《针灸穴名解》："本穴在承扶穴之下，委中之上，两穴相距折中之处。其处肌肉丰盈，故名之以'殷'。其治为腰痛不可俯仰，且难伸举，因恶血汇注致股肿等证。其功用在于通泻，故名之以'门'。其体则'殷'，其用则犹'门'，故名'殷门'。即于丰腴之处宣其瘀滞之气也。湿痹之证，多生于肌肉丰盈之处，本穴与焉。"

38 浮郄

【出处】《黄帝明堂经》。

【别名】无。

【穴义】浮，浅薄；郄，孔隙。本穴位于委阳上一寸，股二头肌腱内侧的间隙处，与上一穴殷门相比，穴处肌肉浅薄，故名"浮郄"。

【定位】腘横纹上1寸，股二头肌腱的内侧缘。

【主治】①便秘；②股腘疼痛，麻木。

【释义摘录】

《医经理解》："脉至殷门又浮折而上也。"

《古法新解会元针灸学》："浮郄者，三阳之气輶輶至门而返浮于上冲三寸，夫下而归经，故名浮郄。"

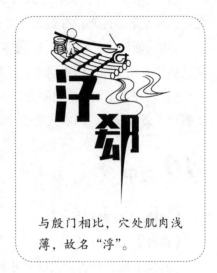

与殷门相比，穴处肌肉浅薄，故名"浮"。

《针灸穴名释义》："浮，指浮竹。郄，孔隙。谓穴位所在有浮竹之象。"

《针灸穴名解》："郄，大隙也。本穴穴位扩大，而功用浮泛，故名'浮郄'。"

《针灸腧穴通考》："腘，古作'郄'，《灵枢》'腘中'，马王堆出土文献《阴阳十一脉灸经》作'郄中'；《素问·刺禁论》'刺郄中大脉'，即刺腘中大脉也。《内经》中可找到大量这类用例。本穴在郄（腘）之上，故曰浮郄。"

39 委阳（三焦下合穴）

【出处】《灵枢·本输》。

【别名】无。

【穴义】委，曲折，大腿和小腿屈曲而形成腘窝。穴在腘横纹外侧端，外为阳，故名"委阳"。

【定位】腘横纹上，股二头肌腱的内侧缘。

【主治】①腹满，小便不利；②腰背痛，腿足痛。

【释义摘录】

《医经理解》："委阳，在承扶下六寸，与

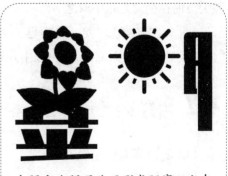

大腿和小腿屈曲而形成腘窝，穴在腘横纹外侧端，外为阳，故名。

殷门并，出于腘中外廉两筋间，为足太阳之别络，手少阳之辅俞，故谓是委折间之阳穴也。"

《经穴解》："委，犹旁也。以本经之支，直行者结殷门，此穴乃溢而上，既结浮郄之穴，而又下结此穴，有委之之义，故曰委阳。"

《古法新解会元针灸学》："委阳者，因浮郄反上轻浮与三焦之气相接，至委阳而稍平，斜伏委托于阳，而生阴络，故名委阳。"

《经穴释义汇解》："委阳为足太阳之别络，位在足太阳经之前，足少阳经之后，出于腘中外廉两筋间，因喻穴居委中之外侧寸许，并可委曲而取之，外为阳，故名委阳。"

40 委中（合穴，膀胱下合穴）

【出处】《灵枢·本输》。

【别名】无。

【穴义】委，曲折，大腿和小腿屈曲而形成腘窝；中，中间。本穴在腘窝中央，因其所处部位故名"委中"。

【定位】腘横纹中点。

【主治】小腹痛，小便不利，遗尿；腰背痛，下肢痿痹。

【释义摘录】

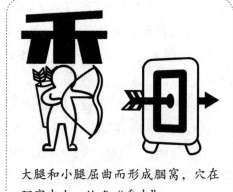

大腿和小腿屈曲而形成腘窝，穴在腘窝中央，故名"委中"。

《医经理解》："委中，在腘中央约文动脉陷中，正当足膝委折之中也。"

《针灸穴名释义》："委，委曲顺从貌，亦卧倒之意。中，指中间。即俯身卧倒屈曲膝关节而在腘窝之正中取之。"

《针灸穴名解》："委，委顿也，又委屈也。猝触此穴，令人下肢委顿，立即跪倒。《灵枢经》谓：'委而取之'。更以本穴在膝腘窝正中，委曲之处，故名'委中'。"

41 附分（手、足太阳经交会穴）

【出处】《黄帝明堂经》。

【别名】无。

【穴义】附，依附；分，分支。本穴是足太阳膀胱经背部第二侧线的第一个穴位，第二侧线为膀胱经分支，依附于第一侧线，两条侧线并行而下，故名"附分"。

【定位】第 2 胸椎棘突下，后正中线旁开 3 寸。

【主治】肩背拘急，颈项强痛，肘臂麻木。

【释义摘录】

《医经理解》："言附于背部，又分为二行也。背部二行去脊中各三寸半。"

《经穴解》："穴名附分者，此太阳支别之络下行者也。"

《古法新解会元针灸学》："附分者，诸阳斜屈而为经，足太阳之气独盛，故能上下循环。附者，附于脊肉相分，肺之上部两旁，连项附内廉，故名附分。"

《经穴释义汇解》："穴在第二椎下附项内廉两旁各三寸处，处在背部膀胱脉之第二行之分枝上，故名附分。"

《针灸穴名释义》："附，依附，附属；分，分别，分行，指足太阳互相依附之内外两行，在此分行而下也。"

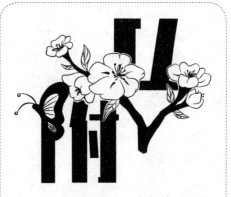

本穴是足太阳膀胱经背部第二侧线的第一个穴位。第二侧线为分支，依附于第一侧线。

42 魄户

【出处】《黄帝明堂经》。

【别名】无。

【穴义】本穴位于第三胸椎棘突下两侧，与肺俞平，为肺气出入之门户，主治虚劳、肺痿、咳嗽、气喘等肺疾。肺藏魄，故名"魄户"。

【定位】第 3 胸椎棘突下，后正中线旁开 3 寸。

【主治】①咳嗽，气喘，肺痿；②肩背痛，颈项强痛。

【释义摘录】

《医经理解》："魄户，肺之户也。肺藏魄，在第三椎下。"

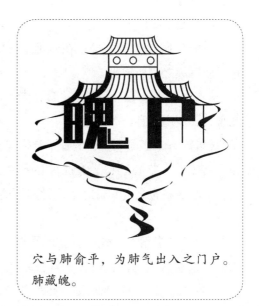

穴与肺俞平，为肺气出入之门户。肺藏魄。

《经穴解》："穴名魄户者，肺藏魄者也，此穴横直肺俞，内穴为系肺之原，此穴乃肺之户也，其主皆肺病。”

《古法新解会元针灸学》："魄户者，在肺俞两旁，因肺藏魄，故名魄户。"

《经穴释义汇解》："肺者，气之本，魄之处，藏魄，故名魄户。"

《针灸穴名解》："本穴与肺俞平，肺藏魄也，故名'魄户'。即附于肺，而分道下行者也。治虚劳、肺痿、喘满、呕逆，及肩膊胸背相连而痛。"

43 膏肓

【出处】《千金要方·针灸下·杂病第七》。

【别名】膏肓俞。

【穴义】中国古代医学称心尖脂肪为"膏"，心脏和横膈膜之间为"肓"，"膏肓"指心下膈上的部位，是药力达不到的地方。本穴与心包之背俞穴"厥阴俞"相平，用于治疗各种慢性虚损的疾病，故名"膏肓"。

【定位】第4胸椎棘突下，后正中线旁开3寸。

【主治】①咳嗽，气喘，盗汗，肺痨；②遗精；③羸瘦虚损。

【释义摘录】

《医经理解》："膏肓俞，在四椎下五椎上，是膏脂肓膜之气所输也。"

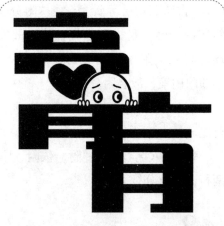

膏肓，指心下膈上的脂膜，是"攻之不可，达之不及，药不至"的狭隘部位，难以施治。本穴近心膈，故名。

《古法新解会元针灸学》："膏肓者，心与肺连，心之膏黄脂幔裹，心阳藏其中，因此禁针，灸之最宜，故名膏肓。"

《经穴释义汇解》："心附着于脊之第五椎。膏肓在第四椎下，近五椎上，两旁相去脊中各三寸，临心。心下为膏，心下膈上曰肓，穴处心膈之间，为膏脂，肓膜之气所输；又喻疾在肓之上，膏之下，针药不能及，而以此穴灸之，即能见效，故名膏肓，或膏肓俞。"

《针灸穴名解》："本穴平于厥阴俞……《春秋》晋景公病，请医缓诊治。景公夜梦二竖子议避医缓之治，逃避于膏肓之间处也。本穴外景，上有肺之魄户，下有心之神堂，本穴居二者之间，即医缓所谓'肓'之上，'膏'之下也，故名'膏肓俞'。"

44 神堂

【出处】《黄帝明堂经》。

【别名】无。

【穴义】本穴位于第五胸椎棘突下两侧，与心俞平，为心气留住而深居之处，主治心疾诸证。心藏神，故名"神堂"。

【定位】第5胸椎棘突下，后正中线旁开3寸。

【主治】①咳嗽，气喘，胸闷；②腰背痛。

【释义摘录】

《医经理解》："神堂，在五椎下。心藏神也。"

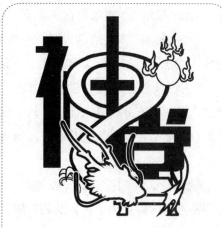

穴与心俞平，为心气留住而深居之处。心藏神。

《经穴解》："此穴横与心俞平直，心藏神者也，故其横旁之腧，则曰神堂。"

《古法新解会元针灸学》："神堂者，心为君主之官，神明出于心焉，穴居心俞之旁，经气朝会之堂，故名神堂。"

《经穴释义汇解》："心形如未敷莲花……附着于脊之第五椎，神堂在第五椎下两旁各三寸，应心。心者，生之本，神之变也。心藏神，心为明堂，又经气留住而深居之穴位称堂，穴为心神留住之处，主心疾，故名神堂。"

《针灸穴名释义》："神，是象征君主的阳气。堂，是高大明敞的居室。指其犹如心君用事的明堂。"

45 譩譆

【出处】《素问·骨空论》。

【别名】无。

【穴义】譩，同"噫"；譆，同"嘻"，均为语气叹词，表示叹息或者悲痛。本穴位于第六胸椎棘突下两侧，风邪客于足太阳状态下按压取穴，病人常有畏痛之譩譆声，故名"譩譆"。

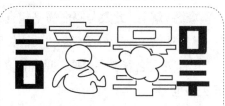

语气叹词。伤风时按压本穴患者常有畏痛之譩譆声。

【定位】第6胸椎棘突下，后正中线旁开3寸。

【主治】①咳嗽，气喘；②疟疾，热病；③肩背拘急引胁。

【释义摘录】

《医经理解》："噫嘻，在六椎下。令病者呼噫嘻，其动应手，是穴也。"

《经穴解》："穴在肩膊内廉，夹六椎下两旁，相去脊各三寸，正坐取之，以手重按，使病人大言谵语谵语，则穴应手，方是其处。"

《古法新解会元针灸学》："谵者，欢也；语者，心悦也。有事侥幸而成之曰谵语。背之六椎两旁三寸，有穴而动，故名谵语也。"

《针灸穴名释义》："谵语，哀痛声。按压取穴时，病人常有畏痛之谵语声，因而得名。"

《针灸穴名解》："'谵'通'噫'，伤痛声；'语'通'嘻'，悲恨声。治大热汗不出，劳损不得卧，温疟久不愈，及胸腹闷胀、肩背胁肋痛、鼻衄等症。"

46 膈关

【出处】《黄帝明堂经》。

【别名】无。

【穴义】本穴位于第七胸椎棘突下两侧，与膈俞平，内应膈肌，为胸腹交关之隔界；主治嗳气、呃逆，同膈俞。因名"膈关"。

【定位】第7胸椎棘突下，后正中线旁开3寸。

【主治】①呕吐，呕逆，嗳气；②胸闷，腰背痛。

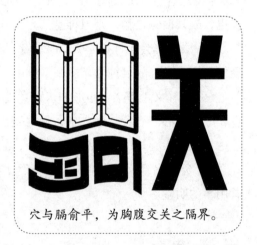

穴与膈俞平，为胸腹交关之隔界。

【释义摘录】

《医经理解》："膈关，在七椎下，是膈之关也。"

《经穴解》："此穴与膈俞横平相直，俱在七椎下，故曰膈关。"

《古法新解会元针灸学》："关清、膈浊，气血出入之关也，故名膈关。"

《针灸穴名释义》："膈，见膈俞条。关，关口，关格。指穴如胸膈之关口，且可开通关格也。"

《针灸穴名解》："本穴内应膈肌，与膈俞平，为胸腹交关之隔界，因名'膈关'。"

47 魂门

【出处】《黄帝明堂经》。

【别名】无。

【穴义】本穴位于第九胸椎棘突下两侧，与肝俞齐平。肝藏魂，穴为肝魂出入之门户，主治胸胁胀痛等肝疾，故名"魂门"。

【定位】第9胸椎棘突下，后正中线旁开3寸。

【主治】①呕吐，泄泻；②胁痛，背痛。

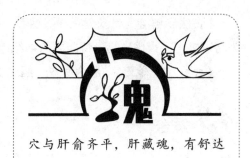

穴与肝俞齐平，肝藏魂，有舒达之功。

【释义摘录】

《采艾编》："魂门，九节各开三寸，肝藏魂也。"

《经穴解》："此穴横直平与肝俞等，肝藏魂者也，故此穴亦肝俞之部分，而名曰魂门。"

《古法新解会元针灸学》："……独阳无生，独阴无存，魂门在肝俞之旁，又因肝藏魂，居九椎之旁，亦应帝都九数之门，故名魂门。"

《针灸穴名释义》："魂，为人身阳气之精。门，见云门条，又为守护之意。魂门者，肝阳出入之门与护卫肝阳之处也。"

48 阳纲

【出处】《黄帝明堂经》。

【别名】无。

【穴义】本穴位于第十胸椎棘突下两侧，与胆俞齐平。胆为"中正之官"，比喻胆主决断，维持公正，为正气之纲纪，正气相对邪气为"阳"，故名"阳纲"。主治身热消渴、食不下、目黄等少阳枢机不利之证，同胆俞。

【定位】第10胸椎棘突下，后正中线旁开3寸。

【主治】①肠鸣，泄泻，食饮不化；②小便黄赤。

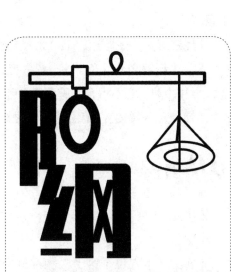

穴与胆俞齐平，胆为"中正之官"，为正气之纲纪。

【释义摘录】

《医经理解》："阳纲，在十椎下。胆为甲木，是阳气之纲领也。"

《经穴解》："此穴横直与胆俞平，胆为少阳，乃三阳之始，故曰阳纲。"

《古法新解会元针灸学》："阳纲者，肝之阳为胆，胆又为中正之官，决断出焉，肝为将军之官，谋虑出焉，恃胆阳为纲纪，故名阳纲。"

《针灸穴名释义》："胆为将军，胆主决断。肝胆依辅，阳刚之气得以伸张矣。"

49 意舍

【出处】《黄帝明堂经》。

【别名】无。

【穴义】本穴位于第十一胸椎棘突下两侧，与脾俞齐平，为脾气所居，主治腹胀、泄泻等脾疾。脾藏意，故名"意舍"。

【定位】第 11 胸椎棘突下，后正中线旁开 3 寸。

【主治】①腹胀，泄泻，消渴；②发热；③目黄。

【释义摘录】

《采艾编》："意舍，十一节各开三寸，脾主意。"

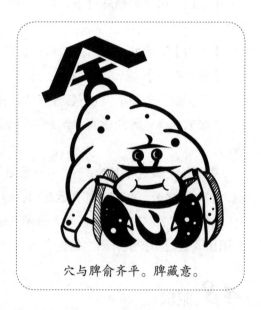

穴与脾俞齐平。脾藏意。

《经穴解》："思莲子议曰：'此穴与脾俞相对，横直相平。'脾藏意，故曰意舍。"

《古法新解会元针灸学》："意舍者，意之舍出形于外也。又因脾藏意与志，而土生金，心气冲动，意不得舍，脾藏而舍于外，故名意舍。"

《针灸穴名释义》："意舍为脾俞之附属，犹如脾气休息留止之处也。"

50 胃仓

【出处】《黄帝明堂经》。

【别名】无。

【穴义】本穴位于第十二胸椎棘突下两侧，与胃俞齐平，主治腹满、食不下等胃病。胃为仓廪之官，故名"胃仓"。

【定位】第 12 胸椎棘突下，后正中线旁开 3 寸。

【主治】①胃痛，腹胀，水肿，小儿食积；②腰背痛。

【释义摘录】

《采艾编》："胃仓，十二节各开三寸，仓廪之舍。"

《经穴解》："此穴与胃俞横直平对，故曰胃仓。"

《古法新解会元针灸学》："胃仓者，胃为仓廪之官，五味出焉。在胃俞之旁，故名胃仓。"

《针灸穴名释义》："指其犹如胃府之仓库。横居胃俞之外，为胃俞之附属，可与太仓（中脘）互观。"

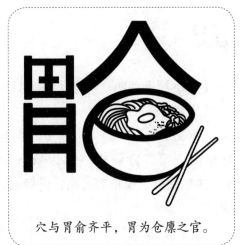

穴与胃俞齐平，胃为仓廪之官。

51 肓门

【出处】《黄帝明堂经》。

【别名】无。

【穴义】肓，肓膜，五脏之间的薄膜组织，如胸膜、腹膜。人体肓膜之间，为三焦之气往来的通道。本穴位于第一腰椎棘突下两侧，与三焦俞齐平，是三焦之气往来出入之门户，故名"肓门"。

【定位】腰部。第1腰椎棘突下，后正中线旁开3寸。

【主治】①腹痛，痞块；②产后诸证。

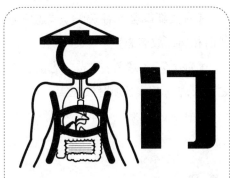

肓膜为三焦之气往来的通道。穴与三焦俞齐平，是三焦之气往来出入之门户。

【释义摘录】

《医经理解》："肓门，在十三椎下。肓膜也，人身肓膜之间，为三焦之气所往来，故谓之肓门也。"

《采艾编》："肓门，十三节各开三寸，前为肓俞。"

《古法新解会元针灸学》："肓门者，膈之门也，是精气生育之根源，三焦之所属，上通膏肓，下通胞肓，皆精气发源阴阳朝会之处，邪弗能伤。"

《经穴释义汇解》："肓，此处指腹部之肓膜。门，见云门条。指其有如诸肓门户之意。"

52 志室

【出处】《黄帝明堂经》。

【别名】精宫，神关。

【穴义】志，意志、记忆；室，居室。本穴与肾俞齐平，肾藏志，穴为肾气留住之所，主治腰痛、遗精等肾疾，同肾俞，故名"志室"。

【定位】第2腰椎棘突下，后正中线旁开3寸。

【主治】①遗精，阳痿，小便不利；②腰背痛。

穴与肾俞齐平，肾藏志。主治腰痛、遗精等肾疾。

【释义摘录】

《经穴解》："此穴与肾俞穴横直平对，肾藏志者也，故曰志室。"

《古法新解会元针灸学》："志室者，肾为作强之官，伎巧出焉。肾为藏志之室，与肾俞相通，故名志室。"

《针灸穴名释义》："志，志向，意志；此指肾之精气。室，人物所居之处，亦充实之意。志室者，必须肾气充实，意志方能发挥。"

《针灸穴名解》："本穴与肾俞穴平。肾藏志也，肾属水，水之精为志，因名之为'志室'。"

53 胞肓

【出处】《黄帝明堂经》。

【别名】无。

【穴义】胞肓，指包绕膀胱的脂膜。本穴位于第二骶后孔两侧，与膀胱俞齐平，主治膀胱诸疾，故名"胞肓"。

【定位】横平第2骶后孔，后正中线旁开3寸。

【主治】①癃闭；②肠鸣，腹胀，便秘；③腰脊痛。

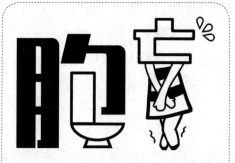

指包绕膀胱的脂膜。穴与膀胱俞齐平，主治膀胱诸疾。

【释义摘录】

《医经理解》:"胞肓,在十九椎下,是膀胱脂膜之间也。"

《采艾编》:"胞肓十九节各开三寸。膀胱之胞,此其系属也。"

《经穴解》:"此穴横平与膀胱俞相对,为足太阳本经脉气所发。胞者,指膀胱而言也;肓者,膈也。膀胱有下口无上口,亦犹上之膈膜,不与上下相通之义同。其溺乃用下焦之气以渗入者,故亦曰肓也。此穴主渗入之原本,故曰胞肓也。"

《古法新解会元针灸学》:"胞肓者,与膏肓、肓门同胞之属于上焦中下三膈也,故名胞肓。"

《针灸穴名解》:"胞,即胞宫。肓,即脂膜。胞宫位于小肠、直肠、膀胱各脏器之间,四围脂膜包绕,故名'胞肓'。"

54 秩边

【出处】《黄帝明堂经》。

【别名】无。

【穴义】秩,秩序,有条理;边,边缘。足太阳膀胱经背部诸穴皆依次排列,秩序井然,本穴位于二十一椎两侧,背部第二侧线的最后一穴,当边缘处,因名"秩边"。

【定位】横平第4骶后孔,后正中线旁开3寸(骶管裂孔旁开3寸)。

【主治】①痔疾,便秘,小便不利,阴痛;②腰骶痛,下肢痿痹。

膀胱经背部诸穴秩序井然,本穴为第二侧线最后一穴,故名。主治腰骶疼痛、痔疾等。

【释义摘录】

《医经理解》:"秩边,在二十椎下。言列于边行也。"

《采艾编》:"秩边,似云如衣之边,此为裕也。"

《经穴解》:"此穴横与中膂俞相对,中膂者,乃夹脊两行肉也,督脉行于脊之正中,而两旁膂肉夹之。内为夹脊两行之脂膜,所以裹系诸脏腑。外所列太阳左右两行各脏腑俞穴,左右秩秩然成行列,而下至此穴,而太阳在背之穴尽,故名曰秩边,命名之义昭然矣。"

《古法新解会元针灸学》:"秩边者,从头至背下依秩序次列而下,至背俞终,旁通之边际,故名秩边。"

55 合阳

【出处】《黄帝明堂经》。

【别名】无。

【穴义】足太阳膀胱经一条支脉"从腰中，下夹脊，贯臀，入腘中"；另一条支脉"从髆内左右别下贯胛，夹脊内，过髀枢，循髀外后廉下合腘中"。本穴在腘横纹下，为太阳经两条支脉相合之处。故名"合阳"。

【定位】腘横纹下2寸，腓肠肌内、外侧头之间。

【主治】①疝气，崩漏；②腰背痛，下肢痿痹。

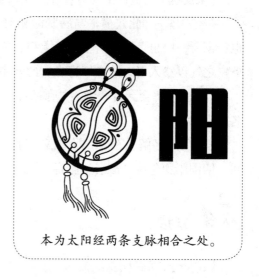

本为太阳经两条支脉相合之处。

【释义摘录】

《医经理解》："合阳，在膝腘约文下二寸；太阳之脉，一支从腰中下夹脊，贯臀入腘；一支从髆内左右下，贯胛，夹脊，循髀外后廉下合腘中。此则太阳二支之合也。"

《采艾编》："合阳，腘下二寸，上分至委中而合，此下委中二寸，言膀胱所合也。"

《经穴解》："太阳直行之支别者，旁行过髀枢之支别者，俱合委中，过膝之后而下行，故曰合阳，以太阳两脉合而得名也。"

《古法新解会元针灸学》："合阳者，合者会合也，足太阳经从头至足而下，手阳明金生水，手足阳金生水，手足阳明相交而合于阳，随气分而分经络，筋交逆行委中，生克制化，交经相通，手阳相合足阳于阴部，故名合阳。"

《针灸穴名解》："物体以凹陷为阴，凸突为阳。本经之气至此，即出于凹陷之阴，而抵于凸突之阳也。其所治症，多为腰脊腿腹寒热，偏于湿滞之症。"

56 承筋

【出处】《黄帝明堂经》。

【别名】腨肠，直肠，真肠。

【穴义】承，承接；筋，经筋。本穴位于腓肠肌肌腹中，为足太阳经筋所结之处，且主治小腿拘急挛痛、转筋等筋病，故名"承筋"。

【定位】腘横纹下5寸，腓肠肌两肌腹之间。

【主治】① 痔疾；② 腰痛，小腿拘急疼痛。

【释义摘录】

《医经理解》："言承于足膝后两筋之下也。"

《采艾编》："承筋，其承者，胁筋，言阳陵泉为筋之会，此当其下廉承之也。"

《经穴释义汇解》："穴在腨肠中央凹陷处，言承于足膝后两筋之下，故名承筋。"

《针灸穴名释义》："承，见承光条。筋，经筋，筋肉。指其位于足太阳经筋所结之处，且全身躯体筋肉之重，此处可以承担也。"

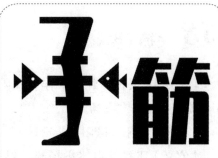

穴在腓肠肌肌腹中，为足太阳经筋所结之处，且主治筋病。

57 承山

【出处】《黄帝明堂经》。

【别名】鱼腹，肉柱，肠山，伤山，玉柱。

【穴义】承，承载、承受；山，指躯体之高重。穴在腓肠肌两肌腹分开的下端凹陷中，犹如身处山麓之峡谷中，可承载一身如山之重，故名"承山"。

【定位】腓肠肌两肌腹与肌腱交角处。当伸直小腿或足跟上提时，腓肠肌肌腹下出现尖角凹陷中。

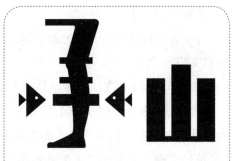

穴在腓肠肌肌腹下凹陷中，承载一身，如山之重。

【主治】①痔疾，便秘；②腰背痛，小腿拘急疼痛。

【释义摘录】

《医经理解》："言承载一身，如山之重也。"

《经穴解》："此穴在腿肚之下上，视腿肚之隆，而高有山象，又有下垂之象，故曰承山。"

《古法新解会元针灸学》："承山者，承于上阳气之起伏，肉峰之高秀，得山川之美，通谷达野，故名承山。"

《针灸穴名释义》："承，见承光条。山，指躯体之高重。人身高大沉重如山，腨肠之分肉足可承受也。穴在腨肠分肉之间，当挺身直立时，则分肉更为明显。《金针梅花诗钞》承山条'两腨任重可承山'。与承筋、承扶其义相近。"

58 飞扬（络穴）

【出处】《灵枢·经脉》作"飞阳"，《黄帝明堂经》始作"飞扬"。

【别名】飞阳，厥阳，蚕扬。

【穴义】飞扬，有飞举扬起，斜行别出，脱离正轨之意。本穴为足太阳膀胱经的络穴，经气由此别走足太阴肾经，沟通两经，故可治疗两经病变，如尿路感染、肾炎、膝胫无

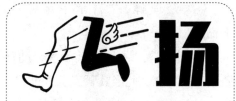

本穴常用于治疗腿软无力，针刺此穴能使人扬步似飞。

力，故名"飞扬"。此外，本穴是治疗腿软无力的常用穴，因此也形容针刺此穴能使人扬步似飞。

【定位】昆仑直上7寸，腓肠肌外下缘与跟腱移行处。

【主治】①头痛，眩晕；②鼻衄；③痔疾；④腰腿疼痛。

【释义摘录】

《黄帝内经太素》："足太阳之别，名曰飞阳，此太阳络，别走向少阴经，迅疾如飞，故曰飞阳也。"

《医经理解》："飞扬，在足外踝上七寸，足太阳之络，谓有飞而走少阴者也。"

《古法新解会元针灸学》："飞扬者，走足太阴之经水过胜，飞扬而起，从上而下，激急冲出如细条，故名飞扬，而生太阳经之脉络也。"

《经穴释义汇解》："穴在足外踝上七寸。为足太阳之络，谓有飞而走足少阴经；又喻针此穴能扬步似飞，故名飞扬。"

59 跗阳（阳跷脉郄穴）

【出处】《黄帝明堂经》。

【别名】附阳，付阳。

【穴义】跗，同"附"，依附。本穴在足外踝上三寸，跗骨阳侧；又因本穴为阳跷脉之郄穴，阳跷脉过此穴而上行，有阳跷附太阳之穴而生之意，故名"跗阳"。

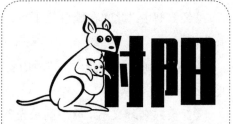

阳跷脉过此穴而上行，有阳跷附太阳之穴而生之意。

【定位】昆仑直上3寸，腓骨与跟腱之间。

【主治】①头痛；②腰骶痛，下肢痿痹，

足踝肿痛。

【释义摘录】

《医经理解》："附阳，在足外踝上三寸，筋骨之间，太阳前、少阳后，是足两阳脉之相附而行者也。"

《经穴解》："此穴将近少阳，已有附阳之义，而阳跷之脉，又以为郗而上行，故曰附阳，言阳跷附太阳之穴而生也。"

《经穴释义汇解》："穴在足外踝上三寸，筋骨间，跗骨之阳侧；又因本穴附于太阳经与少阳经之间，阳跷脉过此返附其中，三阳相扶，故名跗阳或附阳。"

《针灸穴名释义》："跗，足背。阳，指上方，外方。穴在小腿下端外侧、足背之上方，有如足跗之阳也。"

《针灸穴名解》："本穴在足三阳交近处，位于足少阳、足阳明之后，相与附丽而行，故名'附阳'。"

60 昆仑（经穴）

【出处】《灵枢·本输》。

【别名】 外昆仑，上昆仑，足太阳，巨阳。

【穴义】 昆仑，山名。古人以昆仑山为最高山峰，此处用来比喻外踝骨高突状如昆仑。穴在外踝高点的后方，故名"昆仑"。

【定位】 外踝尖与跟腱之间的凹陷中。

【主治】 ①头痛，目痛，鼻衄；②滞产；③癫痫；④颈项强痛，腰痛，足踝肿痛。

穴在外踝高点的后方，外踝骨高突状如昆仑。

【释义摘录】

《医经理解》："言骨起如昆仑也。"

《经穴解》："中国之山，无大于昆仑者，太阳自睛明而下，所过之穴，其骨而峙起者，无如外踝之大也，既至小指之至阴为井而上行，亦无大于外踝者，故名以昆仑焉。凡《内经》不言名，而止言取太阳之经者，即此穴也。"

《古法新解会元针灸学》："昆仑者，上有踝骨，旁有跟骨，下有软骨，高起如山，足太阳之经水，有气质升高促阳而返下之象，故名昆仑。"

《针灸穴名解》："考足外侧踝突，较其他踝突为高。古人眼界未宽，以昆仑为最高山峰，故取喻本穴为'昆仑'。"

61 仆参

【出处】《黄帝明堂经》。

【别名】安邪。

【穴义】仆，古之卑称；参，参见。古时仆人参见主人，行屈膝礼，手指垂处，正当其穴，故名"仆参"。

【定位】昆仑直下，跟骨外侧，赤白肉际处。

【主治】①癫痫；②腰痛，下肢痿软，腿痛转筋，足跟肿痛。

【释义摘录】

《医经理解》："仆者卑称也。仆参，言立于下参乘者也。"

《采艾编》："仆参，至卑之地，如仆，此其恭随也。"

《经穴释义汇解》："穴在跟骨下凹处，阳跷之本。仆，附也。穴为膀胱脉之腧穴，受阳跷脉所参附；又古之卑称为仆，因喻古时仆人参见主人，行屈膝礼，手指垂处，正当其穴，故名仆参。"

《针灸穴名释义》："有仆人参见主人之象。仆，侍从也。参，拜见也。必须使小腿屈曲有如参拜，方可便于取穴。"

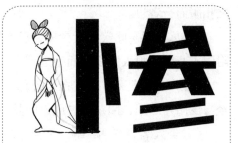

古时仆人参见主人，行屈膝礼，手指垂处，正当其穴。

62 申脉（八脉交会穴，通阳跷脉）

【出处】《黄帝明堂经》。

【别名】鬼路，阳跷。

【穴义】本穴名有两层含义。其一，申，申时，指下午三点到五点。该时段是气血流注于足太阳膀胱经的时段，故名"申脉"。其二，申，通"伸"，有屈伸之意；脉，指阳跷脉。本穴为八脉交会穴之一，通阳跷脉，为阳跷脉所出。阳跷脉司下肢运动，是维持下肢屈伸等正常功能活动之脉，本穴主治腰背强直、关节屈伸不利、转筋等肢体功能障碍，

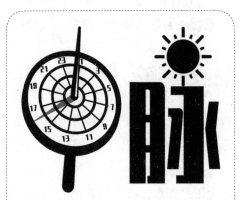

本穴是阳跷脉的起点，申时（15至17时）是阳跷脉气血流注于足太阳膀胱经的时段，故名。

故名"申脉"。

【定位】外踝尖直下，外踝下缘与跟骨之间凹陷中。

【主治】①失眠，头痛，眩晕，癫狂痫；②腰腿痛。

【释义摘录】

《医经理解》："申，伸也。申脉在足外踝下五分，为阳跷脉所生，阳跷自足上行，故谓脉之申而上者也。"

《采艾编》："膀胱经属申位，故言申脉。"

《经穴解》："太阳标为巨阳，本为寒水，故曰在上则为阳，在下则为水。水之长生在申，故此穴在足踝之下，以申脉名之，言其水所生之源也，其下穴即曰金门，亦金生水之义也。"

《古法新解会元针灸学》："申脉者，申即深也，阳跷脉生于足之深下也，故名申脉。"

《针灸穴名释义》："申，同伸，同呻；又十二时之一。脉，经脉。指其可治经脉之屈伸不能及气郁而呻诸病，且可内应膀胱之本府也。

申，伸也，又展也。申脉为阳跷脉所生，太阳主一身之表，故能治屈伸不能、筋脉拘挛诸病。

申，呻也。肾在志为呻，张隐庵曰：'呻者伸也。'肾气在下，故声欲太息而伸出之。肾与膀胱为表里，在气郁不伸及气郁而呻者，申脉与复溜同取，每可收效。

申，申时。十二时与十二脏腑相应，申时正是膀胱之时。故申脉穴可以认为是膀胱本府之穴。"

63 金门（郄穴）

【出处】《黄帝明堂经》。

【别名】关梁。

【穴义】金，五行之一。本穴的前一穴为申脉，申支属金，足太阳膀胱脉申时气血注此门户，故名"金门"。又金从革，有沉降、肃杀、收敛之性。太阳经至此穴，临于垂末，将与少阴之气交接，犹时届暮秋，金风肃起，阳和之气转变为萧瑟之阴，故曰"金门"。

【定位】外踝前缘直下，骰骨下缘凹陷中。

【主治】①头痛；②小儿惊风；③腰痛，

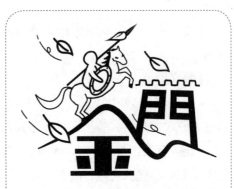

太阳经至此，临于垂末，将与少阴之气交接，犹时届九秋，金风肃起，变为萧瑟之阴。

下肢痿痹，足踝肿痛。

【释义摘录】

《医经理解》："金者水所从出。金门，在足外踝下一寸，足太阳郄，是寒水所生之门也。"

《古法新解会元针灸学》："此穴在足方寸之中，会阳维通于阳金阳跷出入之门，故名金门。"

《经穴释义汇解》："穴为足太阳膀胱脉之郄，穴之上一寸是申脉，申支属金，足太阳膀胱脉申时气血注此门户，故名金门。"

《针灸穴名释义》："金，为肺金之气。门，见云门条。金门者，意为息风利水之门户也。"

《针灸穴名解》："金，禁也，又兵象也。本穴在申脉穴前方，太阳经至此，临于垂末，将与少阴之气交接，犹时届九秋，金风肃起，遏化阴和之气一变而为萧瑟之阴，故曰'金门'。"

64 京骨（原穴）

【出处】《灵枢·本输》。

【别名】 无。

【穴义】 京，大。足外侧第五跖骨基底部分有显著突起，古称"京骨"，本穴在京骨处，故名"京骨"。

【定位】 第5跖骨粗隆前下方，赤白肉际处。

【主治】 ①头痛；癫痫；②颈项强痛，腰腿痛。

古称足外侧第五跖骨基底部为"京骨"。穴在京骨处。

【释义摘录】

《经穴解》："物之大者，多以京称之，小指后之骨，无有大于此者，故曰京骨，而膀胱之原穴在其下，故指京骨以志其穴。"

《经穴释义汇解》："京，大也。位在足外侧大骨下。又京作原，古通用，京即原字。穴为足太阳膀胱脉之原，故名京骨。"

《针灸穴名解》："京，巨也。此骨弓形而上凸，古称'京骨'。本穴在京骨下缘，故名之为'京骨'。如腕骨处穴名'腕骨'，束骨处穴名'束骨'者，意同。"

65 束骨（输穴）

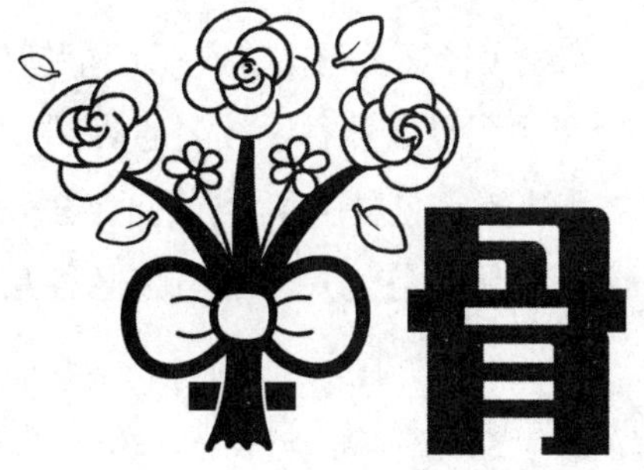

【出处】《灵枢·本输》。

【别名】无。

【穴义】束，收束。穴在第五跖骨小头后下方，由京骨至本穴，第五跖骨渐成收束状，故名"束骨"。

【定位】第 5 跖趾关节的近端，赤白肉际处。

【主治】①头痛，眩晕；②癫狂病；③颈项强痛，腰腿痛。

【释义摘录】

《医经理解》："在足小指外侧本节后陷中，是骨之收束处也。"

《采艾编》："束者何也？言历京骨至此有筋脉以之束也。"

《经穴释义汇解》："穴在足小指外侧，本节后凹陷处，喻为骨之收束处，故名束骨。"

《针灸穴名释义》："束，束缚，收束。骨，指趾骨。穴位如趾骨之束，又能收束骨节缓纵诸病也。"

由京骨至本穴，第五跖骨渐成收束状。

66 足通谷（荥穴）

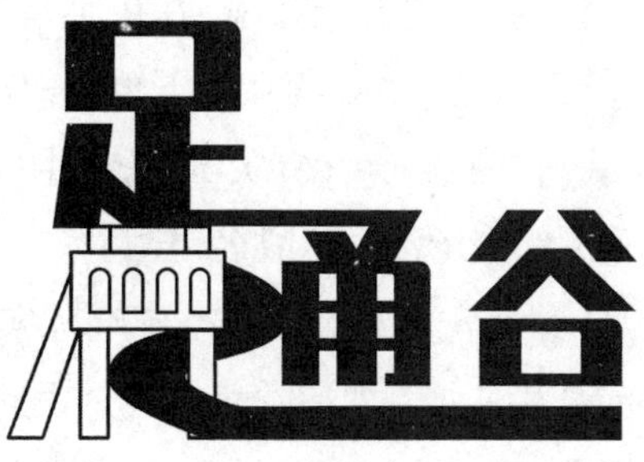

【出处】《灵枢·本输》。

【别名】无。

【穴义】通，通过；谷，山谷。穴在足外侧第五跖趾关节前下方凹陷处，形似山谷；穴为荥穴，所溜为荥，如同经气出于井而流注通过于此，为了与腹部同名穴通谷（足少阴肾经）相区别，故名"足通谷"。

【定位】第 5 跖趾关节的远端，赤白肉际处。

【主治】①头痛，颈项强痛；②鼻衄；③癫狂。

穴在足外侧第五跖趾关节前下方凹陷处，如同经气流注于山谷中。

【释义摘录】

《医经理解》："在足小指外侧，本节前陷中，太阳所溜，是其气所通也。"

《经穴解》："谷者，水流之处；通者，水之初流未畅，资此穷以通之也。太阳为寒水，此其本也。"

《经穴释义汇解》："穴在足小指外侧，本节前凹陷处，喻为足太阳脉气所过并又通于肾足少阴经之然谷，故名通谷。"

《针灸穴名释义》："通，通畅，疏通。谷与穀通。功能除结积留饮、胸满食不化，为足部通胀消谷之穴，可与腹通谷互参。"

67 至阴（井穴）

【出处】《灵枢·本输》。

【别名】无。

【穴义】至，到达；阴，指足少阴肾经。穴在足小趾端，足太阳膀胱经脉气由此交接足少阴经，表示阳气已尽，阴气将起，故名"至阴"。

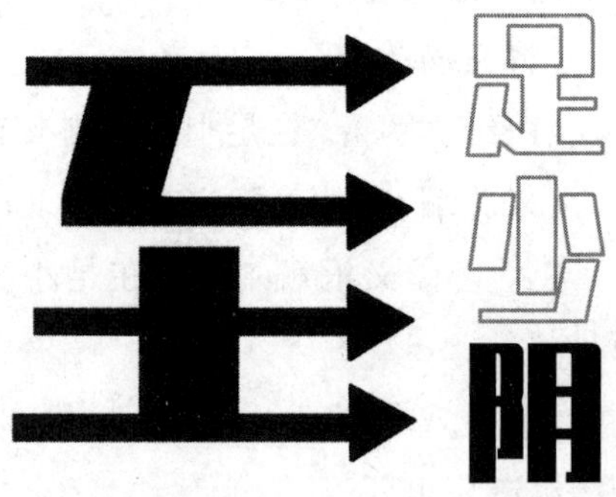

【定位】小趾末节外侧，趾甲根角侧后方0.1寸。

【主治】①胎位不正，滞产；②头痛，目痛，鼻塞，鼻衄；③足膝肿痛。

足太阳膀胱经脉气由此交接足少阴经。

【释义摘录】

《医经理解》："至阴，在足小指外侧端，指之小，阳之尽，故谓至阴也。"

《经穴解》："以其在最下也，故曰至阴。以其将传于少阴经也，亦曰至阴。"

《古法新解会元针灸学》："至阴者，足太阴之根，深通于少阴也，从阳而至于阴分，由独阴斜交于涌泉，故名至阴。"

《针灸穴名解》："本经自申脉穴以下，有阳极反阴、动极生静之意，故以'至阴'二字名其末穴。即谓本经之气，由此复行于阴分也。即《素问·阴阳离合论》所谓'太阳根于至阴'之义也。"

第九章

足少阴肾经穴

1 涌泉（井穴）

【出处】《灵枢·本输》。

【别名】地冲。

【穴义】涌，上涌，涌出；泉，水自地出。本穴居足心凹陷处，为足少阴肾经之井穴，脉气初出犹如泉水涌出，故名"涌泉"。

【定位】屈足卷趾时足心最凹陷中。

【主治】①发热，心烦，惊风；②咽喉肿痛，咳嗽，气喘；③便秘，小便不利；④足心热，腰脊痛。

【释义摘录】

《医经理解》："涌泉，在足心陷中。少阴所出，为井，故谓如泉之涌出于下也。"

穴为肾经井穴，脉气初出犹如泉水涌出。

《经穴解》："穴名涌泉者，此穴受太阳、少阴之交，而趋足心，又将上行，肾为水也，故为泉，自足下上行，有涌之象也，故曰涌泉。"

《古法新解会元针灸学》："涌泉在下，而泉出之正也，故名涌泉。又名地冲者，膀胱与肾分壬癸二水而相通，天一生水，以养万物，水落深渊于地，而生泉。人之血气在筋脉经络流通者，亦如水之在于地中流通，水之源为泉，流而成川。山下之泉曰滥泉，正而涌出者曰涌泉。"

《经穴释义汇解》："涌泉者，足心也，即穴居足心凹陷之处。本穴为肾少阴经之井穴。肾属水，喻穴为泉水初出之处，犹如泉之涌出于下，故名涌泉。"

2 然谷（荥穴）

【出处】《灵枢·本输》。

【别名】然骨，龙渊，龙泉。

【穴义】本穴名有两层含义。一从古代解剖命名。古称舟骨粗隆为"然骨"，本穴当然骨下缘凹陷中，故名之。其二，然，通"燃"；谷，山谷。本穴属荥火，在足内侧舟骨下凹陷处，犹如龙雷之火燃于谷间。观本穴所治，凡肾火衰微所生种种虚证，如遗精、阴挺、不孕不育等皆可取之，以振奋阳气，故名"然谷"。

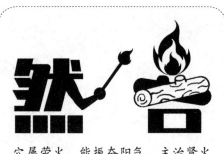

穴属荥火，能振奋阳气，主治肾火衰微诸症。

【定位】足舟骨粗隆下方，赤白肉际处。

【主治】①咳血，咽喉肿痛；②消渴，黄疸，泄泻；③月经不调，阴挺，阴痒，遗精，阳痿；④小儿脐风；⑤足跗肿痛。

【释义摘录】

《医经理解》："然谷，在足内踝前起大骨下陷中，挨骨而求。穴如火之燃于谷间也。"

《经穴解》："穴名然谷者，火之始灼曰然，此穴接涌泉之脉上行，涌泉为木，然谷为火，水之所溜为谷，故曰然谷。"

《古法新解会元针灸学》："然骨者，在足下空谷之中，通于心脾，有龙临深渊之性。一名然谷，故又名龙渊。"

《针灸穴名释义》："然，指然骨。然骨，古代解剖名。谷，见合谷条。穴在然骨下方有如山谷之凹陷处，故名。"

3 太溪（输穴、原穴）

【出处】《灵枢·九针十二原》《灵枢·本输》。

【别名】吕细。

【穴义】太，大；溪，指山间的流水。穴为足太阴肾经输穴，本经经气起于涌泉之泉，出于然谷之谷，至本穴则经气渐盛，犹如山间之溪。且本穴位于内踝和跟腱之间深大的凹隙中，故名"太溪"。

【定位】内踝尖与跟腱之间的凹陷中。

【主治】①遗精，阳痿；②月经不调；③咳嗽，气喘，咳血，胸痛；④咽喉肿痛，齿痛；⑤消渴，便秘；⑥腰背痛，下肢冷痛。

【释义摘录】

《医经理解》："太溪在足内踝后五分，跟骨上动脉陷中，少阴所注，故谓之溪。以其为原，故称之为太也。"

《经穴解》："穴名太溪者，肾为人身之水，自涌泉发源，尚未见动之形，溜于然谷，亦未见动之形，至此而有动脉可见。溪乃水流之处，有动脉则水之形见，故曰太溪。溪者，水之见也；太者，言其渊不测也。"

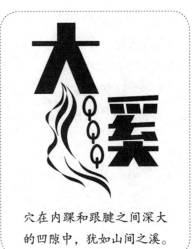

穴在内踝和跟腱之间深大的凹陷中，犹如山间之溪。

《针灸穴名解》："古法诊脉，三部九候，本穴为三部九候之一，取本穴以诊少阴经疾患。玩本经各穴大意，起于涌泉之泉，出于然谷之谷，本穴则犹溪涧之溪也。且本穴出于内踝之后，凹隙大深之处，故名'太溪'。人身脏器最深潜者，莫过于肾，本穴由阳经传来，由足下通之，亦太溪之意也。"

4 大钟（络穴）

【出处】《灵枢·经脉》。

【别名】无。

【穴义】本穴名解有二。其一，钟，通"踵"，足后跟部为踵。穴当足跟部，故名。其二，钟，注也，聚也。穴为足少阴肾经之络穴，是足少阴大络别注之处，经脉在此聚而分之，故名"大钟"。

【定位】内踝后下方，跟骨上缘，跟腱附着部前缘凹陷中。

【主治】①癃闭，便秘；②咳血，气喘；③痴呆，嗜卧；④腰背痛，足跟痛。

穴为络穴，是足少阴大络别注之处。

【释义摘录】

《医经理解》："足少阴络别走太阳者。钟，聚也，经脉之聚而分处也。"

《经穴解》："穴名大钟者，言其部分之形也，其穴在内踝后，有细动脉应手，在太溪之上，其形空悬如钟，所以吸肾脉之上行者，故曰大钟。"

《古法新解会元针灸学》："大钟者，即足跟之踵，上体之阳气钟聚贯足踵中，其足后跟大如覆盅，故名大钟。"

《经穴释义汇解》："钟，注也，聚也。穴在足跟后冲（踵）中，是少阴大络别注之处，亦是经脉之聚而分之处，故名大钟。"

5 水泉（郄穴）

【出处】《黄帝明堂经》。

【别名】无。

【穴义】本穴为足少阴肾经之郄穴，为肾经之气血深聚之处，犹如深处的水源，故名"水泉"。

【定位】太溪直下1寸，跟骨结节内侧凹陷中。

【主治】①月经不调，痛经，阴挺，小便不利；②目视不明。

【释义摘录】

《医经理解》："水泉，在足内踝下太溪下一寸。为少阴之郄，故谓是水所出也。"

《采艾编》："水泉，为原，犹言涌泉也，涌为井，此为原，外踝下跟为仆恭于泉在地也。"

穴为郄穴，肾之气血深聚之处，犹如深处的水源。

《古法新解会元针灸学》："溪水从上而折下，冲泉而反上。水泉者，是肾水所生之泉也，故名水泉。"

《针灸穴名解》："本穴为足少阴之'郄'。郄，大穴也。人身泉穴多在于郄，犹水源出于地下也。其所治症，为月事不调、小便淋漓等症，诸关于水泉者。取本穴犹疏水之极源也。故名'水泉'。"

6 照海（八脉交会穴，通阴跷脉）

【出处】《黄帝明堂经》。

【别名】阴跷，太阴跷，漏阴。

【穴义】照，光照。足少阴肾经属水，然谷为肾经之荥火穴，犹如水中龙火，本穴临近然谷，犹如龙火光芒照在海面上，故名

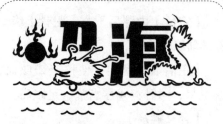

本穴临近肾经荥火穴"然谷"，犹如龙火光芒照在海面上。

"照海"。

【定位】内踝尖下 1 寸，内踝下缘边际凹陷中。

【主治】①失眠，目赤肿痛，咽干，咽痛；②月经不调，赤白带下，阴挺，癃闭，疝气；③癫痫。

【释义摘录】

《医经理解》："照海，在足内踝骨下一寸。其地如海之大，穴如火之焰于海也。"

《经穴解》："穴名照海者，以此穴又折而上，俯视涌泉、水泉，有海之象焉，而穴居其上，有以上照下之义，故名曰照海。"

《古法新解会元针灸学》："照海者，照是明照也；海者百川水之所归也。因水泉为肾阴，然谷为肾阳，水火相照而明，化跷脉与肾共命门水火通照于血海、气海等，故名照海。"

《针灸穴名解》："江海为百谷之王。泉虽幽迁，终归于海。所云照者，因肾为水火之脏，又古说水中有火，本穴达之，故名'照海'。"

7 复溜（经穴）

【出处】《灵枢·本输》。

【别名】昌阳，外命，伏白，复白。

【穴义】复，恢复；溜，同"流"。本穴名解有二。一从穴位循行命名。本经之脉，从足心斜走内踝后绕行，经大钟、水泉而合于照海，然后斜走至本穴后恢复直行之正（水顺势直流而为正），故名"复溜"。二从穴位功用命名。本穴主治汗证、水肿、泄泻等水液分布障碍的疾病，有通调水道、维护与恢复水液正常流动之功，故名。

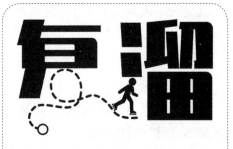

肾经从足心斜走内踝后绕行，然后斜走至本穴后返还直行之正。

【定位】内踝尖上 2 寸，跟腱的前缘。

【主治】①腹胀，泄泻；②多汗，无汗，水肿；③腰背痛，下肢痿痹。

【释义摘录】

《采艾编》："复溜，言汗出不止，溜而可复，水病不渗，复而可留也。"

《经穴解》："此穴承照海之脉而上行，流而不居，故曰复溜。又脉绝者，取此穴则脉生，亦有复溜之义。与交信穴共居一处，止隔一条筋，亦有复溜之义，乃肾经离踝上行之第一穴也，其脉动而不休，故为经。"

《古法新解会元针灸学》："复溜者，泉水入渠涌海成潮，而越阴渠，潮下，复溜而归经，故名曰复溜。"

《针灸穴名释义》："复，通複，通伏，又通澓。溜，见温溜条。指其功能通调水道，维护与恢复水液之正常流行。"

8 交信（阴跷脉郄穴）

【出处】《黄帝明堂经》。

【别名】无。

【穴义】信，五德之一，古人以仁、义、礼、智、信"五德"配属"五行"，信属土，脾亦属土，因此此处代指足太阴脾经。本穴虽属足少阴肾经，但却位于脾经循行线上，肾经由本穴交会至脾经三阴交，因此具有藏血、统血之功，可用于治疗月经不调、崩漏等月信之疾，故名"交信"。

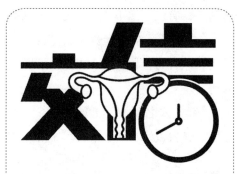

本穴常用于治疗月经不调等月信之病。

【定位】内踝尖上2寸，胫骨内侧缘后际凹陷中。

【主治】①癃闭，疝气痛引股膝，月经不调；②泄泻，便秘。

【释义摘录】

《医经理解》："交信，在足内踝上二寸，与复溜相并，前傍骨是复溜，后傍筋是交信，二穴以相交为信也。"

《采艾编》："交信，信之为言伸也，少阴前太阴后交伸而上行也，交者三阴之交也。"

《古法新解会元针灸学》："交信者，精气相交，去而复来，女子为经，故名交信。"

《经穴释义汇解》："因肾经之脉从此穴交会到脾经之三阴交穴去，脾属土，在五德中主信，故命名为交信。"

9 筑宾（阴维脉郄穴）

【出处】《黄帝明堂经》。

【别名】无。

【穴义】筑，建筑；宾，宾客，此处代指宾客住的屋子。穴属足少阴肾经，又为阴维之郄穴。穴以足少阴脉为主，阴维脉为客，犹如在足少阴经上筑一宾舍，迎阴维脉之来临，故名"筑宾"。

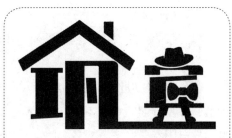

穴为阴维之郄穴。本穴以肾经为主，阴维脉为客，犹如在肾经上筑一宾舍，迎阴维脉之来临。

【定位】太溪直上5寸，比目鱼肌与跟腱之间。

【主治】①癫痫，吐舌；②呕吐；③疝气；④小腿疼痛。

【释义摘录】

《医经理解》："宾，当作膑，膝腨也。筑宾，在足内踝后上六寸腨分中，言行则腨间筑动也。"

《经穴解》："足少阴肾之经，而阴维始于此，有宾之象焉。维者，所以维内防出也，有墙之象，有筑之义，故曰筑宾。"

《古法新解会元针灸学》："筑宾者，筑是足内踝之上七寸着地之十也，同身寸之一尺也。宾者因阳跷脉主阴经，阴维脉主阴络，共护阴之经络，同在足少阴共事而异行，与内关经脏相交，络脉相通，故名筑宾。又因内关为阴维之主穴，心包为络脉之根原，卫气之所宗，于膻中；内关为心包之主络，所郄在筑宾，肉如筑基之坚，阴维之郄如外来者，为宾，结于踝上，故另有筑宾一说也。"

《针灸穴名解》："古'宾'与'膑'通。人当腿部努力时，则本穴处坚强坟起，如有所筑者。筑，杵也。本穴有利于膑骨，犹筑之使坚实也。故治腨痛、足痛，因名'筑宾'。"

10 阴谷（合穴）

【出处】《灵枢·本输》。

【别名】无。

【穴义】阴，指内侧；谷，山谷。本穴在膝关节内侧，半腱肌与半膜肌肌腱之间，其处凹陷形如山谷，故名"阴谷"。

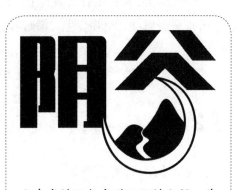

穴在半腱肌与半膜肌肌腱之间，其处凹陷形如山谷。

【定位】在腘窝内侧，屈膝时，当半腱肌肌腱与半膜肌肌腱之间。

【主治】①阳痿，小便不利，月经不调，崩漏；②癫狂；③腰脊痛，少腹、前阴、膝股引痛。

【释义摘录】

《医经理解》："阴谷，在膝下内辅骨后，大筋下小筋上，按之动脉应手，是少阴所会之谷也。"

《经穴解》："此穴为少阴经所入，冲脉由上而下行者，亦由于此。阴维脉由下而上行者，亦由于此，并本经之上行者，俱入于此穴。谷，言其深也；阴，言众阴之所聚也，故曰阴谷。"

《古法新解会元针灸学》："阴谷者，谷能通，谷能传远，两筋间如谷之穴在于阴筋之分，故名阴谷。"

《针灸穴名解》："本穴在膝腘阴侧稍下，凹僻中，故名'阴谷'。"

11 横骨 （足少阴经、冲脉交会穴）

【出处】《黄帝明堂经》。

【别名】下极，屈骨，曲骨。

【穴义】横骨，指两股之间的横起之骨，即耻骨，本穴位于耻骨上方，与任脉之曲骨齐平，故名"横骨"。

【定位】脐中下 5 寸，前正中线旁开 0.5 寸。

【主治】少腹胀痛，小便不利，遗尿，遗精，阳痿，疝气。

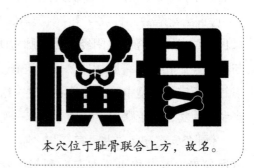

本穴位于耻骨联合上方，故名。

【释义摘录】

《医经理解》："横骨，一名下极，在阴上横骨中，在盲俞下五寸，夹中行五分。"

《经穴解》："肾经由骨后廉直上，行至此穴，则横入里行，故曰横骨。"

《古法新解会元针灸学》："横骨者，横于阴上之骨，横上为少腹，下即交骨，故名横骨。"

《针灸穴名解》："本穴位于横骨上缘，因名'横骨'。"

12 大赫 （足少阴经、冲脉交会穴）

【出处】《黄帝明堂经》。

【别名】阴维，阴关。

【穴义】本穴名解有二。其一，赫，指盛。穴处为冲脉、足少阴之会，脉气盛大，故名"大赫"。其二，赫，有炎热炽盛之意。穴与中极相平，与胞室精室相应，其治证多属子宫、阴器之虚证，如阴挺、阳痿等，有助热生阳之功，故名"大赫"。

【定位】脐中下4寸，前正中线旁开0.5寸。

【主治】遗精，阳痿，阴挺，带下，阴囊挛缩。

【释义摘录】

《医经理解》："赫，盛也，大赫，在气穴下一寸。一名阴维，一名阴关。为冲脉少阴之会。阴气之盛也。"

《经穴解》："穴名大赫者，前名横骨之穴，部分犹在骨际，至此穴，初入腹中，内之所藏，深广不测，故曰大赫。"

《古法新解会元针灸学》："大赫者，精气阜聚，大兆民生，故名大赫。"

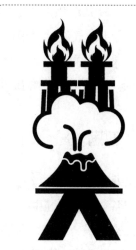

本穴有助热生阳之功，故名。

《针灸穴名解》："赫，盛也，明也。《素问·五常政大论》曰'火曰赫曦'，《诗·大雅》云'赫赫明明''赫赫炎炎''王赫斯怒'，俱为隆盛奋发之意。本穴平于中极穴，为足少阴脉气所发，与胞宫精室相应，蕴有赫赫之势。其所治症，多为子宫阴器局部之虚病，有助热生阳之功。即龙雷在下，水中发火之意。亦即《庄子》所谓'赫赫出乎地'也。故名'大赫'。"

13 气穴（足少阴经、冲脉交会穴）

【出处】《黄帝明堂经》。

【别名】胞门，子户。

【穴义】气，元气。关元为元阴元阳交关之处，本穴位于关元穴旁，为元气生发之处，亦为纳气要穴，故名"气穴"。

【定位】脐中下3寸，前正中线旁开0.5寸。

【主治】①月经不调，带下；②不孕；③腹痛引腰脊。

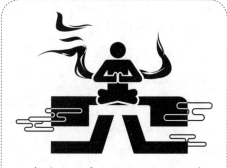

穴在关元穴旁，是下丹田之所在，纳气要穴。

【释义摘录】

《医经理解》："气穴，在四满下一寸，一名胞门，正当膀胱下口，为水气所出也。"

《经穴解》："穴名气穴者，以冲脉上行，而此穴其始。"

《经穴释义汇解》："穴在四满下一寸，正当膀胱下口，为水气所出；又穴为肾脉之腧穴，'肾主纳气'，是为纳气之穴，亦谓肾气归聚之穴，故名气穴。"

《针灸穴名解》："本穴与关元穴平。关元穴为人身元气交关之处，本穴与之挨近，故功能亦与略同。养生家凝神入气穴，即在于此。因名'气穴'。"

14 四满（足少阴经、冲脉交会穴）

【出处】《黄帝明堂经》。

【别名】髓府，髓中。

【穴义】满，饱满，胀满。本穴为足少阴肾经进入腹部后的第四个穴位，当小腹饱满之处，且主治"脐下积、疝瘕"（《针灸甲乙经·经络受病入肠胃五脏积发伏梁息贲肥气痞气奔豚第二》）诸胀满之症，故名"四满"。

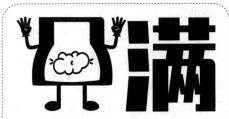

穴为肾经进入腹部后的第4个穴位，且主治"脐下积、疝瘕"诸胀满之症。

【定位】脐中下2寸，前正中线旁开0.5寸。

【主治】①月经不调，带下，遗精，遗尿；②泄泻，腹痛，积聚，水肿。

【释义摘录】

《医经理解》："四满，在中注下一寸，直膀胱中水气所四满也。"

《采艾编》："四满，血气食积水湿，凡人胀满此可治也，意其所治而命之也。"

《经穴解》："穴名四满者，盖足少阴之经，自横骨入腹，至此穴为四，而适当小腹饱满之处，乃大肠回叠层积之所，故曰满也。又小肠、大肠、膀胱、广肠，皆在其内，其数亦为四，故曰四满。"

《针灸穴名释义》："四，数字；又通驷，指驷星。满，盈满，胀满，又指小满节。言地气充盈上与驷星相应，且能治腹部四面膨胀满肿诸病也。"

《针灸穴名解》："本穴与任脉之石门穴，及足阳明经之大巨穴相平。内应脐下方寸，为全身精气凝聚之处。故本穴别名'髓府'。又以其处为大肠、小肠、膀胱、精室四夹之隙，受四者严密围壅，故名'四满'。"

15 中注（足少阴经、冲脉交会穴）

【出处】《黄帝明堂经》。

【别名】无。

【穴义】中，内部；注，注入。本穴名解有二。本穴在脐周，对应肠道，肾之精气由本穴向内注入，从而以肾水通润肠道之燥，主治腹中积热、大便坚燥等热证，故名"中注"。其二，本穴内应胞宫、精室，是肾之精气注入胞中之处，故名。

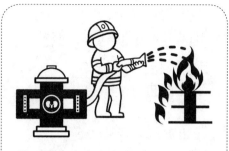

肾之精气由本穴向内注入，从而以肾水通润肠道之燥热。

【定位】脐中下 1 寸，前正中线旁开 0.5 寸。

【主治】腹痛，便秘。

【释义摘录】

《医经理解》："中注，在肓俞下一寸。值膀胱上，水气所中注也。"

《经穴解》："穴名中注者，乃人腹之上下，以脐为中，肓俞仅夹脐旁一寸，而此穴乃肓俞之下，为肓俞之所注，故曰中注。中注，自上而下之名，肾经自下而上，何亦以注名也？经无有不升降，升者其气，降者其血，故亦曰注也。"

《古法新解会元针灸学》："中注者，肾脉依任脉而化冲脉，注阴交于胞中，故名中注。"

《针灸穴名解》："本穴与任脉之阴交穴及足阳明之外陵穴相平。内应胞宫、精室。为肾水精气之集中。而肾之精气，又借本穴以达胞中。因名'中注'。"

16 肓俞（足少阴经、冲脉交会穴）

【出处】《黄帝明堂经》。

【别名】无。

【穴义】肓，肓膜，五脏之间的薄膜组织。穴在脐旁，内有腹膜，并与足太阳膀胱经肓门穴前后相应，故名"肓俞"。

【定位】脐中旁开 0.5 寸。

【主治】腹痛，便秘。

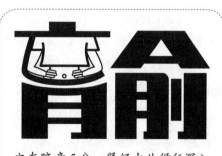

穴在脐旁 5 分，肾经由此循行深入肓膜，与背部肓门前后相应。

【释义摘录】

《医经理解》："肓俞，肓膜之俞也。值脐旁，在商曲下一寸。"

《采艾编》："肓俞，背有肓门，言肾所注也。"

《古法新解会元针灸学》："肓俞者，胞之膜，肓由是而过，上通胸膈之部，连系带脉，主肓之原，包裹脐中，故名肓俞。"

《经穴释义汇解》："穴在商曲下一寸，直脐旁五分，属肓膜之俞；又称本穴系指肾脉由此循行深入肓膜之意，故名。"

17 商曲 （足少阴经、冲脉交会穴）

【出处】《黄帝明堂经》。

【别名】无。

【穴义】本穴位于上腹部，内应肠，大肠属金，金在音为商；且肠有屈曲之象，故名"商曲"。

【定位】脐中上 2 寸，前正中线旁开 0.5 寸。

【主治】腹痛，泄泻，便秘，积聚。

【释义摘录】

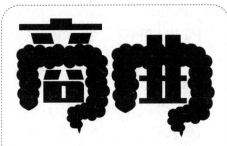

本穴内应肠，大肠属金，在音为商，且肠有屈曲之象。

《医经理解》："商，大肠金也。商曲，在食关下一寸，正腹肠之曲折处也。"

《经穴解》："此穴在脐上第一穴，夹中行任脉水分穴一寸五分，正大、小肠会处，自此际渗入膀胱，而为溺便，谷之渣秽，则自阑门而传送于大肠，肺属金，大肠亦属金，金为商，故曰商曲。"

《古法新解会元针灸学》："商曲者，胃之下肠之曲处，通水湿运输糟粕之发原处，通畅津液，故名商曲。"

《针灸穴名解》："商为秋金气令，于六气为阳明。本穴内景在胃与大肠之间，胃肠俱具屈曲之象，故名之以'曲'。胃与大肠俱属阳明燥金之经，俱具喜燥恶湿之性，俱具秋商肃敛之气。故曰'商曲'。商，言穴之性能；曲，言穴之内在地位。且本穴与足阳明之太乙门穴平。乙，亦曲屈也，又鱼肠也。"

18 石关 （足少阴经、冲脉交会穴）

【出处】《黄帝明堂经》。

【别名】石阙。

【穴义】本穴名解有二。其一，石，形容坚硬；关，指人体重要的孔窍。本穴善治大便不通、心下硬满、气淋等坚满充实之证，故名"石关"。其二，石，通食。本穴在胃脘处，为饮食之关，故名。

【定位】脐中上 3 寸，前正中线旁开 0.5 寸。

【主治】腹痛，便秘，多唾，嗳气。

【释义摘录】

《医经理解》："食关，值胃脘，是饮食之关也。"

《采艾编》："上治心满，下治泄泻，此为坚固之关也。"

《古法新解会元针灸学》："石关者，水谷出下脘，仗水分以分清浊，以水土之精化石质，关助小大肠，与分化之扶助力，故名石关。"

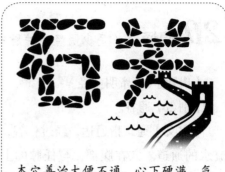

本穴善治大便不通、心下硬满、气淋等坚满充实之症。

《针灸穴名解》："本穴平于任脉之建里穴，及足阳明之关门穴。其所应证，多为坚满充实之证，如大便不通、心下硬满、哕、噫、腹痛、气淋、小便黄、脏有恶血、血上冲，多属肝脾范畴之郁结证。石，犹病之坚；关，喻治之通也。本穴与任脉之'石门'意义不同。'石门'意在体，'石关'意在用也。"

19 阴都（足少阴经、冲脉交会穴）

【出处】《黄帝明堂经》。

【别名】食宫，通关。

【穴义】都，有汇聚之意。本穴属于足少阴肾经，肾为阴中之阴，但其处内应胃脘，为饮食入内存积之处，故名"阴都"。

【定位】脐中上 4 寸，前正中线旁开 0.5 寸。

【主治】腹痛，腹胀，肠鸣。

【释义摘录】

《医经理解》："阴都，一名食宫……谓之阴都者主肾经而言，谓之食宫者主胃分而言也。"

《采艾编》："阴都，少阴肾之都会也。"

《古法新解会元针灸学》："阴都者，脾胃为中

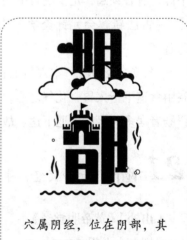

穴属阴经，位在阴部，其处正当胃脘部，为水谷汇聚之处。

宫，饮食入内存积，故有食宫之说，足少阴之会于胃之两旁胃经之中，如通邑之都会，故名阴都。"

《针灸穴名解》："幽，隐也，冥也。幽都，即阴都也。本穴秉少阴之气，外平中脘穴，内应胃弯。胃主中气，宜常充盈。故名'阴都'。"

20 腹通谷（足少阴经、冲脉交会穴）

【出处】《黄帝明堂经》。

【别名】通谷。

【穴义】通，指通达，经过；谷，为山间流水的通道。穴在腹部，与任脉的上脘穴相平，当胃脘之上部，是饮食通行之道路。且本穴主治腹痛、腹胀、呕吐，心痛、心悸等局部病症，有上通下达之功，故名"腹通谷"。

【定位】脐中上5寸，前正中线旁开0.5寸。

【主治】腹痛，腹胀，腹中积聚，呕吐。

【释义摘录】

《医经理解》："通谷，在幽门下一寸陷中，夹上脘，通冲也。冲脉足少阴之会也。"

《经穴解》："谷者，水所行之地，有虚象焉，穴以谷名，正胃中脘之旁，胃属土而中虚，有谷象焉，足少阴自下而上行，同冲脉以过之，故曰通谷。"

《古法新解会元针灸学》："通谷者，即胃门两旁有耳中空，含有收纳之气，故名通谷。"

《针灸穴名解》："本穴与上脘穴平。有关气向上通也。《内经》谓谷道通于脾，即水谷由食道下行入胃，化气之后，脾气散精，周布全身，即幽者通之也。本穴治症，关于胃肠者居多，且能上通下达。故名'通谷'。"

穴在腹部，主治局部病症，有上通下达之功。

21 幽门（足少阴经、冲脉交会穴）

【出处】《黄帝明堂经》。

【别名】上门。

【穴义】幽，幽暗、沉静，均为阴象，此处指"两阴交尽"。具体来讲，足少阴肾经入腹后与冲脉并行而上，冲脉在本穴与肾经交会后散于胸中，肾经也由腹部之阴而至胸廓之阳，如阴阳交界之门，故名"幽门"。

【定位】脐中上6寸，前正中线旁开0.5寸。

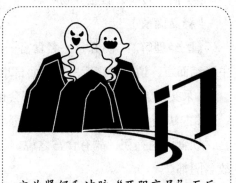

穴为肾经和冲脉"两阴交尽"而后散于胸部之处，如阴阳交界之门。

【主治】腹痛，腹胀，呃逆，呕吐，泄泻。

【释义摘录】

《医经理解》："幽门，一名上门，夹巨阙两旁陷中。谓之上门者，以居胃上口也；谓之幽门者，以其属少阴经，是幽阴之门也。凡自横骨至幽门，皆去中行各五分也。"

《采艾编》："幽门，幽隐之第一门也。"

《古法新解会元针灸学》："幽门者，六腑精气、谷气、清气、阴阳冲和之气，会合从幽门而入膈上，以安五脏换五脏浊气而出。隔绝混乱清阳之气，所入五脏以阳养阴，清净而贞。深入之门，故名幽门。"

《经穴释义汇解》："穴在巨阙两旁各五分凹陷处，当冲脉至胸中散处，属冲脉、肾经交会之穴。因两阴交尽称幽，故以为名。"

22 步廊

【出处】《黄帝明堂经》。

【别名】无。

【穴义】步，行走；廊，走廊。本穴与任脉"中庭"穴相平，足少阴肾经由本穴自腹走胸，沿胸骨两侧循行，犹如步入庭堂两侧的游廊，故名"步廊"。

【定位】第5肋间隙，前正中线旁开2寸。

【主治】①咳嗽，气喘，胸胁胀满；②呕吐。

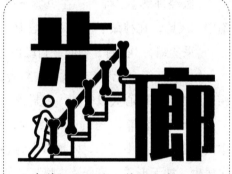

穴在第5肋间隙，肾经由本穴循行于肋骨犹如步入游廊。

【释义摘录】

《医经理解》："廊，堂下屋也。步廊，在神封下一寸六分陷中，夹中行二寸，言此已步于堂之廊庑也。"

《采艾编》："步廊，止步于膺，此为廊腋。"

《经穴释义汇解》："足太阳膀胱经从足走胸，本穴系由腹部之幽门穴转而向上走胸，犹如即此而步入胸之廊庑。……穴喻肾脉之通道，故名步廊。"

《针灸穴名解》："步，度量也。廊，侧屋也。本穴在膈上，与任脉之中庭穴平。本经左右两线，夹任脉，沿胸骨两侧，各肋骨歧间是穴，犹中庭两侧，房廊相对也。两侧穴位，排列整齐，如有尺度，故曰'步廊'。"

23 神封

【出处】《黄帝明堂经》。

【别名】无。

【穴义】神，心藏神，此处代指心；封，藏。本穴在内对应心，在外与任脉之膻中穴相平，膻中为心包之宫城，比喻本穴犹如封藏心神之处，故名"神封"。

【定位】第4肋间隙，前正中线旁开2寸。

【主治】①咳嗽，气喘，胸胁胀满；②呕吐，食欲不振；③乳痈。

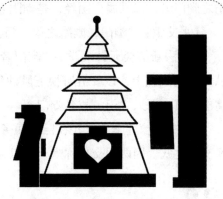

穴在第4肋间隙，在内对应心，比喻本穴犹如封藏心神之处。

【释义摘录】

《医经理解》："神封，在灵墟下一寸六分陷中，灵墟，在神藏下一寸六分陷中，神之封，灵之墟，皆心君之居也。"

《采艾编》："神封，神明之封疆也。"

《古法新解会元针灸学》："神封者，因心藏神，出于膻中，肾之神水上朝，与相火相通，而真阳降心火以安神，有封锁之力，故名神封。"

《针灸穴名解》："封，阜也，又闭而藏之也；又界也，国界曰封疆，地界曰封堆。本穴与任脉之膻中穴平。内景膻中为心主之宫城。横膈以上为胸腔，胸腔最喜空旷，神之居也。神无形质，喜居清虚境界，故名曰'神封'。犹云神识封藏之处也。"

24 灵墟

【出处】《黄帝明堂经》。

【别名】灵墙。

【穴义】灵，同"神"；墟，居处、场所。本穴在第3肋间隙，对应心脏，犹如心之居处，故名"灵墟"。穴名的含义和治症与神封相同。

【定位】第3肋间隙，前正中线旁开2寸。

【主治】①咳嗽，气喘，胸胁胀满；②呕吐；③乳痈。

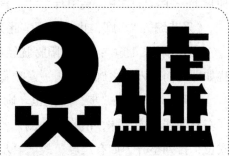

穴在第3肋间隙，对应心脏，犹如心之居处。

【释义摘录】

《医经理解》："神封，在灵墟下一寸六分陷中，灵墟，在神藏下一寸六分陷中，神之封，灵之墟，皆心君之居也。"

《采艾编》："灵墟，灵妙之墟址也。"

《古法新解会元针灸学》："灵墟者，阳气化神，阴气化灵，肾阴之精华藏于胸肉墟起中，故名灵墟。"

《经穴释义汇解》："灵，神也。穴在心旁，主心疾，心藏神。又'墟'，有君居处之义，穴在心君居处之旁，故名灵墟。"

25 神藏

【出处】《黄帝明堂经》。

【别名】无。

【穴义】本穴在第 2 肋间隙，对应心脏，犹如封藏心神之处，故名"神藏"。穴名的含义和治症与神封、灵墟相同。

【定位】第 2 肋间隙，前正中线旁开 2 寸。

【主治】①咳嗽，气喘，胸胁胀满；②呕吐，食欲不振。

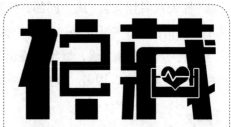

穴在第 2 肋间隙，对应心脏，犹如封藏心神之处。

【释义摘录】

《医经理解》："神藏，则君主之室矣，在或中下一寸六分陷中。"

《经穴解》："此穴乃近心之所，而心之神藏于其内，故曰神藏。"

《古法新解会元针灸学》："神藏者，是阴能生阳化神，五脏之阴灵化神，通识觉，神藏于胸中，故名神藏。"

《针灸穴名解》："本穴与任脉之紫宫穴平。胸腔为清虚之府，故有'玉堂''紫宫'之名。譬如人居清净之地，则神识为之清朗。本穴在紫宫穴之侧，灵墟穴之上，犹神灵内守，得其安居也，故名'神藏'。"

26 或中

【出处】《黄帝明堂经》。

【别名】或中。

【穴义】或，形容有文采的。肺为华盖，相傅之官。"相傅"指宰相，宰相多才识

广博、文采风流，故以"彧"喻肺。本穴在内对应
肺脏，在外平任脉之华盖穴，且主治咳嗽、气喘，
胸胁胀满等肺疾，故名"彧中"。

【定位】第1肋间隙，前正中线旁开2寸。

【主治】咳嗽，气喘，痰多，胸胁胀满。

【释义摘录】

《医经理解》："彧，文貌，肺为华盖，相傅之
官，是文郁之府也。府者，君相之所藏。"

《古法新解会元针灸学》："彧中者，彧人不倦，
中藏水火，上朝天池，下通丹田，或上或下，皆与
任脉相通，故名彧中。"

穴在第1肋间隙，内对应
肺脏，肺为华盖；在外平
任脉之华盖穴。

《针灸穴名释义》："彧，同郁，畅顺貌。中，指
胸中，又指情志，参中渚条。谓其功能宽胸理气，使胸怀舒畅也。"

《针灸穴名解》："彧，繁华茂盛也。本穴平任脉之华盖穴，且居神藏穴之上。神明
内藏，彧乎其中矣，因名'彧中'。所治多为痰喘满闷之证，亦即病气彧于中也。"

27 俞府

【出处】《黄帝明堂经》。

【别名】无。

【穴义】俞，通"输"，传输；府，内府。本经
之气从足至胸，于此处输于内府，胸为肺之府，且
主治咳嗽、气喘等胸满之证，故名"俞府"。

【定位】锁骨下缘，前正中线旁开2寸。

【主治】①咳嗽，气喘，胸痛；②呕吐。

【释义摘录】

《医经理解》："府者，君相之所藏。俞府，谓肾
气之传输于府者也。"

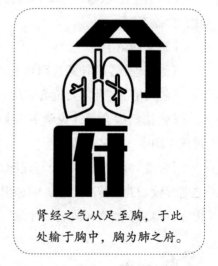

肾经之气从足至胸，于此
处输于胸中，胸为肺之府。

《经穴解》："俞者，输也，足少阴之经自涌泉而
上输至此穴，肾经之穴已尽，故曰俞府。"

《古法新解会元针灸学》："俞府者，俞者过也，府者会也，足少阴之交于手厥阴，
而络终会过于此，故名俞府也。"

《针灸穴名解》："俞，输也；府，内也。本穴平任脉之璇玑穴。'璇玑'具转动灵活

之意。本穴借血气灵运，而促本经之气，输之内府，故名'俞府'。简言之，即有关内府之腧穴也。治嗽而不得息，及诸胸满之证，用以输达内郁之气，及有关神识意志作用者。"

第十章
手厥阴心包经穴

1 天池

【出处】《灵枢·本输》。

【别名】天会。

【穴义】天，天部，指腰以上的部位；池，水池。穴居天位，穴处凹陷似池，故名"天池"。

【定位】第4肋间隙，前正中线旁开5寸。

【主治】①咳嗽，气喘，痰多，胸闷，胸痛；②腋下肿，瘰疬。

穴居天位，穴处凹陷似池。

【释义摘录】

《医经理解》："天池，池为水所钟，泉为水所出，心主脉行于上，故高而言天也。"

《经穴解》："三焦主气，此经主血，血之所行，有水象焉，故曰天池。"

《古法新解会元针灸学》："天池者，天一生水，而注池沼，过胁之肉陷处，故名天池。"

《针灸穴名解》："穴在胸廓。为人体清虚境界。本穴与天溪、乳中穴相平，承足少阴内行络心之气，转注而来，穴近乳房。乳房为储藏乳汁之所，故喻之为'池'。以其在胸，故名'天池'。天池亦含清凉解热之意，治胸满热郁之证，如腋下肿、上气、寒热、目眈眈、臂痛、疟疾等证。"

2 天泉

【出处】《黄帝明堂经》。

【别名】天湿。

【穴义】天，指腰以上的部位；泉，水出之处。穴在上肢臂内侧，居天位，手厥阴心包经沿此穴下行，似泉水下流，故名"天泉"。

【定位】腋前纹头下 2 寸，肱二头肌的长、短头之间。

【主治】①心痛，咳嗽，胸胁胀痛；②臂痛。

【释义摘录】

穴为本经入臂后的最高处，心包经下行似泉水下流。

《医经理解》："池为水所钟，泉为水所出，心主脉行于上，故高而言天也。"

《经穴解》："此穴在本经初入臂而下行，自中冲而视之，乃最高焉。天池在胸，有停水之象，故曰天池。此穴乃注水而下行，故曰天泉。"

《古法新解会元针灸学》："天泉者，天部之泉，根通于肾经，如泉之居下，而冲上入支流也，故名天泉。又名天湿者，言腋下居天部，常有津津湿液，显于外，如天阴时之潮湿，故又名天湿。"

《经穴释义汇解》："泉为水所出，心主脉循此穴下行，似泉水下流。穴在曲腋下去臂二寸，居天位，又借用天上星名天泉，故名为天泉。"

3 曲泽（合穴）

【出处】《灵枢·本输》。

【别名】无。

【穴义】曲，弯曲，本穴在手肘内侧凹陷处，屈肘可得，故以"曲"名。泽，指水汇聚的地方。本穴是手厥阴心包经之合穴，比喻经气在此汇聚，故名"曲泽"。

【定位】肘横纹上，肱二头肌腱的尺侧缘凹陷中。

【主治】①心痛，心悸，善惊；②胃脘痛，

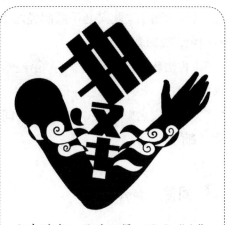

穴在肘内，屈肘可得，故名"曲"；穴为合穴，经气所聚，故名"泽"。

吐血，呕吐；③发热，口干；④肘臂痛。

【释义摘录】

《医经理解》："曲泽，在手肘内廉横纹陷中筋内侧动脉，是肘内曲处也。"

《经穴解》："水所聚者为泽，此穴乃在肘臂曲折之处，故曰曲泽。又为本经所入为合水，亦为泽象。"

《古法新解会元针灸学》："肘臂相交之曲中，血从三阴而入曲泽，润手臂之经筋，为肘内部之大血管，润关荣筋，故名曲泽。"

《针灸穴名解》："本穴在曲肘横纹正中凹陷处。平于曲池及尺泽穴，故名'曲泽'。"

4 郄门（郄穴）

【出处】《黄帝明堂经》。

【别名】无。

【穴义】郄，通"隙"，缝隙。本穴为手厥阴心包经的郄穴，处于桡骨与尺骨的间隙，两侧如门，故名"郄门"。

【定位】腕掌侧远端横纹上5寸，掌长肌腱与桡侧腕屈肌腱之间。

【主治】①心痛，心悸，心烦，胸痛；②咳血，吐血，衄血。

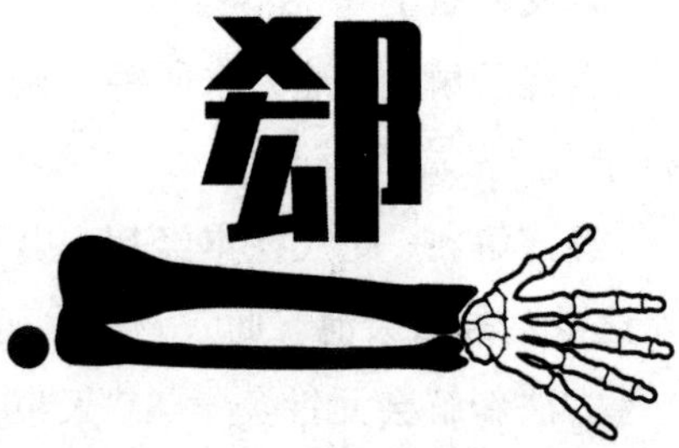

穴为郄穴，在桡骨与尺骨的间隙，两侧如门。

【释义摘录】

《医经理解》："手厥阴郄也，在掌后去腕五寸。"

《经穴解》："此穴乃手厥阴经之郄也，界在手少阴、手太阴两脉之间，而有郄焉，有门象，故曰郄门。"

《古法新解会元针灸学》："由经郄入分肉间，两筋相夹分肉相对，如门之状，故名郄门。"

《针灸穴名解》："穴在前膊两筋间，掌后去腕五寸处，两筋夹隙中，其穴深大，故称'郄门'。"

5 间使（经穴）

【出处】《灵枢·本输》。

【别名】鬼路，剑巨。

【穴义】间，中间，穴在掌后三寸两筋间凹陷处，故以"间"名。使，臣使。心为"君主之官"，心包为心之外围，有代心受邪、替君行令之功，故为"臣使之官"。本穴为手厥阴心包经经穴，主治心神失常，癫病癫痫，故以"使"名。其定位从"间"，主治从"使"，故名"间使"。

【定位】腕掌侧远端横纹上3寸，掌长肌腱与桡侧腕屈肌腱之间。

【主治】①心痛，心悸，心烦；②胃脘痛，呕吐；③癫，狂，痫；④失音；⑤热病，疟疾。

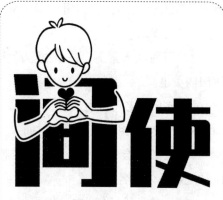

本穴有代心受邪之功，主治癫病癫痫等精神失常。

【释义摘录】

《医经理解》："在掌后横纹上三寸两筋间陷中，包络为臣使之官，此则行与两筋间也。"

《经穴解》："此穴在两阴经之间，而本经乃心主臣使之官，故曰间使。"

《古法新解会元针灸学》："间接分肉经络之间，使经络通手足太阴，因肉主脾，生金味辛通肺，火生土益脾，虚者补之火为土母，实者泻肺土之子为金，因此于脾肺相通，故名间使。"

《针灸穴名释义》："穴在两筋之间，为臣使用命及君臣相间行事之处。"

《针灸穴名解》："间，夹隙之中间也，又间隔也。使，使令也，又治事也……因名'间使'。"

6 内关（络穴；八脉交会穴，通阴维脉）

【出处】《灵枢·经脉》。

【别名】无。

【穴义】内，指代方位；关，联络、关要。内关为手厥阴心包经之络穴，联络手少阳三焦经，且位于前臂掌侧，与"外关"互为内外，故名"内关"。

【定位】腕掌侧远端横纹上2寸，掌长肌腱与桡侧腕屈肌腱之间。

【主治】①心痛，心悸，胸闷；②胃脘痛，

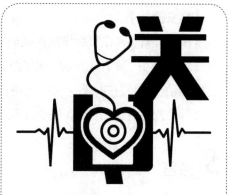

穴为八脉交会穴，通阴维脉，主治胃、心、胸诸疾。

呕吐，呃逆；③癫，狂，痫；④上肢痹痛。

【释义摘录】

《黄帝内经太素》："手心主至此太阴少阴之内，起于别络，内通心包，入于少阳，故曰内关也。"

《经穴解》："穴名内关者，第四穴名郄门，而间使穴在于其中，既过门，而复有关焉。内者，与外相对也，皆离肘而入掌骨节交经之处，有关象焉，故曰关。"

《古法新解会元针灸学》："阴维脉所发，是心包经之络脉，通乎任脉，关于内脏，血脉之连络，故名内关。"

《针灸穴名释义》："内，指胸膈之内及前臂之内侧。关，关格，关要。内关，病名。穴居前臂内侧之冲要，可以通胸膈关塞诸病也，与外关相对。"

7 大陵（输穴、原穴）

【出处】《灵枢·九针十二原》《灵枢·本输》。

【别名】鬼心，手心主。

【穴义】陵，丘陵。穴在掌后两筋间凹陷处，因其隆伏较大，掌骨犹如大山，故名"大陵"。

【定位】腕掌侧远端横纹中，掌长肌腱与桡侧腕屈肌腱之间。

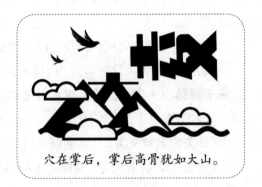

穴在掌后，掌后高骨犹如大山。

【主治】①胸胁痛，心痛，心悸；②胃脘痛，呕吐，吐血；③癫，狂，痫；④上肢痹痛；⑤疮肿。

【释义摘录】

《医经理解》："在掌后横纹两筋间，言掌骨如大陵也。"

《经穴解》："陵者，土也，以此穴为本经之输穴，故曰陵。又其穴在掌后骨下，其上骨肉丰隆，而穴在其下，故曰大陵。"

《针灸穴名释义》："大，高大；陵，丘陵。穴在掌后高骨形如丘陵之下方也。"

8 劳宫（荥穴）

【出处】《灵枢·本输》。

【别名】掌中，五里，五星。

【穴义】劳，劳动，劳作。本穴名解有二。其一，穴位于手掌中央，手为劳动的主要器官，故以"劳"名。"宫"是帝王之居室。"劳宫"意指本穴位于手心，为心神所居之宫阙。其二，心包性属相火，本穴为手厥阴心包经之荥火穴，为火经火穴，主治口疮、口臭等心经热证和癫痫、昏迷等神志病，代心而劳，故名"劳宫"。

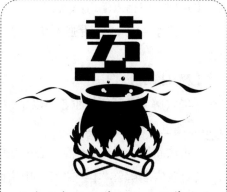

穴为心包经之荥火穴，故尊称为"宫"，喻心神所居之宫阙。

【定位】横平第3掌指关节近端，第2、3掌骨之间偏于第3掌骨。握拳屈指时，中指尖下是穴。

【主治】①口疮，口臭；②鹅掌风；③癫，狂，痫；④心痛，心烦；⑤呕吐，吐血；⑥热病，口渴。

【释义摘录】

《医经理解》："在掌中央动脉中，人劳倦则掌中热，故此为劳宫也。"

《经穴解》："人劳于思，则此穴之脉大动，盖以此穴为本经之火，心劳则火动，火动则脉大动于此穴，故曰劳宫。"

《古法新解会元针灸学》："手掌四周位列八卦，手居中宫，手十四节，仗中宫之真空神力，任劳而不倦，勤劳而功成。故名劳宫。"

《经穴释义汇解》："劳，勤也。穴为心包络之荥火穴，臣使之官，代心主之官行政而劳，故名劳宫。"

《针灸穴名解》："劳，操作也；宫，中室也。手任劳作，穴在掌心，因名'劳宫'，即劳动中心主力也。"

《针灸穴名释义》："劳，病苦也。《淮南·精神》：'使人之心劳。'《论语·为政》：'有事弟子服其劳。'手司劳作，穴在掌心，因其所在与功用而得名。"

9 中冲（井穴）

【出处】《灵枢·本输》。

【别名】无。

【穴义】中，指代方位，中指；冲，冲出。穴在手中指之端，为手厥阴心包经经气冲出之处，故名"中冲"。

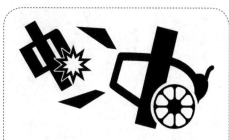

穴在中指之端，为心包经经气冲出之处。

【**定位**】中指末端最高点。

【**主治**】①中风，舌强不语；②神昏；③心痛，心烦；④中暑，热病；⑤小儿惊风。

【**释义摘录**】

《经穴解》："穴名中冲者，以中指而得名，言心包之脉，在两阴之间，而直冲于手中指之端也，故曰中冲。"

《古法新解会元针灸学》："心阳从中指直而冲出也，故名中冲。"

《针灸穴名解》："本经之气，中道而行，直达手中指之端，故名中冲。"

第十一章
手少阳三焦经穴

1 关冲（井穴）

【出处】《灵枢·本输》。

【别名】无。

【穴义】关，指出入的要道；冲，要冲，重要的地方。因本穴为手厥阴心包经与手少阳三焦经表里出入之枢纽，故名"关冲"。

【定位】第4指末节尺侧，指甲根角侧上方0.1寸。

【主治】①头痛，耳鸣，耳聋，咽喉肿痛；②目翳；③热病，口渴，唇干。

本穴为手厥阴心包经与手少阳三焦经表里出入之枢纽。

【释义摘录】

《医经理解》："关冲，少阳之冲，本经之关界也。"

《经穴解》："三焦经行手太阳、手阳明两脉之中，有关象焉，冲而上行，故曰关冲，以与包络之中冲者对，彼以在手太阴、手少阴之中，故曰中冲。"

《古法新解会元针灸学》："关冲者，关乎上而通下，从下而冲上，达于上中下，头腰腿也。内关于脑胸，外关于肢体，三焦经络从四肢外侧始发之根，故名关冲。"

《经穴释义汇解》："因喻穴为少阳之冲，本经之关界，又是心包至此之关会，故名关冲。"

2 液门（荥穴）

【出处】《灵枢·本输》。

【别名】腋门，掖门。

【穴义】液，津液。"三焦者，决渎之官，水道出焉"，液门为手少阳三焦经之荥水穴，刺激本穴可治疗咽痛、目涩等伤津之证，故以"液"名。门，取繁体"門"之形。穴在小指与无名指间凹陷处，似"門"字形。故名"液门"。

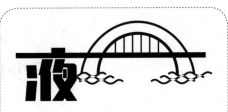

穴为荥水穴，主治伤津之症，故名"液"；穴在小指与无名指间凹陷处，似"门"字象形。

【定位】第4、5指间，指蹼缘上方赤白肉际凹陷中。

【主治】①头痛，目赤，耳鸣，耳聋，咽喉肿痛；②热病，疟疾；③手臂肿痛。

【释义摘录】

《医经理解》："两户曰门。液门，少阳所溜，谓是液泽之门也。"

《经穴解》："液者，水之称也，本经为火而主气，本穴乃水穴也，则亦液而已，在歧骨之间，有门象焉，故曰液门。"

《古法新解会元针灸学》："液门者，阳经之精液，血津出入之门，故名液门。"

《经穴释义汇解》："门（門），繁体从二户象形。穴在小指次指间凹陷处，小指次指之间似'門'字象形。穴为手少阳脉之所溜，犹似液泽之门，故名液门。"

《针灸穴名释义》："液，指水液，腋部。门，见云门条。谓穴能主液所生病与腋部诸病也。"

3 中渚（输穴）

【出处】《灵枢·本输》。

【别名】无。

【穴义】中，指代方位；渚，水中之小洲。"三焦者，决渎之官，水道出焉"（《素问·灵兰秘典论》），三焦水道似江，穴居其中如渚，故名"中渚"。

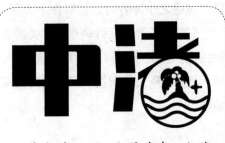

三焦水道似江，穴居其中，如渚（水中小洲）。

【定位】第4、5掌骨间，第4掌指关节近端凹陷中。

【主治】①头痛，目痛，耳鸣，耳聋，咽喉肿痛；②肩背、肘臂痛，手指不能屈伸；③热病。

【释义摘录】

《医经理解》："小洲曰渚。指腕中间，其陷者有如渚焉，故谓中渚。"

《经穴解》："渚者，水所留之称也，中乃三焦之脉，行乎两经之中也，故曰中渚。"

《古法新解会元针灸学》："中渚者，约束经皮膜阳气，回折入经脉之中。其旺于春，仗依肾原与中土相扶助而生万物，充实经络，以防天地之厉气，如中风中暑之害，故名中渚。"

《经穴释义汇解》："渚，遮也，能遮水使旁回也。三焦者，决渎之官，水道出焉。穴为三焦脉之木穴，木能遮水，使水旁回，而穴居手小指次指本节后间凹陷处，如《诗·召南》载：'江有渚。'三焦水道似江，穴居其中，如渚，故名中渚。"

《针灸穴名释义》："中，指人身元气之根本，又指心神情志。渚，水中之小洲。言心神情志之气在此集结如洲渚也。"

4 阳池（原穴）

【出处】《灵枢·本输》。

【别名】别阳。

【穴义】穴在手背腕上凹陷处，其处凹陷如池，背为阳，故名"阳池"。

【定位】腕背侧远端横纹上，指伸肌腱的尺侧缘凹陷中。

【主治】①手腕痛，肩臂痛；②疟疾；③口干。

【释义摘录】

《医经理解》："手背为阳，腕骨之上，有如池焉，故谓阳池。"

《经穴解》："水之所聚者为池，此穴上自关冲，至腕陷中，有聚象，故曰池，阳指三焦而言也。"

穴在手背腕上凹陷处，其处凹陷如池。

《经穴释义汇解》："穴为手少阳脉之原穴，位于手背腕上凹陷处，其处凹陷如池，背为阳，故名阳池。"

《针灸穴名释义》："为手少阳脉气所过之原穴，犹如水之停积于池也。"

5 外关（络穴；八脉交会穴，通阳维脉）

【出处】《灵枢·经脉》《灵枢·根结》。

【别名】 无。

【穴义】 外，指代方位；关，联络，关隘，关要。外关为手少阳三焦经之络穴，为手少阳、手厥阴互相联络关要之处，且位于前臂背侧，与"内关"互为内外，故名"外关"。

穴位于前臂背侧，与内关相对。

【定位】 腕背侧远端横纹上2寸，尺骨与桡骨间隙中点。

【主治】 ①耳鸣，耳聋；②胸胁痛；③上肢痹痛。

【释义摘录】

《医经理解》："外关在腕后二寸两筋间，正与内关相通，手心主为阴血之关，手少阳为阳气之关也。"

《经穴解》："外关者，对内关而言也，此穴在八法中，以为通带脉，而与足少阳胆经之临泣穴通阳维，为男女主客相应。"

《古法新解会元针灸学》："外关者，阳经之络脉，主阳经之阴，与手厥阴经络相交，内外二关，脏腑相会膻中。内关主阴维脉，维于诸阴之交。外关主阳维脉，维于诸阳之会，关乎阳经，通阴达神经于外而开阳经之关节，故名外关。"

《经穴释义汇解》："穴为手少阳之络，在腕后二寸凹陷处，别行心主外关，此与内关相对而属外，故名外关。"

《针灸穴名释义》："外，指前臂外侧。关，关隘，关要。指穴居前臂外侧之要冲，又与内关相对，为手少阳厥阴互相联络关要之处。"

6 支沟（经穴）

【出处】《灵枢·本输》。

【别名】 飞虎。

【穴义】 支，同肢，指上肢；沟，狭长之低洼处。穴为手少阳三焦经经穴，位于腕后三寸两骨（桡骨与尺骨）之间的凹陷处，犹如水注于沟中，故名

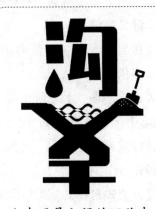

穴在两骨之间的凹陷中，经气运行犹如水注于沟中。

"支沟"。

【定位】腕背侧远端横纹上 3 寸，尺骨与桡骨间隙中点。

【主治】①耳鸣，耳聋，失音；②瘰疬；③胁肋痛；④呕吐，便秘；⑤热病。

【释义摘录】

《医经理解》："古者穿地为沟，支沟在腕后三寸两骨间陷中，其支脉直透厥阴之间使，故谓其之行如水之注入于沟也。"

《经穴解》："沟者，水之所行也，此穴在手臂之外，如木有枝，故曰支沟。"

《古法新解会元针灸学》："支沟者，手臂表面两筋如沟，肘前曰支，故名支沟。"

《针灸穴名释义》："支，支持；又同肢，指上肢。沟，狭长之低洼处。穴在上肢尺桡两骨间之沟中，又须支臂取之。支肘屈臂，手掌向内，则尺桡两骨之沟自见，穴在沟端，故名。"

7 会宗（郄穴）

【出处】《黄帝明堂经》。

【别名】无。

【穴义】会，会聚；宗，宗本。穴位于腕后三寸，支沟穴旁五分，三阳络之前。三焦经脉气经由支沟会聚本穴后行入三阳络，从而沟通手三阳经气，故名"会宗"。

【定位】腕背侧远端横纹上 3 寸，尺骨的桡侧缘。

【主治】①耳聋；②癫痫；③上肢肌肤疼痛。

三焦经气汇聚本穴后，方转入三阳络，犹系统之支别。

【释义摘录】

《医经理解》："会宗，手少阳郄，是经气所会宗也。"

《采艾编》："会宗，腕后三寸空中一寸前后为支曰络，此为会合之宗门也。"

《经穴释义汇解》："穴在腕后三寸空中，即支沟穴之尺侧旁约五分处，为手少阳之郄，是经气会宗所在，故名会宗。"

《针灸穴名释义》："会，聚会，会合。宗，宗主，宗派。指穴为前臂各派阳脉会合之宗主。穴位斜出本经之外，联系三阳，绾罗诸脉，会宗之名，其义可通。"

8 三阳络

【出处】《黄帝明堂经》。

【别名】通间。

【穴义】络，联络。三阳络位于手少阳三焦经、手太阳小肠经、手阳明大肠经阳气联络交会之处，故名"三阳络"。

【定位】腕背侧远端横纹上4寸，尺骨与桡骨间隙中点。

【主治】①耳聋，暴喑，齿痛；②腰胁痛，上肢痹痛。

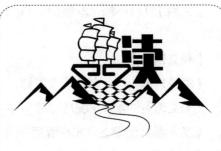

手三阳经阳气联络交会之处。

【释义摘录】

《医经理解》："是三阳络脉所交也。"

《经穴解》："手太阳、阳明俱有络，与本经会于此穴，故曰三阳络。"

《古法新解会元针灸学》："手足三阳之经与三焦相交而通阴，手之三阳化阴而通大交脉，三阳聚结，会宗而化阳络之郊，故名三阳络。"

《针灸穴名释义》："三阳，指手太阳、阳明、少阳三经。络，联络，维系。与手三阳经皆有联系之意。"

9 四渎

【出处】《黄帝明堂经》。

【别名】无。

【穴义】渎，大川。古人将长江、黄河、淮河和济水称为"四渎"，且四条大川均流入大海。本穴前穴为"三阳络"，手三阳阳气交会之处；后穴为本经合穴"天井"，以"四渎"命名，比喻本穴汇聚溪流为大川而后流入大海。

比喻本穴汇聚溪流为大川而后流入大海。

【定位】肘尖下5寸，尺骨与桡骨间隙中点。

【主治】①耳聋，齿痛；②手臂疼痛。

【释义摘录】

《医经理解》："四渎，在肘前五寸外廉陷中，江河淮济为四渎，谓是水所注者也。"

《古法新解会元针灸学》："四渎者，手足名四肢，经络发于五脏六腑而通四海。手少阳会膻中，为气聚之海；散络胸中，上通于脑，为髓海；生于命门，为血海；与足少阳气相交，合于宗筋而通胃，为水谷之海。渎者独也，独通四海，故名四渎。"

《经穴释义汇解》："穴在肘前五寸外廉凹陷处，为三焦脉之腧穴。三焦者，中渎之府，决渎之官，穴通水道，于三阳络之后，故名四渎。"

《针灸穴名解》："渎，为沟渠之大者，本穴前穴为三阳络，则犹汇细流而为巨川也。古称江、淮、河、济四水为'四渎'，以其有润通之力也。本穴治证，多以润通为务。"

10 天井（合穴）

【出处】《灵枢·本输》。

【别名】无。

【穴义】本穴为手少阳三焦经的合穴，五行属土。"三焦者，水道出焉"，土地出水之处为"井"。且本穴位于尺骨鹰嘴之上，两筋之间凹陷如"井"，又居天位，故名"天井"。本穴常用于治疗瘰疬、瘿气，有行气解郁之功，可谓手臂上的"消气穴"。

【定位】肘尖上1寸凹陷处。

【主治】①胸痛，心痛；②耳聋，偏头痛；③癫痫；④瘰疬，瘿气；⑤胸胁痛，肩臂痛。

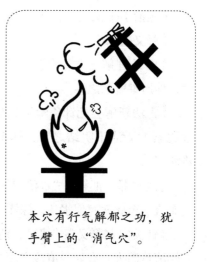

本穴有行气解郁之功，犹手臂上的"消气穴"。

【释义摘录】

《医经理解》："穴地出水曰井。天井，言其高也。"

《古法新解会元针灸学》："天井者，肘后叉骨空孔中如井，有阳气相生，故名天井。"

《经穴释义汇解》："天井者，土也。土，地之体也。地出水曰井。三焦者，水道出焉，亦含'井'义。穴在肘外大骨之后，两筋间凹陷处，居天位，又应天井星名，故名天井。"

《针灸穴名释义》："天，指上肢。井，深凹有水之处。天井，水名，星名，又地形名。言经气如井水之清净，而穴位亦有井之形象也。"

11 清冷渊

【出处】《黄帝明堂经》。

【别名】清泠泉，青灵。

【穴义】清冷渊，古代之水名。清，使清澈，引申为清热；渊，深潭也。手少阳三焦经之脉气血流注至此穴，似水注入深潭。此穴名三字，富有寒泉凛冽之意，临床上毒热之病均可以取此，故名"清冷渊"。古法种痘，取清冷渊、消泺二穴，以其能透解郁热之毒。[1]

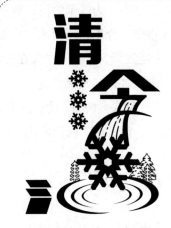

穴名三字富有寒泉凛冽之意，寓意本穴透解郁热之功。

【定位】肘尖与肩峰角连线上，肘尖上 2 寸。

【主治】①头痛，目痛，胁痛；②上肢痹痛。

【释义摘录】

《医经理解》："清冷渊，言其深也，在肘上二寸，伸肘举臂取之。"

《古法新解会元针灸学》："清冷渊者，清者远秽也，冷者灵也，渊者深通源也。穴含原素，清洁于阴结之灵，达深渊之中，解先天遗毒，通身体构造之根原，故名清冷渊。"

《经穴释义汇解》："水治曰清；泠为水名；渊，潭名。三焦者，水道出焉，三焦脉气血流注至此穴，似水注入深潭；又应古水名清冷渊，故以为名。"

《针灸穴名释义》："清冷，清澈凉爽之意。渊，深水，深潭。清冷，又为水名。言穴能清热泻火，有如入清冷之深渊也。"

12 消泺

【出处】《黄帝明堂经》。

【别名】消烁，消铄，消沥。

【穴义】消，消散；泺，水名。本穴善解热，有清三焦热邪的功效，犹如清凉之水

---

① 《痧疹辑要·引种》："《泰西方鉴》云：'种疹法，先于患者发疹最多处部，以铍针微刺之，急将绵一片，浸取其血。尔后就种者上徐徐刺之，令血流漓，凡一刻顷，乃取彼浸血绵贴其疵上，直紧绑之，放置三日许，而后撤去。但要其针疵不深不浅，一适其宜；贴绵间不长不短，惟中其时。'霖按，此即泰西牛痘法也，由清冷渊、消泺等穴引出命门伏毒。"

能消散暑热，故名"消泺"。"泺""止泺"亦为中药"贯众"之别名，此药苦涩，清热解毒，与本穴同功。

【定位】肘尖与肩峰角连线上，肘尖上5寸。

【主治】①齿痛；②头痛，颈项疼痛。

【释义摘录】

《医经理解》："泺，陂泽也。消泺，言水所消注处也。"

《经穴释义汇解》："消，散也。泺，泊名。穴在肩下三寸，肘尖约去六寸，臂外骨内肘斜分间，为三焦脉之腧穴。三焦是全身水液通行的路径，三焦脉流注此穴，似水流入于散泊之中，故名消泺。"

《针灸穴名释义》："消，消除，消渴。泺，水名。言穴用如清凉之水，能清热解渴也。"

《针灸穴名解》："消，放散而消化也。泺（《集韵》音历，即药名'贯仲'也），此药善能解热，功同本穴，故名之为'消泺'。"

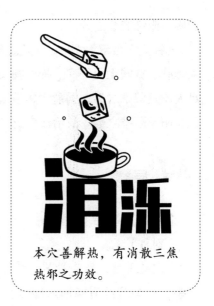

本穴善解热，有消散三焦热邪之功效。

13 臑会

【出处】《黄帝明堂经》。

【别名】臑髎。

【穴义】臑，上臂部。穴在三角肌的后下缘，臂臑肉不着骨之处，为手少阳、阳维交会之处，故名"臑会"。

【定位】当肘尖与肩髎的连线上，肩髎下3寸，三角肌的后下缘。

【主治】①瘿气，瘰疬；②上肢痿痹。

【释义摘录】

《医经理解》："少阳阳维之会，肩下臑肉处也。"

《经穴释义汇解》："穴在肩前廉之肩端三寸宛宛中，肩下臑肉处，即上肢的上节内侧，三角肌后缘处，为手阳明、手少阳结脉之会，故名臑会。"

《针灸穴名释义》："臑，见臂臑条。会，见会宗条。穴与臂臑及臑俞相近，又为手

穴在上臂臑部，手少阳经、阳维脉交会之处。

少阳、阳维交会之处。"

《针灸穴名解》："穴在臂臑之侧，臑俞穴之下，三臑穴位傍近，因名'臑会'。治肩项瘿肿、臂酸无力等症。推'臑会'之意，为三臑之会穴。如臂臑穴属手阳明经，为手足太阳及阳维之会；臑俞穴属手太阳经，为手太阳及阳维之会；臑会属手少阳经，为手足少阳及阳维之会。故治症广泛。"

14 肩髎

【出处】《黄帝明堂经》。

【别名】无。

【穴义】髎，意为骨节空隙处。上臂外展平举，肩关节部肩峰前后即可呈现出两个凹陷窝，前者为肩髃，后者为肩髎，两穴相配治臂痛肩重，不能扬举，故名"肩髎"。

【定位】肩髃后方，当臂外展时，于肩峰后下方呈现凹陷处。

【主治】肩痛、活动受限。

【释义摘录】

《医经理解》："在肩端臑下陷中，斜举臂取之，是肩骨空也。"

《经穴释义汇解》："髎，与窌同。窌，空穴也。穴为三焦脉之空穴，位在肩端臑上，故名肩髎或肩窌。"

《针灸穴名释义》："泛指为肩部之凹陷处。"

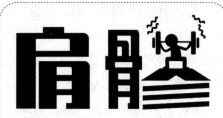

上臂外展时穴在肩峰后凹陷处，主治臂痛肩重，不能扬举。

15 天髎

【出处】《黄帝明堂经》。

【别名】无。

【穴义】髎，指骨间空隙处。穴居胸腔极上，为天部，位于肩胛骨上角骨际凹陷处，故名"天髎"。

【定位】肩胛骨上角骨际凹陷中。

【主治】肩臂痛，颈项强痛。

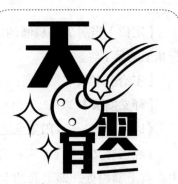

穴居天部，肩胛骨上角骨际凹陷处。

【释义摘录】

《医经理解》："在肩缺盆中愁骨际陷者中，是天部之骨空也。"

《古法新解会元针灸学》："独得天之积阳气，在肩井后一寸，故名天髎。"

《经穴释义汇解》："髎，音寥，骨空处也。穴在肩缺盆中上愁骨之间凹陷处，即肩井与曲垣二穴之间，因穴属天部的骨空，故名天髎。"

《针灸穴名释义》："天，指人体的上部。髎，见肘髎条。穴当肩背之间，以其位置较高而言。"

16 天牖

【出处】《灵枢·本输》。

【别名】无。

【穴义】天，天部；牖，窗户。本穴可开通耳目壅塞之气，治疗目视不明、耳聋等，犹如人体天部之窗牖，故名"天牖"。

【定位】横平下颌角，胸锁乳突肌的后缘凹陷中。

【主治】①目视不明，耳聋，咽喉肿痛；②头痛，眩晕；③瘰疬；④颈项强痛。

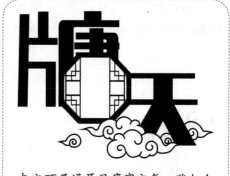

本穴可开通耳目壅塞之气，犹如人体天部之窗牖。

【释义摘录】

《医经理解》："牖以通气，耳为天部之窗牖也。"

《古法新解会元针灸学》："天牖者，阳气属天，项筋向阳处，故名天牖。"

《针灸穴名释义》："天，见天髎条。牖，墙上通风采光的洞口。言穴能开通耳目壅塞之气，如人身上部之窗牖也，与天窗同义。"

《针灸穴名解》："窗开旁墙曰牖。所以助明也，与天窗穴意同。穴在颈侧，有如旁墙之窗，故名'天牖'。以文义揆之，所治者当为头面颈项诸疾也。"

17 翳风

【出处】《黄帝明堂经》。

【别名】无。

【穴义】翳，遮蔽；风，指代风邪。穴位于耳后凹陷处，"翳风"比喻耳朵像屏障一样能为之遮风。又因本穴可驱风邪，善治风证，是治疗面瘫、面肌痉挛的常用穴，故名"翳风"。

【定位】乳突下端前方凹陷中。

【主治】①耳鸣，耳聋；②口眼㖞斜，口噤；③颊肿，瘰疬；④咽喉肿痛，音哑。

【释义摘录】

《医经理解》："在耳后尖角陷中，按之引耳中。翳，蔽也，言以耳为之蔽风也。"

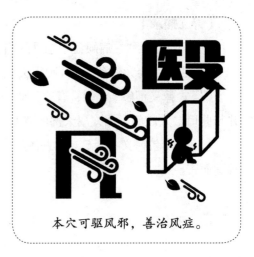

本穴可驱风邪，善治风症。

《经穴解》："此穴在耳之下后，乃无物遮蔽之所，风之自后者，如风池、风府之穴，皆常中风之所也，故曰翳风。"

《古法新解会元针灸学》："翳风者，两耳如翳，两完骨如屏，所谓为挡前后之风，开口空孔中，为风眼。邪乘开口易冲入空窍。开口前有耳，后有完骨，下有颊骨护之，故名翳风。"

《针灸穴名释义》："风，风邪。穴当衣领上缘，正为屏蔽风邪之处。"

18 瘛脉

【出处】《黄帝明堂经》。

【别名】资脉。

【穴义】瘛，通"瘈"，指瘛疭抽搐；脉，指青络脉。本穴在耳根后青络脉形如鸡爪处，主治小儿惊风等惊痫瘛疭诸证，故名"瘛脉"。

【定位】角孙与翳风沿耳轮弧形连线的上2/3与下1/3的交点处。

【主治】小儿惊痫，瘛疭，头痛，耳鸣，耳聋。

本穴主治小儿惊风等惊痫瘛疭诸症。

【释义摘录】

《医经理解》："瘛，牵掣也。谓耳后之络脉牵引处也。"

《采艾编》："耳本后鸡足青络。《外台》禁灸，《明堂》许灸二壮。鸡足所形而名之也。"

《古法新解会元针灸学》："血脉越经而生狂络，遇急热则作跳动、耳赤。如耳干或枯黑，知其阳气不达，肾原虚亏，瘛形也。故名瘛脉。"

《经穴释义汇解》："穴在耳根后鸡足青络脉，即耳后青络脉形如鸡爪处。瘈，牵掣之意，喻耳后之络脉牵引处，主瘈疭，故名瘈脉。"

《针灸穴名释义》："瘈，瘈疭。脉，指筋脉及耳后的青脉。是治疗筋脉瘈疭的耳后青脉。"

19 颅息

【出处】《黄帝明堂经》。

【别名】颅囟，阳维。

【穴义】穴在耳后间青络脉处，耳以报息，比喻此为头颅呼吸之处，故名"颅息"。

【定位】角孙至翳风沿耳轮弧形连线的上2/3 与下 1/3 交点处。

【主治】①耳鸣，头痛；②小儿惊风。

【释义摘录】

穴在耳后，耳以报息，比喻此为头颅呼吸之处。

《医经理解》："耳以报息，谓头颅之报息处也。"

《采艾编》："颅息，耳后间青络脉，足少阳脉气所发。庄子曰：'真人之息以耳段为头息脉会也。'"

《古法新解会元针灸学》："颅息者，头颅近耳之脉，通于呼吸之息，故名颅息。"

《经穴释义汇解》："穴在耳后间青络脉，耳以报息，喻此为头颅之报息处。穴又主喘息，故名颅息。"

《针灸穴名释义》："颅，颅脑，头颅。息，安息，休息，又是塞满之意。谓穴能醒脑安神，治头目昏沉如塞诸病也。"

20 角孙（手少阳经、足少阳经、手阳明经交会穴）

【出处】《黄帝明堂经》。

【别名】无。

【穴义】角，指耳上角；孙，分支，指孙脉。穴在耳角上方，耳轮向耳屏对折时，当耳尖直上入发际处，有太阳经、少阳经的孙脉会于此，故名"角孙"。

【定位】耳尖正对发际处。

【主治】齿痛，颊肿，目翳。

【释义摘录】

《医经理解》："在耳上角外间，发际之下，开口有孔，足太阳、少阳孙脉之会于耳角者也。"

《经穴解》："名角孙者，当在耳角之下也。"

《古法新解会元针灸学》："角者，耳廓上角也，孙者，络于下也。即耳廓内上角稍下开口空中，故名角孙。"

《经穴释义汇解》："穴在耳廓中间上，发际下，即耳轮向耳屏对折时，耳廓上端的尖端处。因喻太阳、少阳经的孙脉会于耳，故名角孙。"

《针灸穴名释义》："角，指头角，角星，又指东方阳春升发之气。孙，幼小、微弱之意。谓穴当头角未成之处，且有角星之象，又如春气在头、初生而未盛也。"

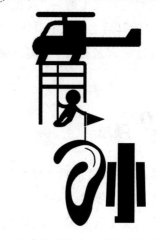

穴在耳角上方，是手太阳经与手少阳经孙脉交汇之处。

21 耳门

【出处】《黄帝明堂经》。

【别名】无。

【穴义】耳，指耳窍；门，指出入之门户。本穴在耳前耳屏上切迹前凹陷处，本经支脉"从耳后入耳中"，再由本穴出走耳前，故名"耳门"。

【定位】耳屏上切迹与下颌骨髁突之间的凹陷中。

【主治】①耳鸣，耳聋，齿痛；②颊肿，颈肿。

本经支线"从耳后入耳中"，再由本穴出走耳前。

【释义摘录】

《医经理解》："当耳之门，在耳前起肉，当耳缺陷中。"

《经穴解》："以穴在耳门旁，故曰耳门。"

《古法新解会元针灸学》："耳门者，肾气朝耳之所入，三焦之原气合于胆之所出，连系于脑，通知觉而达听闻声音，辨别善恶，入于神系，阴复出阳复入，识觉声分别之门，通耳出入阳阴之机关，故名耳门。"

《经穴释义汇解》:"穴在耳前起肉当耳缺者,即耳珠上的缺口处,顾名思义,为耳之门户,故曰耳门。"

《针灸穴名释义》:"穴居外耳道口,功能聪耳助听,有如声音入耳之门户。"

22 耳和髎(手少阳经、足少阳经、手太阳经交会穴)

【**出处**】《黄帝明堂经》。

【**别名**】和髎。

【**穴义**】和,音声调和;髎,骨间空隙。本穴主治耳聋等一切耳疾,使耳能听五音之和,且穴在耳郭根前方凹陷处,故名"耳和髎"。

【**定位**】鬓发后缘,耳廓根的前方,颞浅动脉的后缘。

【**主治**】头痛,耳鸣,牙关紧闭。

【**释义摘录**】

《医经理解》:"耳听音声之和而为锐骨之空也。"

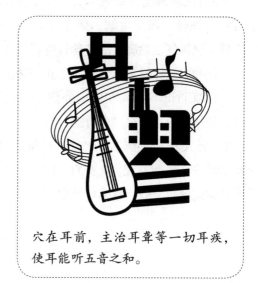

穴在耳前,主治耳聋等一切耳疾,使耳能听五音之和。

《采艾编》:"和髎,耳门前兑发下横动脉。手太阳脉气所发,耳前审知声音之穴隙也。"

《经穴释义汇解》:"髎,与窌同。窌,空穴也。穴为三焦脉之空穴,位在耳前兑发下横动脉,即鬓发后下缘颞浅动脉横过处。耳不听五声之和为聋,肾和则耳能闻五音,穴主治耳聋等一切耳疾,使耳能闻(听)五音,故名耳和髎或和髎。"

23 丝竹空

【**出处**】《黄帝明堂经》。

【**别名**】目髎。

【**穴义**】本穴名解有二。其一,丝,细小的;竹,竹叶;空,凹陷,孔穴。本穴在眉稍外侧凹陷处,眉毛聚集形如竹叶,故名"丝竹空"。其二,弦乐器为"丝",管乐器为"竹","丝竹"合用泛指音乐。眉毛细长弯曲,如箫如弓弦,即穴位处如同箫管或者弓弦上的孔眼,故名。

【**定位**】眉梢凹陷中。

【**主治**】①头痛,眩晕,目赤肿痛,眼睑瞤动;②癫痫、目上视。

【释义摘录】

《医经理解》："在眉后陷中，以耳常听丝竹之音也。"

《经穴解》："此穴虽在目旁，而实通耳之窍以听声者，故曰丝竹空。"

《古法新解会元针灸学》："丝竹空者，目之系有细丝，藏于青润，如在竹之中，连结于目，通风气之轮廓，故名丝竹空。"

《针灸穴名解》："丝，细络也；空，孔窍也；眉犹竹叶。本穴在眉梢外侧端，穴下孔窍，细络旁通，故名'丝竹空'。"

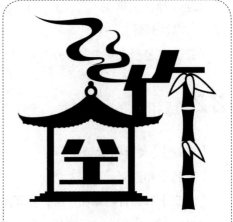

穴在眉梢外侧凹陷中，眉毛聚集形如竹叶。

《经穴释义汇解》："丝竹，音乐之总称，丝谓琴瑟，竹谓箫管。穴在眉后凹陷处，其穴似箫管之孔。孔与空通，又穴近耳，以此喻耳常闻丝竹之音，故名丝竹空。"

第十二章
足少阳胆经穴

1 瞳子髎（手太阳经、手少阳经、足少阳经交会穴）

【出处】《黄帝明堂经》。

【别名】前关，后曲。

【穴义】瞳子，目珠，为目之精华所在；髎，缝隙。因穴在目眦旁，骨隙中，有明目之功，故名"瞳子髎"。

【定位】目外眦外侧 0.5 寸凹陷中。

【主治】①头痛；②目赤肿痛，内障，青盲，目翳，流泪。

【释义摘录】

《经穴解》："穴名瞳子髎者，以穴在目锐眦后五分，此穴之内与瞳仁相近，故曰瞳子髎。"

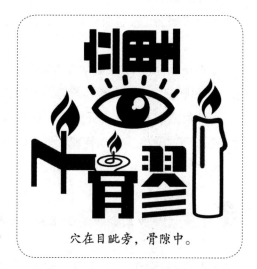

穴在目眦旁，骨隙中。

《古法新解会元针灸学》："瞳子髎者，因肾主骨，化精生于瞳；肝主筋，化精为子。五脏六腑之精华注于目，分五轮八廓，各有部位。手足少阳与手太阳三脉之精华，偏行阳之孔窍，注目之神，遇风热目外皆即赤，穴居目骨眶之边髎，故名瞳子髎。"

《针灸穴名释义》："穴近眼球，横直瞳孔，有明目之功，有如瞳子之孔窍也。"

《针灸穴名解》："目之精华在瞳子，故称目珠为瞳子。穴在目外角，骨隙中，因名瞳子髎。"

2 听会

【**出处**】《黄帝明堂经》。

【**别名**】听呵，后关。

【**穴义**】听，听觉；会，会聚。本穴位于耳前，且主治耳聋耳鸣等诸耳疾，为司听之汇，故名"听会"。

【**定位**】耳屏间切迹与下颌骨髁状突之间的凹陷中。

【**主治**】①耳鸣，耳聋；②齿痛；③下颌关节脱位；④口眼㖞斜。

【**释义摘录**】

《经穴解》："穴名听会者，以此穴专主乎听事，故曰听会。"

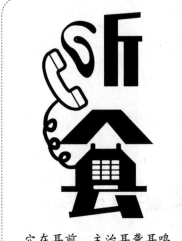

穴在耳前，主治耳聋耳鸣诸证，如司听之汇。

《古法新解会元针灸学》："听会者，司听之神系，会和肝脏之魂，会意其若何。听知其所为，故名听会。"

《针灸穴名释义》："听，指听觉，听力。会，都会，聚会。穴在耳前，主治耳病，为耳部脉气之聚会，亦如管理听觉之都会处也。"

《针灸穴名解》："本穴为司听之汇，而名听会。"

3 上关（手少阳经、足少阳经、足阳明经交会穴）

【**出处**】《素问·气穴论》《灵枢·本输》。

【**别名**】客主人。

【**穴义**】关，开阖之枢机，这里指牙关。"上关"与"下关"相对而言，下关在颧骨弓下，本穴在颧骨弓上，故名"上关"。又因本穴为手足三条阳经之会，少阳为主，阳明为客，如宾主之相聚，故又名"客主人"。

【**定位**】颧弓上缘中央凹陷处。

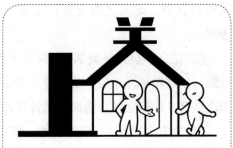

穴为三经之会，足少阳为主，手足阳明为客，如宾主之聚，又名"客主人"。

【**主治**】①耳鸣，耳聋，聤耳，齿痛，口眼歪斜；②下颌关节脱位，功能紊乱；③癫痫病。

【释义摘录】

《医经理解》："客主人，一名上关，在耳前上廉起骨端，开口有孔乃取之。手足三阳诸脉之会，如客与主人之相聚也。"

《经穴解》："穴名客主人者，手少阳为火，而生胃土，足少阳为木，而克胃土。土木有相克之理，而胃经自下而上会十一穴，有客与主人之义，故曰客主人。"

《古法新解会元针灸学》："客主人者，手足少阳为主经穴，手足阳明为客，胃之谷气上朝化神，权作主人，故名客主人。又名上关者，上腭骨开合之关，故又名上关。"

《经穴释义汇解》："耳前曰关，穴在耳前上廉起骨端，故名上关；又因穴为手足三阳诸脉之会，少阳为主，阳明为客，如客与主人相聚，故又名客主人。"

《针灸穴名释义》："上，下之对。关，见下关条。穴在耳前下颌关节之颧弓之上方，与下关相对。"

4 颔厌（手少阳经、足少阳经、足阳明经交会穴）

【出处】《黄帝明堂经》。

【别名】无。

【穴义】颔，额角；厌，合。咀嚼食物时，额角合动处为本穴之所在，故名"颔厌"。

【定位】从头维至曲鬓弧形连线（其弧度与鬓发弧度相应）的上 1/4 与下 3/4 的交点处。取穴时，先定头维和曲鬓，从头维沿鬓角凸至曲鬓作一弧线，于弧线之中点定悬颅，在头维与悬颅之间定颔厌。

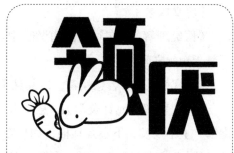

当咀嚼食物时，下颌骨运动，引动本穴所在处颞肌。

【主治】①目外眦痛，耳鸣；②偏头痛，眩晕。

【释义摘录】

《医经理解》："在耳前曲角下颞颥上廉。颔，含也。厌，揜也，上曰颥，下曰颔，颔以含物，此则上以揜下处也。"

《经穴释义汇解》："穴在耳前曲角颞颥上廉，约当悬颅、头维两穴之间。颔，额角也。厌，合也。喻额角合动处即穴之所在，故名颔厌。"

《针灸穴名释义》："颔，腮颔。厌，是极与止的意思，又与餍通。指穴在颔部的边缘与咽食牵动所止之处。"

《针灸穴名解》："人当嚼咽食物时，颔下与颞颥俱动，是颔下与本穴有牵合也，因名'额厌'。古'厌'与'靥'通，又引也，意即额动，引及本穴亦动也。以其近于上关穴，故所治略同于'上关'。"

5 悬颅

【**出处**】《黄帝明堂经》。

【**别名**】无。

【**穴义**】悬，悬空；颅，头颅。本穴名解
有二。其一，本穴悬于头颅之侧，因部位而
得名；其二，头晕时人自觉两足无根，头如
悬空，本穴位于颅侧，主治头晕目眩，故名
"悬颅"，因功用而得名。

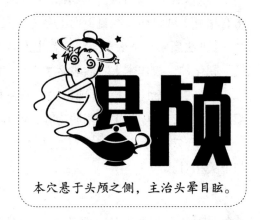

本穴悬于头颅之侧，主治头晕目眩。

【**定位**】从头维至曲鬓弧形连线（其弧度
与鬓发弧度相应）的中点处。

【**主治**】①偏头痛引目、颌、齿痛；②热病。

【**释义摘录**】

《医经理解》："在耳前曲角颞颥中。囟前为发际，发际前为额颅，额厌居上，此则
下悬于额颅之间也。"

《经穴解》："穴名悬颅者，以其悬于头颅之侧，故曰悬颅。"

《古法新解会元针灸学》："悬颅者，悬系偏阳半之头颅中，耳上外廓尖上，发际下
肉部，上不及发，下不及耳根，如悬在头颅部，故名悬颅。"

《针灸穴名解》："本穴在颞颥动脉处，承额厌穴之气下行，即犹头上经气悬行于颅
侧也。沿皮刺之，可治悬晕，此症如人在悬空晃动，病者自觉两足无根，头晕如身悬
也。故名'悬颅'。所治为头痛、牙痛、身热、烦满等症。穴在颅侧，因治病功能而得
名也。"

6 悬厘（手少阳经、足少阳经、足阳明经交会穴）

【**出处**】《黄帝明堂经》。

【**别名**】无。

【**穴义**】厘，毫厘，形容距离小。本穴位于颅侧，与"悬颅"距离很近，只差毫
厘，主治头目眩晕、头痛等，与悬颅相同，故名"悬厘"。

【**定位**】从头维至曲鬓弧形连线（其弧度与鬓发弧度相应）的上 3/4 与下 1/4 的交

点处。

【主治】①偏头痛，目痛；②热病。

【释义摘录】

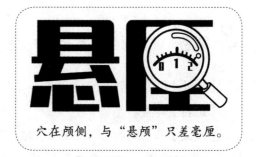

穴在颅侧，与"悬颅"只差毫厘。

《医经理解》："在耳前曲角颞颥下廉。言于悬颅只争毫厘也。"

《古法新解会元针灸学》："悬厘者，耳廓外角上，斜向后，外角不及发际，悬于头部，与悬颅分曲角上下之别，差之毫厘，相隔如山。厘者里也，双足履步，司前脑之阳力，贯于足而能步履，故名悬厘。"

《经穴释义汇解》："穴在头部曲角颞颥下廉，同悬颅只争毫厘，故名悬厘。"

《针灸穴名解》："扬雄云：'荷天冲，提地厘。'言犹荷天之道，提地之理，则而效之也。又悬者，提也；厘者，理也，含有纠偏矫正之义。后人纠正事物之差，多曰厘正。凡头侧之穴，多治偏风、头痛、喎噼、烦心、耳鸣之症。循经取效也。本穴之上，有天冲穴。故本穴取地厘之意，以与相对。因名'悬厘'。"

7 曲鬓（足少阳经、足太阳经交会穴）

【出处】《黄帝明堂经》。

【别名】无。

【穴义】本穴位于鬓发弯曲处，故名"曲鬓"。

【定位】耳前鬓角发际后缘与耳尖水平线的交点处。

【主治】头痛，齿痛，颊肿，口噤。

【释义摘录】

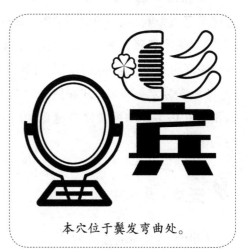

本穴位于鬓发弯曲处。

《经穴解》："耳上发际，鼓颔则不动。耳微前发际，鼓颔则有动处，穴名曲鬓，则在耳上微前，不在正耳上矣"

《古法新解会元针灸学》："曲鬓者，两颊上额发肉相交之处，为鬓。颊耳上崖岸发之曲处，故名曲鬓。"

《经穴释义汇解》："因喻穴居面颊耳上方崖岸发之曲处，故名曲鬓。"

《针灸穴名释义》："指穴当鬓角之弯曲处。"

8 率谷（足少阳经、足太阳经交会穴）

【出处】《黄帝明堂经》。

【别名】蟀谷。

【穴义】本穴名解有二。其一，率，沿着，顺着；谷，山谷。此穴自曲鬓循耳而上，形如山谷，故名"率谷"。其二，率，率领，表率。全身以"谷"命名的穴位中，仅有率谷高居头上，犹如诸"谷"之表率，故名。

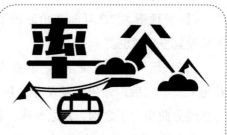

胆经自曲鬓循耳而上到达此穴，形如山谷。

【定位】耳尖直上入发际 1.5 寸。

【主治】①偏头痛，眩晕，呕吐；②小儿惊风。

【释义摘录】

《医经理解》："在耳上入发际一寸五分，嚼牙取之，足太阳少阳之会。肉之大会曰谷。率，循也，言循耳上而为肉会也。"

《经穴解》："此穴在曲鬓之上，有跃然上行之势，故曰率谷。"

《古法新解会元针灸学》："率谷者，在天盖骨、颞额骨、鬓蝶骨，三骨之角相接处。表率骨空在头偏部，率少阳经曲屈如蛇行，通三叉神经结于三骨之空中，故名率谷。"

《针灸穴名释义》："率，率领，表率之意。全身以'谷'命名的各穴均在肢体，仅有率谷高居头上，有如诸谷穴之表率。"

《针灸穴名解》："本穴在侧头骨与颞颧骨合缝处……谷，喻两骨之合缝也，因名此合缝为率谷。"

9 天冲（足少阳经、足太阳经交会穴）

【出处】《黄帝明堂经》。

【别名】无。

【穴义】天，天位，此处指头部；冲，通。本穴在耳后入发际 2 寸，与通天相直，与足太阳经气相交，故借星名"天冲"来比喻其气通于天上。且本穴主治头痛、癫痫、牙龈肿痛等头面部疾病，以"通"的作用为主，

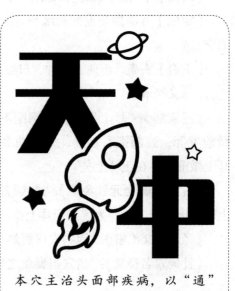

本穴主治头面部疾病，以"通"为用。

故名"天冲"。

【定位】耳根后缘直上，入发际2寸，即率谷之后0.5寸。

【主治】①头痛，牙龈肿痛；②癫痫。

【释义摘录】

《医经理解》："在耳上入发际二寸，如前三分，言其通行天上也。"

《经穴解》："此穴去率谷而又高矣，有冲上之义，故曰天冲。"

《古法新解会元针灸学》："天冲者，肝阳逆冲于头，与通天相直，与太阳气相交，在耳后入发际上二寸，直于通天，故名天冲。"

《经穴释义汇解》："冲，作通道解。穴在耳上如前三分，因穴居天位，而喻其通行天上，并应天上星名天冲，故名天冲。"

《针灸穴名释义》："天，指头部；冲，要冲。天冲，星座名。借喻为高居头部冲要之地。《广雅·释言》：'天，颠也。'《方言·六》：'颠，上也。'《晋书·天文志》：'天冲为妖星之一。穴在头部之要冲，故名。'"

10 浮白（足少阳经、足太阳经交会穴）

【出处】《素问·气穴论》。

【别名】无。

【穴义】本穴名解有二。其一，浮，浮现；白，白发。当人经常熬夜、失眠、情绪抑郁，则阴血不足，血不养发，肝阳上乘而出现两鬓斑白，并伴有头痛、耳聋、耳鸣等症状，可取本穴治之，故名。其二，浮白，指畅快饮酒，司马光有诗云"须穷今日欢，快意浮大白"（《昔别赠宋复古张景淳》）。本穴主治足不能行、头痛、胸满、吐痰沫等病症，宛如浮大白后的醉酒状态，故名"浮白"。

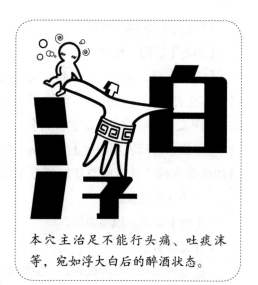

本穴主治足不能行头痛、吐痰沫等，宛如浮大白后的醉酒状态。

【定位】耳后乳突的后上方，从天冲至完骨的弧形连线（其弧度与耳郭弧度相应）的上1/3与下2/3交点处，即耳尖后方，入发际1寸。

【主治】①头痛，目痛，齿痛；②下肢痿痹。

【释义摘录】

《医经理解》："在耳后入发际一寸，白者乾金之气，谓其骨之浮而上者也。"

《古法新解会元针灸学》："浮白者，厥阴之气燥盛，忧愁伤心，厥阴不荣发，乘肝阳上浮两耳上，鬓发斑白，故发入药为血余。《经》言，年六八岁肾气衰，齿脱发堕。肾不养肝，肝阳上浮发白，故名浮白。"

《经穴释义汇解》："浮，作行字解。白，作阴字解。穴在耳后，入发际一寸，因喻本穴在头部循经路线上，上有天冲，下有窍阴，本穴偏行于下，上阳下阴，以白比作阴，故名浮白。"

《针灸穴名释义》："浮，浮游，漂浮，浮越。白，指金气，收敛之意。谓穴能收敛少阳浮越之神气也。浮，漂也，游也，见《广雅·释言》。《素问·生气通天论》：'起居如惊，神气乃浮。'《气交变大论》及《至真要大论》：'少阳之至大而浮。'白为金色，主收藏。少阳风木上干，头目眩晕，神气浮越者，用之得以安定也。"

《针灸穴名解》："本穴治足蹒跚不能行，及耳聋、耳鸣不能听，胸满、咳嗽、吐痰、喉痹、瘿肿、齿痛、吐涎沫等症。病者宛如醉人状态，喻病人如曾浮大白者，本穴可以治此，因名为'浮白'。"

11 头窍阴（足少阳经、足太阳经交会穴）

【出处】《黄帝明堂经》。

【别名】窍阴，枕骨。

【穴义】窍，作"空"字解。穴在头部完骨上、枕骨下，穴处有空，可按而得之，又居头部耳后阴侧空窍处，故名头窍阴。

【定位】耳后乳突的后上方，从天冲到完骨的弧形连线（其弧度与耳廓弧度相应）的上 2/3 与下 1/3 交点处。

【主治】头痛，颈项强痛。

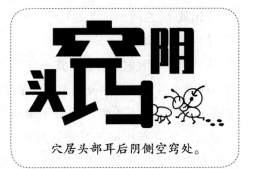

穴居头部耳后阴侧空窍处。

【释义摘录】

《医经理解》："一名枕骨，在完骨上，枕骨下，摇动有空，是髓之会，故谓是阴精所窍也。"

《经穴解》："以此穴有空，可按而得，故曰窍，下浮白而在于阴，故曰窍阴。"

《古法新解会元针灸学》："窍阴者，头为九阳之会而何以生阴窍？因脑后有血属阴，此穴通之，故名窍阴。又名枕骨者，在脑后枕骨两端，与完骨交处之下，故又名枕骨。"

《经穴释义汇解》："窍，作空字解。穴在头部完骨上，枕骨下，摇动有空。是髓之会，故为阴精所窍；又因穴居头部耳后阴侧空窍处，故名头窍阴。"

《针灸穴名释义》："头，相对于足而言。窍，孔窍。阴，指五脏之阴。以穴能治五脏阴窍之病也。目为肝窍，耳为肾窍，舌为心窍，口为脾窍，鼻为肺窍。对头部耳目口舌鼻诸窍之病，本穴均有调摄之功。"

12 完骨（足少阳经、足太阳经交会穴）

【出处】《素问·气穴论》。

【别名】无。

【穴义】完骨，指耳后高骨，即乳突，因颅骨非常坚硬，对脑的保护作用如同城墙一样完备而得名。本穴位于乳突后下方凹陷处，故名"完骨"。

【定位】耳后乳突的后下方凹陷处。

【主治】①头痛，颈项强痛；②咽喉肿痛，颊肿，齿痛；③癫狂；④中风、口眼㖞斜。

【释义摘录】

《医经理解》："在耳后入发际四分，耳后发际高骨谓之完骨也。"

《古法新解会元针灸学》："完骨者，耳后起骨如城郭之完备，护于脑府，中藏神系，通于耳目，故名完骨。"

《针灸穴名释义》："完骨，古代解剖名。即今之颞骨乳突。穴当其处，骨穴同名。"

《针灸穴名解》："完者，全而整也。其处高坚，仅次于强间穴，当头侧外卫之要冲，最须坚固，故名完骨。"

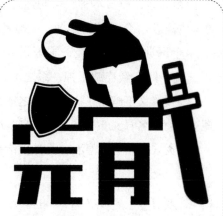

颅骨对脑的保护作用如同首铠。穴在颅骨乳突后下方凹陷处。

13 本神（足少阳经、阳维脉交会穴）

【出处】《黄帝明堂经》。

【别名】无。

【穴义】本，根本；神，元神。头为元神之所在，本穴位于头部，与神庭相平，对应于脑，善治癫痫、小儿惊风、中风昏迷等神不归本的神志病，故名"本神"。

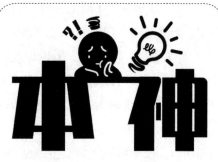

穴在头部，头为元神之所在，善治神志病。

【定位】前发际上 0.5 寸，头正中线旁开 3 寸。

【主治】①头痛，颈项强痛，眩晕；②小儿惊风，癫痫。

【释义摘录】

《医经理解》："脑者人之本，根本之地，人神之所在也。"

《经穴解》："唯木有本，此穴乃本经自完骨外折四，上至于额之上，与督之神庭横直，先取神庭为中，后旁一寸五分，为太阳之曲差，又再旁取一寸五分，为此穴，三穴横列而稍向后，故曰本神，言胆经之神所在也。"

《古法新解会元针灸学》："本神者，本于脑系，通于目系，与足太阳相交于神庭之系。木于识觉，会意神经，国医语云：'肝气痛者，凡有经络筋之处，皆能串到，遂发于肝，出于胆，经连结于神，系之木，故名本神。'"

《经穴释义汇解》："脑者，人之本，主神志病，故名本神。"

《针灸穴名释义》："本，根本，本原。意为穴处为人身元神之根本。"

《针灸穴名解》："善治有关神识诸病，如惊痫、癫风，神不归本等症，故名本神。"

14 阳白（足少阳经、阳维脉交会穴）

【出处】《黄帝明堂经》。

【别名】板眉。

【穴义】阳，此处指头部；白，明亮。本穴在头部前额处，瞳孔直上，主治目疾，使目光明，故名"阳白"。

【定位】眉上 1 寸，瞳孔直上。

【主治】头痛，目痛，目痒，目翳。

【释义摘录】

《医经理解》："在眉上一寸，直瞳子，足少阳、阳维之会，四面光白之地也。"

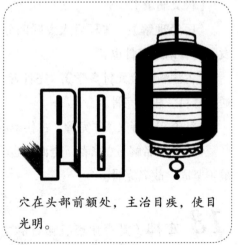

穴在头部前额处，主治目疾，使目光明。

《经穴解》："阳者，少阳也，此穴上不入发，下不入眉，乃在眉发之间，发眉皆黑，而此在其白处，故曰阳白。"

《经穴释义汇解》："白，明也。穴主治目疾，使目光明，故名阳白。"

《针灸穴名释义》："阳，指阳光与头之阳部。白，白色，明白。谓穴能使病目见阳光而明白，及治肺风之眉上生白也。"

《针灸穴名解》："本穴在目上，平明四白之处，故名阳白。"

15 头临泣（足少阳经、足太阳经、阳维脉交会穴）

【出处】《黄帝明堂经》作"临泣"，《针灸资生经》始作"头临泣"。

【别名】无。

【穴义】临，居高临下；泣，流泪。泪从眼出，本穴位于头部发际，瞳孔直上，主治头痛目眩、目赤肿痛、目翳等头目诸疾，故名"头临泣"。

【定位】前发际上 0.5 寸，瞳孔直上。

【主治】①头痛，眩晕；②目痛，流泪，目翳；③鼻塞，鼻渊；④小儿惊风，目上视。

【释义摘录】

《医经理解》："在目上直入发际五分陷中，目者泣之所出，穴临其上，故名也。"

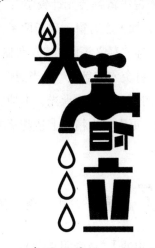

穴在瞳孔直上，主治目疾。泪从眼出，故名。

《经穴解》："此穴正在睛上，故曰临泣。"

《古法新解会元针灸学》："迎风自泪，故名临泣。"

《针灸穴名释义》："头，相对于足而言。临，是监督与治理之意。泪出不止为泣。"

《针灸穴名解》："泣，哭无声也。本穴在前额发际，正当上液之道，酸楚临此，而涕泪乃下，故名临泣。"

16 目窗（足少阳经、阳维脉交会穴）

【出处】《黄帝明堂经》。

【别名】无。

【穴义】本穴位于瞳孔直上，发际上 1.5 寸，主治目赤肿痛、青盲、视物模糊等目疾，其作用犹如开窗通明一样，故名"目窗"。

【定位】前发际上 1.5 寸，瞳孔直上。

【主治】①头痛，眩晕；②目痛，近视。

【释义摘录】

《医经理解》："在临泣上一寸，目气所通也。"

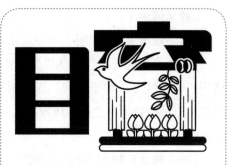

本穴位于瞳孔直上，主治目疾，其作用犹如开窗通明一样。

《采艾编》："目窗，言目上通之窗牖也。"

《经穴解》："穴名目窗者，以此穴正在目之上，刺之目明，如目之有窗者然，故曰目窗。"

《古法新解会元针灸学》："目窗者，目外视而内聪明也，直目向阳之空窍，与顶囟相通，如天之有窗，列于两旁，与目相通，故名目窗。"

《经穴释义汇解》："穴在临泣后一寸，主目疾，是通目气之孔穴，故名目窗。"

《针灸穴名解》："人当回忆往事时，多目睛上视，凝神注脑，则旧时情景历历如见。本穴四周之穴，为承光、本神、临泣、正营诸穴，命名取意，皆关于目。而本穴处四者中间，更为目力精华上达荟萃之处。故本穴治目赤、青盲、白膜覆瞳子诸症，犹开窗通明也。"

17 正营（足少阳经、阳维脉交会穴）

【出处】《黄帝明堂经》。

【别名】无。

【穴义】本穴名解有二。其一，营有营结之意，该穴位于正顶之上，足少阳、阳维两脉之气在此营结，故名"正营"。其二，营，指横线、横路，"南北为经，东西为营"[①]。本穴近于头顶正中百会之横线上，故名"正营"。

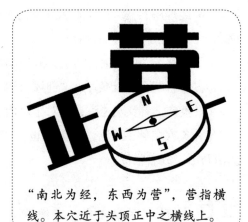

"南北为经，东西为营"，营指横线。本穴近于头顶正中之横线上。

【定位】前发际上 2.5 寸，瞳孔直上。

【主治】①头痛，眩晕；②齿痛。

【释义摘录】

《医经理解》："在目窗上一寸，正顶之上气之营结者也。"

《古法新解会元针灸学》："正营者，足少阳胆经三折于头，正行而下。营为谷气之精华，运于经络，和于五脏，通于阴分。《珍珠囊》云：'目不得血，目不能明。'胆本属阳，而居半营半卫之间，风寒冲入，则寒热往来。虽居最高之位，而与营血相通，故名正营。"

《经穴释义汇解》："穴居正顶之上，谓足少阳、阳维两脉之气所营结，故名。"

《针灸穴名释义》："正，正当、正如之意。营，同荣，指春气。又东西为营。正营，

---

① 《楚辞·九叹》（汉·刘向）："经营原野，杳冥冥兮。"王逸注云："南北为经，东西为营。"

为惊恐状。穴在头顶正中横线上，象少阳升发荣茂之气，功能安神定惊也。营是横线和横路。《楚辞·离世》：'经营原野。'注：'南北为经，东西为营。'穴当头顶正中百会之横线上，对于明确穴位具有一定的指导意义。营有春气在头之象。《礼记·月令》：'孟春之月，日在营室。'正营者，春气在头，脉气荣茂旺盛也。正营，又是惶恐不安之意。《汉书·王莽传》：'人民正营。'正与其功用有关。"

　　《针灸穴名解》："《内经》云：'营主血，目得血则明。'又室之向明者为正室，天子之离宫别馆为营室。人之神智在脑，脑为一身之主宰，犹人世之君主也。本穴有关于脑，犹天子之营室也，故名'正营'。其所治症为头项偏痛、目不明等有关于通明者。"

18 承灵（足少阳经、阳维脉交会穴）

【出处】《黄帝明堂经》。

【别名】无。

【穴义】承，承接。古人认为"举头三尺有神明"，本穴位于发际上 4 寸，因穴居高位可承天之灵，故名"承灵"。

【定位】前发际上 4 寸，瞳孔直上。

【主治】头痛，恶寒，鼻塞，鼻衄。

【释义摘录】

《医经理解》："在正营后一寸，言高可承天之灵也。"

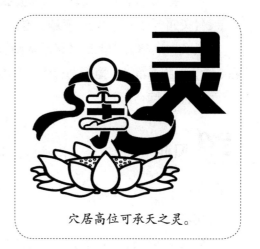

穴居高位可承天之灵。

《经穴解》："此穴与足太阳络却、督经百会穴横直，灵指百会而言，有君象焉，此穴与之横直，有承君之象，故曰承灵。"

《古法新解会元针灸学》："承灵者，承于阴精营血，谷气所化之灵，而行经络筋骨肢膜之间，仗脑府之神系以识觉，故名承灵。"

《针灸穴名释义》："承，见承光条。灵，神灵。脑为神灵之室，头顶骨古称天灵盖。穴在其下旁，乃承受脑神之处也。"

19 脑空（足少阳经、阳维脉交会穴）

【出处】《黄帝明堂经》。

【别名】颞颥。

【穴义】空，空隙。本穴位于枕外隆凸的上缘，其下为脑枕骨之空虚处，故名

"脑空"。

【定位】横平枕外隆凸的上缘，风池直上。

【主治】①目痛，耳聋，鼻衄，鼻部疮疡；②头痛，眩晕，癫狂痫；③发热；④颈项强痛。

【释义摘录】

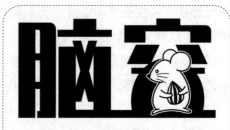

穴在枕外隆凸的上缘，其下为脑枕骨之空虚处。

《医经理解》："一名颞颥，在承灵后一寸五分，夹玉枕骨下陷中，是脑骨之空处也。"

《古法新解会元针灸学》："脑空者，在后脑壳之空处。上有脑，中有脑之总系。连系各经，散络各部，如电网相似，穴居两旁，在后脑交叉大经血管之上，故名脑空。"

《经穴释义汇解》："主脑疾，是通脑之空穴，故名脑空。"

《针灸穴名释义》："脑，颅脑。空，空虚，孔窍。指穴在后脑枕骨下方之空虚处。"

《针灸穴名解》："谚云：'胃常空则病少，脑常空则智多。'吾人运用脑力，必先消除杂念，使脑海澄清，意念乃得专一。本穴内应大小脑之夹间，即脑之间隙处也。脑宜常空，故名'脑空'。"

20 风池（足少阳经、阳维脉交会穴）

【出处】《灵枢·热病》。

【别名】无。

【穴义】本穴位于枕骨下，穴处凹陷似水池，风邪易入，且为治风之要穴，故名"风池"。

【定位】胸锁乳突肌上端与斜方肌上端之间的凹陷中。

【主治】①中风，痫，癫，狂；②眩晕，耳鸣，耳聋；③目赤肿痛，视物不清；④鼻衄；⑤发热，头痛，鼻塞，颈项强痛。

【释义摘录】

穴在枕骨下，穴处凹陷似水池，为治风之要穴。

《医经理解》："在脑空后大筋外发际陷中，夹风府旁二寸，风所从入之地也。"

《古法新解会元针灸学》："风邪易入，而溜注太阳经，内邪一动，即为中风之类，若无内邪而发感冒之类，故名风池。"

《经穴释义汇解》："穴处似池，为治风之要穴，故名风池。"

《针灸穴名释义》："为风邪易于流连和为治风之所当取处。"

《针灸穴名解》："池，喻水之汇储也。本穴为风之所汇，故曰风池。"

21 肩井（手少阳经、足少阳经、足阳明经与阳维脉交会穴）

【出处】《黄帝明堂经》。

【别名】肩解。

【穴义】本穴名解有二。其一，本穴位于肩部正中凹陷处，穴下为胸腔犹如深井，故名"肩井"。其二，井，市井，有四通八达之意。本经通过该穴与诸阳经交会，如同四通八达的交通枢纽，故名"肩井"。

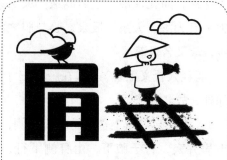

本经通过该穴与诸阳经交会，如同四通八达的井田。

【定位】第7颈椎棘突与肩峰最外侧点连线的中点。

【主治】①颈项强痛，肩背痛；②中风、上肢不遂；③瘰疬；④难产，乳痈，产后缺乳。

【释义摘录】

《医经理解》："肩之深处在肩上陷解中。"

《经穴解》："此穴在肩之上，其下纳五脏，其深不可测，如井然，故曰肩井。"

《古法新解会元针灸学》："居肩部饭匙骨，与大筋，共肩夹骨，连项骨，四骨之间，如井之状，故名肩井。"

《经穴释义汇解》："井，深也。穴在肩上凹陷处，居肩之深处，故名肩井。"

《针灸穴名解》："穴在肩上凹处，故名'肩井'。古有井田之法，'井开四道，而分八宅'。即四通八达也。又古时日中为市，交易者汇通于井，后世称为赶集，又谓通衢为市井。本经通过肩部与诸阳经交会，其所治症极为复杂，有如各病之市集，故名'肩井'。"

22 渊腋

【出处】《黄帝明堂经》。

【别名】泉腋，渊液。

【穴义】渊，深。本穴位于腋下三寸，深藏在腋窝之下，故名"渊腋"。

【定位】第4肋间隙中，在腋中线上。

【主治】①胸胁胀痛，腋下肿；②上肢痹痛。

【释义摘录】

《经穴解》："此穴在腋下，有渊深之意，故曰渊腋。"

《古法新解会元针灸学》："渊液者，在外渊下通于深渊，而化汗液，故名渊液。又名泉液者，因肩腋下有天湿、天泉、极泉，心与胆之汗液而出渊液也，故又名泉液。"

《经穴释义汇解》："穴在腋下三寸宛宛中，腋之深处，故名渊腋。"

《针灸穴名解》："本经起于头侧，注于风池穴，下肩井穴，行于腋下，由身侧下行，结穴于腋下。

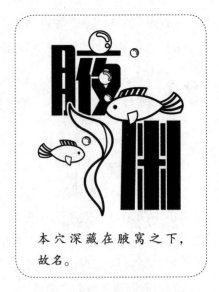

本穴深藏在腋窝之下，故名。

本穴于位则腋，于用则渊，在人身，犹腋下有渊泉也，故名'渊腋'。本穴与天泉、极泉、天溪等穴傍近，故又名'泉腋'。本穴虽浅，所关则深。"

23 辄筋

【出处】《黄帝明堂经》。

【别名】神光，胆募。

【穴义】辄，同"辙"，指车轮压的痕迹。在胁肋两旁大筋如车之有辙也，故名"辙筋"。

【定位】第4肋间隙中，在腋中线前1寸。

【主治】胸中暴满不得卧，气喘。

【释义摘录】

《医经理解》："两车相倚曰辄，辄筋，言倚于筋间也。"

《采艾编》："辄筋，近于肝而以筋名，阳附于阴，此为依辅也。"

《经穴解》："此穴乃本经上胁之筋所行处，故曰辄筋。"

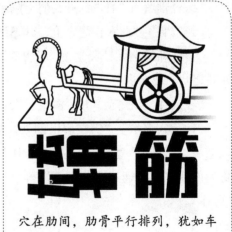

穴在肋间，肋骨平行排列，犹如车轮压过的痕迹。

《古法新解会元针灸学》："辄筋者，在胁肋两旁大筋如车之有辄也。又名神光者，通于神明，光明之大路也。又名胆募者，阳气化阴、阴气出于阳道之膈募相通也。"

《经穴释义汇解》："两车相倚曰辄，辄筋，即说其穴倚于筋间，故名辄筋。"

24 日月（胆募穴，足少阳经、足太阴经之会穴）

【出处】《黄帝明堂经》。

【别名】神光。

【穴义】本穴为胆之募穴。胆为"中正之官，决断出焉"，决断务求明察秋毫，"明"字从日从月，故名"日月"。

【定位】第7肋间隙中，前正中线旁开4寸。

【主治】① 胁痛，多唾，吞酸，呃逆；② 黄疸。

【释义摘录】

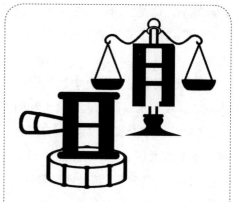

胆募穴。胆主"决断"，务求明察秋毫，"明"字从日从月。

《医经理解》："胆募也，期门下五分第三肋端，横平蔽骨，上直两乳，日月东出，木之华也，胆为甲木，故有神光之称。"

《经穴解》："此穴在肝经期门之下，人身南面而立，此穴正在东西，犹日月出没于东西也，别无所取义焉。"

《古法新解会元针灸学》："日精月华出入也，故名日月。"

《经穴释义汇解》："穴在期门下一寸五分，胆募也。胆者，中正之官，决断出焉，喻决断务求其明，以明察秋毫。'明'字，从日从月，故名日月。"

《针灸穴名解》："《道藏》曰：'日、月者，左右目也。'本穴善治目疾，因名日月，又名神光。神之光，日与月也。"

25 京门（肾募穴）

【出处】《黄帝明堂经》。

【别名】气府，气俞。

【穴义】京，古与"原"通，肾气为人身之原气，穴为肾之募穴，肾脏原气募聚之处，有益肾利水之功，似水道之门户，故名"京门"。

【定位】第12肋骨游离端的下际。

【主治】①腰胁痛；②肠鸣，泄泻，腹胀；

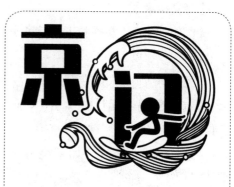

肾之募穴，为肾脏原气聚集之门户，有益肾利水之功。

③小便不利，水肿。

【释义摘录】

《医经理解》："在监骨腰中季肋本夹脊，又曰在脐上五分，旁九寸半，气府、气俞，皆其别名，谓是气所出入之一大门也。"

《经穴解》："其取义于京门者，以此穴在后，为身最虚之处，犹门焉。京者，大也。"

《古法新解会元针灸学》："天一生水，水生木，木之根基连结肾带，木能生火，火为君心，仗阳木以调水火，火水和而土金定，故名京门。"

《针灸穴名释义》："京，与丘同义，高大之土阜；又忧也。门，见云门条。穴位所在犹如胸廓大丘之门，可用以止恐定惊。"

《针灸穴名解》："该处四周隆起。凡四周隆起之处为京，故称京门。"

26 带脉（足少阳经、带脉交会穴）

【出处】《黄帝明堂经》。

【别名】无。

【穴义】本穴是足少阳胆经和带脉的交会穴，主治妇科经带疾患，如带下、月经不调、阴挺、经闭等，故名"带脉"。

【定位】第11肋骨游离端垂线与脐水平线的交点上。

【主治】①月经不调，赤白带下；②少腹疼痛，疝气，腰胁痛。

本穴是胆经和带脉的交会穴。带脉横于腰腹，犹如束带。

【释义摘录】

《医经理解》："在季胁下一寸八分陷中，一云在脐旁八寸半。如带之绕身，管束诸经也。"

《经穴解》："如人束带而前垂，故名带脉。"

《古法新解会元针灸学》："三脉并起而异行，皆与带有连系，带领诸脉，故名带脉。"

《经穴释义汇解》："如带绕身，管束诸经，又主带脉病及妇人经带疾患，故名带脉。"

《针灸穴名释义》："带，指衣带，带下病。脉，经脉。带脉，脉名。穴当带脉之所过，与衣带所系之处，又可治带下病，故名。"

27 五枢（足少阳经、带脉交会穴）

【出处】《黄帝明堂经》。

【别名】无。

【穴义】五，喻五方之位，五居其中。枢，门上的转轴。穴在腹部胆经五穴之中，亦在人身之中。当人转动身体，或者跪拜五体投地时，本穴正当腰部转折处，犹如门上的转轴，故名"五枢"。

【定位】横平脐下 3 寸，髂前上棘内侧。

【主治】①赤白带下，月经不调，疝气；②少腹痛，腰痛，胯痛。

【释义摘录】

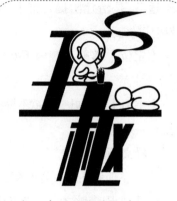

本穴在人体长度折中的地方，当人跪拜时，本穴正当腰部转折处。

《医经理解》："在带脉下三寸，环跳上五寸。一曰水道旁一寸半，足少阳带脉之会，是谓藏气之枢要也。"

《古法新解会元针灸学》："五枢者，上部五形化气过带脉，转枢足之五行气。入十二经十五络相环上下无端，皆不出五行相转枢。带脉之会，足少阳经为枢，故名五枢。"

《经穴释义汇解》："穴在带脉下三寸。五，喻五方之位，五居其中。穴在腹位，腹部胆经五穴上有京门、带脉，下有维道、居髎，五枢居中；穴属藏气之枢要，故名五枢。"

《针灸穴名释义》："五为中数，指人身之中。枢，见天枢条。穴位所在犹如人身中部之枢纽。《易·系词》：'天数五，地数五。'五为中数。穴居人身之中部，可与天枢、大横相应。又'格五'是古代棋戏的一种，至'五'即格不能行，也可以借喻五枢为行走枢要之意。"

《针灸穴名解》："枢，为致动之机。本穴当人身长度之折中，人当扭转身躯，或跪拜五体投地时，本穴正当腰部转折之处。又五者数之中。'五枢'即中枢之意也。"

28 维道（足少阳经、带脉交会穴）

【出处】《黄帝明堂经》。

【别名】外枢。

【穴义】维，维系；道，要道。本穴是足少阳胆经和带脉的交会穴，经脉中只有带脉为横行经脉，是维系诸经脉之要道，故名"维道"，是治疗阴挺、带下、月经不调等经带诸症的常用穴。

【定位】髂前上棘内下 0.5 寸，即五枢内下 0.5 寸。

【主治】①呕吐，食欲不振；②水肿；③腰腿痛。

【释义摘录】

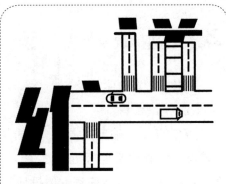

穴为胆经和带脉的交会穴，带脉为横行经脉，是维系诸纵行经脉之要道。

《医经理解》："一名外枢，在章门下五寸三分，是少阳带脉之会，带以维系一身，故谓之维道也。"

《经穴解》："带脉之横束缚诸经也，上下凡三穴，而此穴乃其最下穴也，又向里折斜而下。阳维自循膝外廉，上髀厌，抵少腹侧，会本经于居髎之后，上循胁肋斜上，此正其自下斜上之处，故曰维道。"

《古法新解会元针灸学》："维道者，维护阴阳脉络之道路也。上通子宫带，下通连韧带，经和三焦，行半表半里之间，故名维道。"

《经穴释义汇解》："带以维系一身，维护阴阳脉之道路，故名维道。"

《针灸穴名释义》："维，维系。道，道路。意指穴处为维系与连接下肢之通道。"

29 居髎（足少阳经、阳跷脉交会穴）

【出处】《黄帝明堂经》。

【别名】无。

【穴义】居，蹲；髎，骨间凹陷处。本穴在髋部髂骨上，当人蹲坐时穴位处形成一凹陷，故名"居髎"。

【定位】髂前上棘与股骨大转子最凸点连线的中点处。

【主治】①疝气、腰痛引小腹；②腰腿痛。

【释义摘录】

穴在髋部，当人蹲坐时穴位处形成一凹陷。

《医经理解》："在章门下八寸三分，居腹部监骨上，故曰居髎也。"

《经穴解》："穴在肝经章门穴下八寸三分，监骨上陷中，足少阳、阳跷之会。"

《古法新解会元针灸学》："居髎者，所居监骨上之边髎陷孔，故名居髎。"

《经穴释义汇解》："居，蹲也。髎，与窌同。窌，空穴也。穴在章门下八寸三分，监（髂）骨上凹陷处。取穴时，需蹲而取之，故名居髎或居窌。"

《针灸穴名解》："居，端坐也。本穴在章门穴下四寸处。人当端坐时，则此穴位置在凹隙洼中，以其居则成髎。故名'居髎'。"

30 环跳（足少阳经、足太阳经交会穴）

【出处】《黄帝明堂经》。

【别名】环铫。

【穴义】环，环形；跳，跳跃。本穴位于髋部，取穴时需令患者侧卧，下方的腿伸直，上方的腿屈膝屈髋呈半环形，如跳跃状，故名"环跳"。

【定位】股骨大转子最凸点与骶管裂孔连线的外 1/3 与内 2/3 交点处。

【主治】腰胯痛，下肢痿痹、麻木，半身不遂。

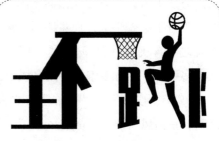

取穴时需令患者屈膝屈髋呈半环形，如跳跃状。

【释义摘录】

《医经理解》："在髀枢中，侧卧伸下足屈上足取之，为环转跳动处也。"

《经穴解》："曰环跳者，骨缝错扣之处，上如环以扣其骨，股之能屈伸往来者，以环故也，跳则走动之象。"

《古法新解会元针灸学》："针之，伸足环从陷处跳起，穴即闭，故名环跳。"

《针灸穴名释义》："环，弯曲。跳，跃起，必须弯身环腿方可便于跳跃。指取穴时之体位及其能治环而难跳之腿病而言。"

《针灸穴名解》："见人当跳跃时，必先蹲身屈其胯膝，则本穴形成半环形之凹隙，因名环跳。"

31 风市

【出处】《肘后备急方·治风毒脚弱痹满上气方第二十一》。

【别名】无。

【穴义】市，集市，指聚集之处。本穴为下肢风邪聚集之处，是祛风之要穴，主治中风偏瘫、震颤麻痹、肌肉抽搐、皮肤瘙痒等，故名"风市"。

【定位】髌底上7寸，髂胫束后缘。

【主治】①半身不遂，腰腿痛，下肢痿痹；②瘙痒。

【释义摘录】

《经穴解》："风之所中，在下体入此穴者多，故曰风市，言风往来之所也。"

《古法新解会元针灸学》："南方之风出而伤头，故南方多头风；北方之风出而伤腿，故北方多寒腿。肝之阳行于半表半里，而主诸风，风市系少阳经穴，地发之风含庚气，起即伤腿。肝阳遇热则失衡，故南方多痿厥，北方多偏枯，故名风市。"

《经穴释义汇解》："位临阴市之旁，为风气所聚之处，是治风之要穴，故名风市。"

《针灸穴名释义》："市，集市，货物集散之处。指穴处易为风邪所集聚，亦为驱散风邪之地也。"

《针灸穴名解》："本穴为治诸风之要穴，犹治疗诸风之市集也，因名风市。"

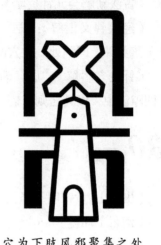

穴为下肢风邪聚集之处，是祛风之要穴。

32 中渎

【出处】《黄帝明堂经》。

【别名】无。

【穴义】渎，大川。在大腿部，足三阳经犹如川渎一样并列顺行，本经循行于股外肌与股二头肌形成的狭长凹陷中，位于足阳明胃经和足太阳膀胱经中间，故名"中渎"。

【定位】髌底上5寸，髂胫束后缘。

【主治】下肢痿痹，半身不遂。

【释义摘录】

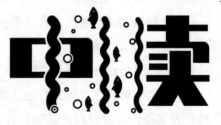

足三阳经犹如川渎一样并列顺行，本经居中。

《医经理解》："在髀骨外膝上五寸分肉间陷中，谓髀骨中之沟渎也。"

《经穴解》："渎者，行水之名，足太阳在其后，足阳明在其前，故曰中渎。"

《古法新解会元针灸学》："中渎者，所居半表中里之中，又系尺折之中，独能通四海，由阳经络行于阴分，故名中渎。"

《经穴释义汇解》："穴在髀骨外，膝上五寸分肉间凹陷处，喻脉气所发，如入髀骨中之沟渎，故名中渎。"

《针灸穴名释义》："中，指中间。渎，参四渎条。指穴在股外侧足太阳、阳明两经之中，形如大川的大沟中。手足少阳上下同气，下肢之中渎与上肢之四渎也有互相应称之意。"

33 膝阳关

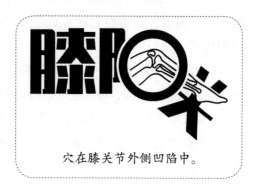

穴在膝关节外侧凹陷中。

【出处】《黄帝明堂经》作"阳关"，《针灸学简编》始作"膝阳关"。

【别名】寒府。

【穴义】阳，肢体外侧为"阳"；关，关节。本穴位于膝关节外侧凹陷中，故名"膝阳关"。

【定位】股骨外上髁后上缘，股二头肌腱与髂胫束之间的凹陷中。

【主治】膝腘肿痛、挛急，小腿麻木。

【释义摘录】

《古法新解会元针灸学》："阳关者，膝关节之外侧，偏重于阳，故名阳关。"

《经穴释义汇解》："穴在阳陵泉上三寸膝部，犊鼻外凹陷处，为足少阳经之关，故名膝阳关。"

《针灸穴名释义》："阳，指人体的外侧。关，见下关条。言穴当膝关节外侧的关要之处。称'膝'者，是区别于腰阳关而言。"

《针灸穴名解》："本穴当膝关节外侧，因名'阳关'。示意阳侧之膝关节也。治风痹膝痛不可屈伸。取此以为通也。"

34 阳陵泉（合穴，胆下合穴，八会穴之筋会）

【出处】《灵枢·邪气脏腑病形》。

【别名】无。

【穴义】陵，山陵；泉，水泉。本穴位于腓骨头前下方凹陷处，腓骨头突起如山陵，穴处凹陷如水泉，且位于小腿外侧，与阴陵泉相对，故名"阳陵泉"。

【定位】腓骨头前下方凹陷处。

【主治】①胁痛，口苦，呕吐，吞酸；②膝肿痛，下肢痿痹、麻木。

【释义摘录】

《医经理解》："与阴陵泉相对，内侧为阴，外侧为阳，在膝下一寸骱骨外廉陷中，故谓是高陵之出泉处也。"

《经穴解》："穴之称陵也，以仅在膝之下，膝有高陵之象焉。故曰陵。阳者，以本经而得名也。泉者，乃本经之脉在此下注，有泉之象焉。"

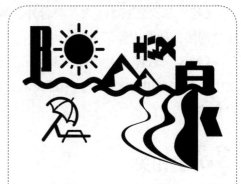

穴在腓骨小头前下方，腓骨头突起如山陵，穴处凹陷如水泉。

《古法新解会元针灸学》："六阳经筋之连系，化精汁，如甘泉，内和脏腑，外润经筋，含天然春日正阳，冲和之气，故名阳陵泉。"

《经穴释义汇解》："因喻穴旁之骨隆起如陵，比作高陵出泉之处，故名阳陵泉。"

《针灸穴名释义》："阳陵，指人体外侧局部隆起处。穴在膝关节外侧隆起处腓骨小头之下方，与阴陵泉对应。"

35 阳交 （阳维脉郄穴）

【出处】《黄帝明堂经》。

【别名】别阳，足髎。

【穴义】交，交会。本穴位于小腿外侧，靠近足太阳、足阳明，又是足少阳胆经与阳维脉的交会穴，故名"阳交"。

【定位】外踝尖上7寸，腓骨后缘。

【主治】①咽喉肿痛；②胸满；③癫狂，抽搐；④下肢痿痹，转筋。

【释义摘录】

《医经理解》："在足外踝上七寸，斜属三阳分肉间，谓斜趋三阳之分而与三阳交也。"

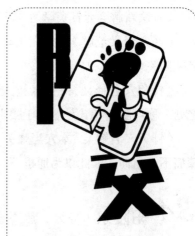

穴在小腿外侧，靠近足太阳、足阳明，又是足少阳和阳维脉之交会穴。

《经穴解》："阳维自下来者，以此穴为郄，而遇少阳过之，此穴两阳相遇，故曰阳交。"

《古法新解会元针灸学》："阳交者，从阳陵内斜，交于阳明，仗阳维之回郄，直交太阳，此三阳之交，故名阳交。"

《针灸穴名解》："本穴为本经与阳维之会。又本穴挨近足太阳、足阳明，故《针灸大成》谓本穴'斜属三阳分肉之间，为阳维之郄'，喻犹足三阳与阳维之交会也。故名'阳交'。本穴与外丘、丰隆、飞扬穴，俱在外踝上七寸许。又本穴治症为寒热痹、喑、嚏、惊、癫、瘛疭等症，及膝足处病，与丰隆、飞扬穴多有相同。因思本穴近旁，或有微细支络，为足三阳之络，以为三阳经脉相互沟通作用。故谓为阳之交也。"

36 外丘（郄穴）

【出处】《黄帝明堂经》。

【别名】无。

【穴义】丘，丘陵。本穴位于小腿外侧，与足阳明胃经的丰隆穴在同一肌肉上，此处肌肉丰满如同丘陵，故名"外丘"。本穴与"阳交"相平，同为郄穴，专治急症，头部、胸胁等胆经循行线上的急性疼痛均可取之。

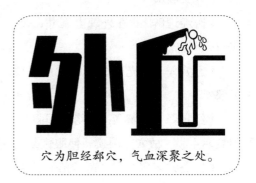

穴为胆经郄穴，气血深聚之处。

【定位】外踝尖上 7 寸，腓骨前缘。

【主治】①胸胁胀满；②癫狂痫；③下肢痿痹。

【释义摘录】

《医经理解》："外丘，外踝上丘聚处也，在外踝上七寸，与阳交差后一寸。"

《古法新解会元针灸学》："外丘者，从阳陵斜下，属于外，起肉如丘，故名外丘。"

《针灸穴名释义》："外，指外侧，又为遗弃之意。丘，见梁丘条。以穴居本经阳交穴之外侧肌肉丰满如丘处而言。外，遗也。《庄子·大宗师》：'参日而后遗[1] 天下。'又，弃也。《吕览·有度》：'则贪污之利外矣。'穴在本经直行路径之外、阳交的外方，如被遗弃，故名。"

《针灸穴名解》："穴在下肢外侧，人当努力时，肌肉隆起之处。与足阳明之丰隆穴，同在一条肉棱，腓骨之后，故与足阳明之丰隆穴，丰满坟起之含意略同。名'外丘'，意其外凸如丘也。"

37 光明（络穴）

【出处】《灵枢·根结》。

---

①　原文为"参日而后能外天下"，疑作者误写。

【别名】无。

【穴义】本穴为胆经络穴，络肝经，主治目痛、夜盲、目视不清等眼疾，使眼睛重见光明，故名"光明"。

【定位】外踝尖上 5 寸，腓骨前缘。

【主治】①目痛，夜盲，近视，目翳；②下肢痿痹。

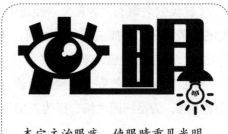

本穴主治眼疾，使眼睛重见光明。

【释义摘录】

《医经理解》："在外踝上五寸，足少阳络别走厥阴者，肝胆之脉上通于目，故谓其穴曰光明也。"

《经穴解》："光明之义，无所发明，岂阳有络以通于阴，以气相通，有光明之可见耶？"

《经穴释义汇解》："光明，即眼也。穴在足外踝上五寸，足少阳络，别走厥阴，少阳厥阴主眼。故穴主眼疾，使眼恢复光明，故以为名。"

《针灸穴名释义》："光，光照。明，明亮。光明，光亮明白与天气清净之意。穴用能使头脑清澈、目见光明也。故光明亦即指双目而言。"

《针灸穴名解》："本穴功在于目，能治目痛、夜盲，故名光明。"

38 阳辅（经穴）

【出处】《灵枢·本输》。

【别名】无。

【穴义】辅，辅骨，指腓骨。本穴位于辅骨的外侧，外为"阳"；且本穴为足少阳胆经之经穴，五行属火，火亦为阳，故名"阳辅"。

【定位】外踝尖上 4 寸，腓骨前缘。

【主治】①咽喉肿痛；②胸胁胀满，腋下肿痛，瘰疬；③下肢痿痹。

本穴位于辅骨（腓骨）的外侧。

【释义摘录】

《医经理解》："外辅骨也，穴在足外踝上四寸，辅骨前绝骨端如前三分。"

《经穴解》："曰阳辅者，乃阳极盛之称，木旺极则生火之义也。"

《经穴释义汇解》："穴为足少阳脉之经火穴，位在足外踝上四寸，因处辅骨之阳侧，故名阳辅。"

《针灸穴名释义》："阳，指小腿的外侧。辅，辅助，辅骨。言穴居小腿辅骨之前外方也。小腿骨古称辅骨，内侧称内辅，外侧称外辅。外辅骨又单指今之腓骨。穴在小腿外侧、腓骨前方，故名。（颧骨亦名辅骨，见颊车条。）"

39 悬钟（八会穴之髓会）

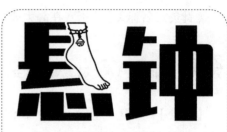

穴在外踝上三寸，当系带脚铃之处。

【**出处**】《黄帝明堂经》。

【**别名**】绝骨。

【**穴义**】本穴位于外踝上三寸，穴下至外踝形如一悬挂的钟，又当系带脚铃之处，故名"悬钟"。

【**定位**】外踝尖上 3 寸，腓骨前缘。

【**主治**】①腹满，不思饮食；②半身不遂，下肢痿痹，足胫挛痛。

【**释义摘录**】

《医经理解》："一名绝骨，在足外踝上三寸，当骨尖前动脉中，谓尖骨下外踝形如悬钟也。"

《经穴解》："穴名悬钟者，以其上悬肉开分如钟形，穴在其内，故曰悬钟。"

《古法新解会元针灸学》："足外侧短骨三寸，尖计三分，名绝骨，穴在内。外踝上三寸上廉，骨悬踵中，故又名悬钟。"

《针灸穴名释义》："悬，悬挂，悬系；又钟锤与钟架均名悬。钟是乐器，又为钟铃。穴效如悬挂之钟，又当系带脚铃之处也。"

《针灸穴名解》："本经沿人体外侧向下循行，本穴位置，未及于足，有如悬象，故名悬钟。"

40 丘墟（原穴）

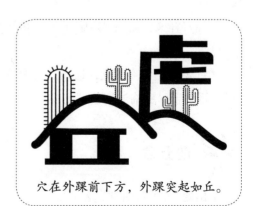

穴在外踝前下方，外踝突起如丘。

【**出处**】《灵枢·本输》。

【**别名**】蹄溪。

【**穴义**】丘墟，大土丘。本穴位于外踝前下方，外踝突起如丘，故名"丘墟"。

【**定位**】趾长伸肌腱的外侧凹陷中。

【**主治**】①胸胁痛，善太息，颈肿，腋下肿；②疟疾；③视物不清，目翳；④小腿酸痛，外踝肿痛，足下垂。

【释义摘录】

《医经理解》："丘墟，在足外踝下如前陷中，盖足部一大丘也。"

《经穴解》："穴名丘墟者，以在外踝前，外踝之骨大而圆，有丘象焉，其穴在前，有墟象焉，故曰丘墟。"

《古法新解会元针灸学》："丘墟者，踝起如丘，大经转毂而墟通之原，故名丘墟。"

《针灸穴名释义》："指穴在高大如丘外踝基底方之空软处。"

41 足临泣（输穴；八脉交会穴，通带脉）

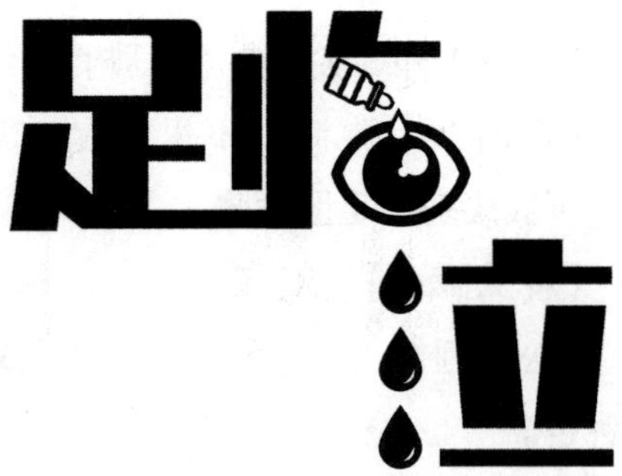

【出处】《灵枢·本输》作"临泣"，《针灸资生经》始作"足临泣"。

【别名】无。

【穴义】本穴位于足背，其气上通于目，主治目赤肿痛、目眩、目涩等目疾，目为泣之所出，与本经"头临泣"主治作用相同，故名"足临泣"。

【定位】第5趾长伸肌腱的外侧凹陷中。

【主治】①偏头痛，眩晕；②胁痛，瘰疬；③膝痛，足痛；④疟疾；⑤月经不调，乳痈。

穴临于足，其气上通于目，主目疾，目者泣之所出。

【释义摘录】

《医经理解》："在足小趾次趾本节后间筋骨缝陷中，足少阳之输，本经有二临泣，在头曰临泣，谓其穴下临于目也，在足亦曰临泣，谓其气上通于目也。"

《古法新解会元针灸学》："临泣者，临其足下而行湿液，水湿居高临下津津浸淫，故名临泣。"

《经穴释义汇解》："穴临于足，其气上通于目，主目疾，目者，泣之所出，故名足临泣。"

《针灸穴名解》："泣，通涩，即凝滞也，故名之以'泣'。以其在足，故曰'足临泣'，示别于'头临泣'也。"

42 地五会

【出处】《黄帝明堂经》。

【**别名**】无。

【**穴义**】本穴名解有二。其一，在足部，足少阳经共有五穴，而肝经之太冲穴有络横连地五会，如木之有根在地，故名"地五会"。其二，地，指地气。风寒暑湿气皆会于地，地气会于足[①]，足五趾易为地之诸气所中之处，故名"地五会"。

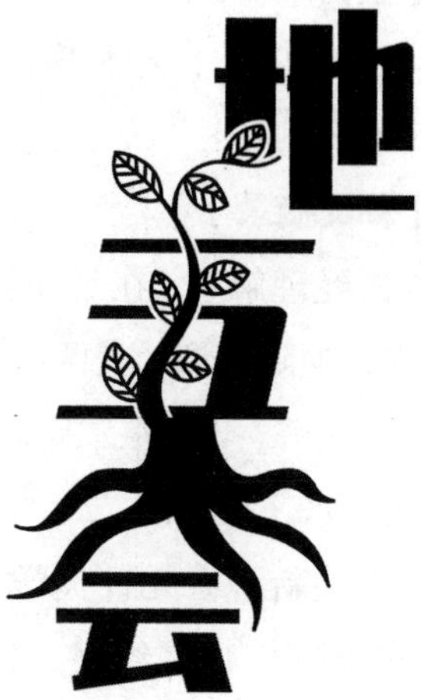

【**定位**】第4、5跖骨间，第4跖趾关节近端凹陷中。

【**主治**】①目赤肿痛；②腋下肿；③乳痈；④足背红肿。

【**释义摘录**】

《医经理解》："五脏之所会也，在足部故曰地，穴在小趾次趾本节后陷中。"

《经穴解》："少阳之穴，在足者有五穴，而肝经之太冲穴，有络横连地五会，如木之有根在地。此穴乃肝经相会之地也，故曰地五会。"

胆经在足部共有五穴，而肝经之太冲穴有络横连地五会，如木之有根在地。

《古法新解会元针灸学》："地五会者，胆属阳木，应于春之正阳，地之春阳正气起，而合五行。五脏之气，朝于原胞中，而生膏泽，故名地五会。"

《经穴释义汇解》："地指足，穴在足小趾次趾本节后间凹陷处，为五脏之气所会，故名地五会。"

《针灸穴名释义》："地，指地气，足部。五，同伍，指五趾与地面风寒暑湿相互为伍之诸气。会，聚会与会合。意为地气会于足，而五趾亦易为地之诸气所中也。"

《针灸穴名解》："凡两经相交处之穴，曰会。本穴为足少阳之气与其他五经之气会合处也。以此之一，会彼之五，足方象地，故称'地五会'。"

43 侠溪（荥穴）

【**出处**】《灵枢·本输》。

【**别名**】无。

【**穴义**】侠，通"夹"。本穴位于足小趾和次趾的夹缝中，穴处犹如狭长的溪流，故名"侠溪"。

【**定位**】第4、5趾间，趾蹼缘后方赤白肉际处。

---

① 《千金翼方》："夫风毒之气皆起于地。地之寒暑风湿皆作蒸气，足当履之，所以风毒之中人也，必先中脚。"

【主治】①热病，头痛，眩晕，颊肿；②耳聋，耳鸣，目赤肿痛；③胁痛，膝股痛，足痛；④乳痈。

【释义摘录】

《医经理解》："在足小趾次趾本节前歧骨间陷中，少阳所溜，盖两指相夹间也。"

《经穴解》："穴在二趾歧骨之间，故曰侠，所溜为荥水，故曰溪。"

《古法新解会元针灸学》："侠溪者，足小趾与次趾歧骨相夹经络，如豀水之形，流其中，故名侠溪。"

《经穴释义汇解》："因喻穴处两指（趾）相夹间如溪，故名侠溪。"

《针灸穴名解》："穴在足小趾次趾趾间夹隙中，故名'夹溪'。"

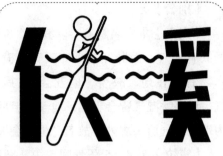

穴在足小脚趾和次趾的夹缝中，穴处犹如狭长的溪流。

44 足窍阴（井穴）

【出处】《灵枢·本输》。

【别名】无。

【穴义】足三阳经循行线路均从头至足，各井穴犹如阳终阴始，阳根于阴。根据根结理论，本穴为少阳经之井穴，根于足部窍阴，且本穴多用于治疗耳聋、耳鸣、舌强、目赤肿痛、头痛等，治症与"头窍阴"大致相同，故名"足窍阴"。

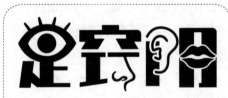

本穴主治耳聋、目赤肿痛、喉痹、头痛等疾，多关于阴脏之窍。

【定位】第4趾末节外侧，趾甲根角侧后方0.1寸。

【主治】①头痛，目赤肿痛，耳鸣，耳聋；②胸胁痛；③足痛。

【释义摘录】

《医经理解》："在小趾次趾端，少阳所出。本经有二窍阴，在首曰窍阴，以其为髓空也；在足亦曰窍阴，以其为足井也。"

《古法新解会元针灸学》："窍阴者，从阳相交于阴也，足少阳与足厥阴相交通于阴窍也，内脏肝胆相连系，外部经络相贯通，气脉表里相交，注于阴卵之关窍，故名窍阴。"

《经穴释义汇解》："足太阳膀胱经、足阳明胃经、足少阳胆经之循行线路均从头至足，各井穴所示犹如阳终阴始，阳根于阴，本穴为少阳经之井穴，根于足部窍阴，故名足窍阴。"

《针灸穴名释义》："本穴对咳逆、喉痹、舌强、口干、耳聋等病有效，与头窍阴的功用有其相近之处。《灵枢·根结》：'少阳根于窍阴，结于窗笼，窗笼者耳中也。'足之窍阴与头之窍阴，更可上下相应矣。《素问·阴阳应象大论》：'阴味出下窍。'注：'味有质，为下流便尿之窍。'对前后阴之阴窍病，当也与有作用。"

《针灸穴名解》："本穴之名'足窍阴'者，以其治症与'头窍阴'大致相同也。"

第十三章
足厥阴肝经穴

1 大敦（井穴）

【出处】《灵枢·本输》。

【别名】大训。

【穴义】敦，厚实，喻大趾趾端最敦厚，形似圆盖之敦器大而厚。本穴在足大趾趾甲根部后外侧 0.1 寸，故名"大敦"。

【定位】大趾末节外侧，距甲根角侧后方 0.1 寸。

【主治】①疝气，睾丸肿痛，前阴痛，少腹疼痛，遗尿，癃闭；②月经不调，子宫下垂；③小儿惊风，癫痫，神昏。

穴在足大趾末节外侧，相比其他四趾大趾最大最厚，形似圆盖之敦器。

【释义摘录】

《医经理解》："敦，厚也，大敦，在足大趾三毛中，谓其指端最敦厚也。"

《经穴解》："木之根在下，须土而后茂，肝之井即木之根也，而与脾土同出足大趾，有土厚而木茂之义，故曰大敦。"

《古法新解会元针灸学》："大敦者，大经气敦厚所生之根本也，足大趾内侧，去爪甲角三毛许，锐肉坚中，故名大敦。"

《经穴释义汇解》："敦，大也，厚也。穴在足大趾端，去爪甲如韭叶及三毛中，即在大趾爪甲根部外侧后二分许从毛际。因喻其趾端最敦厚，形似圆盖之敦器，故名大敦。"

《针灸穴名解》："凡阴气之萃于下者，至博至厚，博厚配地也，故名'大敦'。"

2 行间（荥穴）

【出处】《灵枢·本输》。

【别名】无。

【穴义】行，循行；间，中间。穴在第1、2脚趾间缝纹端，肝经经气自大敦穴循行于两趾之间而至本穴，故名"行间"。

【定位】第1、2趾之间，趾蹼缘的后方赤白肉际处。

穴为荥穴，荥主身热，主治肝阳上亢引起的头晕、高血压等。

【主治】①疝气，少腹疼痛，前阴痛，遗尿，癃闭；②月经不调，带下；③目赤肿痛，口干，口渴，咽喉肿痛；④胁痛，善怒，太息；⑤癫痫；⑥脚膝肿痛。

【释义摘录】

《医经理解》："在大趾歧骨间动脉陷中，言行于两趾之间也。"

《经穴解》："穴名行间者，以其穴在大趾、次趾歧骨间，为肝经初行之所，故曰行间。"

《古法新解会元针灸学》："肝气遇冲逆而发痫风，泄行间，泄肝经怒气，以定痫风，故名行间。"

《经穴释义汇解》："因喻其脉行于两指之间而入本穴，故名行间。"

《针灸穴名解》："行，足之用为行。间，俗称病愈为病间，即病得通而告愈也。犹云：气得行，而病得间也。故曰行间。"

3 太冲（输穴、原穴）

【出处】《灵枢·九针十二原》《灵枢·本输》。

【别名】无。

【穴义】太，大；冲，要冲，要道。本穴为足厥阴肝经的输穴、原穴，所注为输，喻本穴为肝经大的通道所在，也是元气所居之处，脉气盛大，故名"太冲"。

【定位】第1、2跖骨间，跖骨底结合部

穴为冲脉与肝经交会之处，肝主藏血，冲为血海，两者合而盛大。

前方凹陷中，或触及动脉搏动。

【主治】①疝气，前阴痛、少腹肿，癃闭，遗尿；②月经不调，难产；③黄疸，胁痛，腹胀，呕逆；④小儿惊风；⑤目赤肿痛，咽干，咽痛；⑥下肢痿痹，足跗肿痛。

【释义摘录】

《医经理解》："在足大趾本节后二寸陷中动脉，足厥阴所注为输，盖本经之一大冲也。"

《经穴解》："三阴之所交结于脚也，踝上各一行者，此肾脉之下行也，名曰太冲。"

《古法新解会元针灸学》："太冲者，大动脉通胞中冲任，托卫气行经脉，而通营卫，由肾脉、阳明脉、太阴转下冲阳脉、太溪脉，而化太冲脉，三阴直冲而上，故名太冲。"

《经穴释义汇解》："太，大也；冲，通道也。喻本穴为肝经大的通道所在，亦即元气所居之处，故以为名。"

《针灸穴名解》："进步抬足首当其冲，故名之以冲。穴在跗上足大趾次趾歧骨间，以其近于大趾，故名太冲。太，大也。"

4 中封（经穴）

【出处】《灵枢·本输》。

【别名】悬泉。

【穴义】中，中间；封，土堆。本穴位于商丘和丘墟之间，两穴都有土堆之意，本穴犹如立于两封之间。封，亦可理解为封闭。本穴位于内踝前方，胫骨前肌腱内侧凹陷中，穴位犹如被大筋所封闭。故名"中封"。

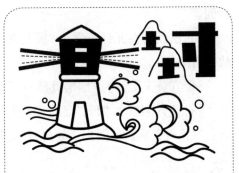

穴在足背胫骨前肌腱与跗长伸肌腱之间凹陷中，穴位犹如被两条大筋所封闭。

【定位】内踝前，胫骨前肌肌腱的内侧缘凹陷中。于商丘与解溪中间处取穴。

【主治】疝气引腰痛、少腹痛，遗精，小便不利。

【释义摘录】

《医经理解》："中封，在足内踝前一寸筋裹宛宛中。盖腕中筋肉封聚处也。"

《经穴释义汇解》："穴在足内踝前一寸，取穴时仰足见凹陷，伸足显筋间，穴为腕中筋肉封聚之处，故名中封。"

《针灸穴名释义》："中，指精神，参中渚条。封，指藏聚，参神封条。意其为精神之藏聚，与情志活动有关。《灵枢·本神》：'随神往来谓之魂。'是神魂即精神情志也。

肝藏魂，故中封者乃肝经之气所聚之处，神与魂之封地也。"

《针灸穴名解》："聚土成凸为封，又土在沟上曰封。《灵枢·经筋》云'厥阴之筋，结于内踝之前'，即商丘、丘墟二凸之间，故名'中封'。犹云中立于两封之间也。"

5 蠡沟（络穴）

【出处】《灵枢·经脉》。

【别名】交仪。

【穴义】本穴名解有二。其一，蠡，啮木之小虫也，毫针尖如蚊虫之喙，穴在胫骨上，用毫针针刺，似虫啮木。其二，蠡亦可理解为"瓢"，一种舀水工具，本穴在内踝上5寸，靠近穴位的腓肠肌形如瓜瓢，胫骨内侧缘形如沟渠，故名"蠡沟"。

【定位】内踝尖上5寸，胫骨内侧面的中央。

【主治】①疝气，睾丸肿痛，小便不利，遗尿；②月经不调，赤白带下，阴痒。

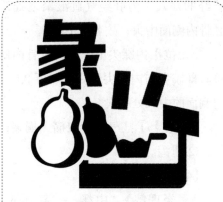

腓肠肌肌肉丰满，形如瓜瓢（蠡），穴在腓肠肌外侧凹陷中。

【释义摘录】

《医经理解》："在足内踝上五寸，足厥阴络别走少阳者。蠡，虫啮木中也，横行直透，惟其所往，其络透于光明之穴，故以蠡象，上行于胻骨之间，故以沟名也。"

《经穴解》："此乃肝经之络，而通胆经者，此经与彼经通，必有窍焉以通之，故曰沟。蠡者，虫也，所以蛀木者，故曰蠡沟。"

《经穴释义汇解》："虫啮木中曰蠡；纵横相交成沟……用毫针针刺，似虫啮木，穴别走少阳，如一分支相交，故曰蠡沟。"

《针灸穴名解》："蠡，水族之阴类也。沟，凹渠之阴象也。喻光明犹明珠，腓肠肌俯覆如蠡（蚌壳），故名为蠡沟。"

《针灸穴名释义》："《广雅·释草》：'匏，瓠也。'《说文》：'匏，瓠也。'段注：'匏，判之曰蠡，曰瓢，曰㪺。'即合之为匏；分之为瓢，为蠡，为㪺（读 jǐn，瓠分为二谓之㪺，即瓢）。《汉书·东方朔传》：'以蠡测海。'杨上善曰：'蠡，瓢勺也。胻骨之内，上下虚处，有似瓢勺渠沟，此因名曰蠡沟。'小腿后方肌肉丰满，其形如瓢，穴在其下际沟中，固形似而得名。又贝壳亦名蠡，形义亦通。"

6 中都（郄穴）

【出处】《黄帝明堂经》。

【别名】中郄。

【穴义】都，有汇聚之意。本穴是足厥阴肝经的郄穴，为肝经气血汇聚之处，且位于胫骨内侧面中央，故名"中都"。

【定位】内踝尖上7寸，胫骨内侧面的中央。即髌尖与内踝尖连线中点下0.5寸、胫骨内侧面的中央处取穴。

【主治】①疝气，少腹痛，崩漏，恶露不尽；②泄泻。

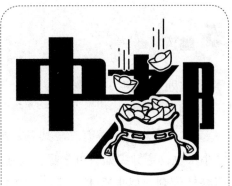

穴为郄穴，是肝经气血汇聚之处，故名"都"。

【释义摘录】

《医经理解》："中都，一名中郄。在足内踝上七寸，当骱骨中，盖足腹间之一都会也。"

《古法新解会元针灸学》："中都者，膝骱骨与髁骨中间，阴阳相聚，故名中都。又名中郄者，阴之支从蠡沟而走阳，从中都而回阴之经中。"

《经穴释义汇解》："都，流水所聚之处。穴在内踝上七寸骱中，为足厥阴郄，因喻肝之气血似水之流聚，穴当胫骨之中部，故名中都。"

《针灸穴名释义》："中，参中封条，又指中间。都，参大都条，又为统帅之意。中都，古官府名，地名。意为穴当小腿之中，为肝经脉气之都会与统帅肝经脉气之郄穴。《后汉·樊准传》：'中都官吏，在京师之官吏也。'多处古地名均有中都之称。以穴位之所在与经气之所聚而比譬命名。"

7 膝关

【出处】《黄帝明堂经》。

【别名】无。

【穴义】关，关节。本穴位于膝关节内侧，主治膝髌肿痛等膝关节诸症，故名"膝关"。

【定位】胫骨内侧髁的下方，阴陵泉后1寸。

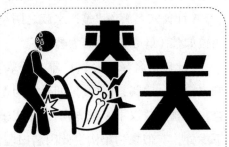

本穴位于膝关节内侧，主治膝髌肿痛等膝关节诸症。

【主治】疝气，少腹痛，膝股痛，下肢痿痹。

【释义摘录】

《医经理解》："膝关，膝之关，在膝盖骨下内侧陷中。"

《经穴解》："穴名膝关者，肝经至此，上行将过膝而入股，上下骨节交折之所，有关之象焉，故曰膝关。"

《古法新解会元针灸学》："膝关者，两腿骨相交之关节也。犊鼻内侧下二寸，是通膝生膏泽之阴关也，故名膝关。"

《针灸穴名解》："穴在膝关节处也。治膝关节病，调其屈伸。后汉刘熙《释名》云：'膝，伸也。可屈伸也。'膝为人身关节之最大者。故名'膝关'。屈膝取之。治膑膝引痛、湿寒历节、咽痛、风痹等症。"

8 曲泉（合穴）

【出处】《灵枢·本输》。

【别名】无。

【穴义】曲，屈曲；泉，泉水。穴在膝盖内侧横纹头上方凹陷中，取穴时需弯曲膝盖，且穴为足厥阴肝经的合穴，五行属水，故名"曲泉"。

【定位】屈膝，当膝关节内侧面横纹内侧端，股骨内侧髁的后缘，半腱肌、半膜肌止端的前方凹陷处。

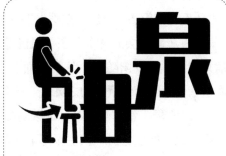

穴在膝盖内侧横纹头上方凹陷中，取穴时需弯曲膝盖。

【主治】①疝气，前阴痛，少腹痛，小便不利；②遗精，阳痿；③妇人腹中包块，月经不调，带下，子宫脱垂，阴痒；④惊狂；⑤膝肿痛，下肢痿痹。

【释义摘录】

《医经理解》："在膝内辅骨下，大筋上，小筋下陷中，屈膝横纹头取之。故谓是屈折间之泉穴也。"

《经穴解》："穴名泉者，以肝经之合穴为水，故有泉之名。曲者，乃以肝经初离膝而上股，正在曲折之地，故曰曲。"

《古法新解会元针灸学》："有泉清自然之升发力，养气含其中，故名曲泉。"

《经穴释义汇解》："穴合水，喻水之高而有来源者为泉，故名曲泉。"

《针灸穴名解》："穴在阴谷穴之前，曲膝横纹内侧端凹处，故名曲泉。"

9 阴包

【出处】《黄帝明堂经》。

【别名】阴胞。

【穴义】包，通"胞"，指子宫、精室等生殖器。本穴位于大腿内侧，内为阴，主治月经不调、腰骶痛引小腹等子宫精室相关疾病，故名"阴包"。

【定位】髌底上4寸，股内侧肌与缝匠肌之间。

【主治】①月经不调，遗尿，小便不利；②腰骶痛引小腹。

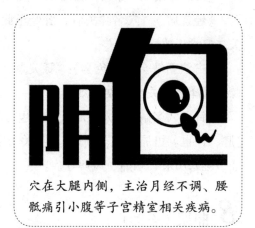

穴在大腿内侧，主治月经不调、腰骶痛引小腹等子宫精室相关疾病。

【释义摘录】

《医经理解》："阴包，在膝上四寸股内廉两筋间虚陷中。盖阴部之虚大有容处也。"

《古法新解会元针灸学》："阴包者，膝股内阴与肉包裹筋槽，中藏阴阳精气，一旦欲火炽动，则少阳随动，从阳络而交于阴，至阴内而阴蕴之气贯睾丸，女子即子宫中，而造精。股阴槽包藏造物之灵气，故名阴包。"

《经穴释义汇解》："穴为足厥阴脉之腧穴，位在膝上四寸，股内廉两筋间。股内廉属阴；包，妊也，引申穴主腹部诸疾及胞宫病，故名阴包或阴胞。"

《针灸穴名释义》："阴，指足三阴经及下腹部。包，包罗，联系，又通胞。与足三阴经及下腹诸部俱有包罗联系之意。足厥阴经由膝关节上行入股内侧，太阴居其前，少阴行其后，故对前阴、下腹以及妇女胞宫诸病，均有包罗在内的治疗作用。"

《针灸穴名解》："包，与胞、脬俱通。本穴在膝上阴侧。治腰尻引小腹痛、遗尿、失精、小便难，诸病之涉及脬者，在女子则有关月经不调、子宫精室者。本穴以功能而得名也。故名阴包。"

10 足五里

【出处】《黄帝明堂经》作"五里"，《针灸资生经》始作"足五里"。

【别名】五里。

【穴义】足，指下肢。里，通理。本穴位于下肢，多用于治理五脏在里诸病，与手五里及手足三里互相应对，故名"足五里"。

【**定位**】气冲直下 3 寸，动脉搏动处。

【**主治**】小腹痛，小便不利，阴挺，睾丸肿痛。

【**释义摘录**】

《医经理解》："五里，在气冲下三寸，阴廉下一寸，阴股中动脉应手。盖五脏之里道也。"

穴在下肢，多用于治理五脏在里诸病。

《古法新解会元针灸学》："五里者，五气之所逾为邻里也。天之轨为十，天之合其运为五，化为天之五气：风、热、湿、燥、寒。地之三百六十为里，化为五行气：木、火、土、金、水；而成五志，为人之五气：怒、喜、思、忧、恐；配于五脏，发于五音，生于五色，食于五谷，识于五味，饲于五畜，乐于五声，常于五动，开于五窍。先天精气之所过，交于内脏，故名五里。"

《经穴释义汇解》："穴在阴廉下，去气冲三寸。里，可作居解。穴正居足厥阴肝经尽处前数第五个穴位；也称五脏之里道，故名足五里。"

《针灸穴名释义》："足，指下肢。五里，指五脏之里。意为此乃下肢与五脏在里诸病有关的孔穴。与手五里及手足三里互相应对。"

《针灸穴名解》："五者数之中，里与理通。即理其中以应于外也。凡肢体病之关于内脏者，本穴可以理之。外因症，多不取此。"

11 阴廉

【**出处**】《黄帝明堂经》。

【**别名**】无。

【**穴义**】阴，外阴；廉，侧边，此处指腹股沟。本穴位于大腿内侧，外阴旁腹股沟中，故名"阴廉"。

【**定位**】气冲直下 2 寸。取穴时，令患者稍屈髋，屈膝，外展，大腿抗阻力内收时显露出长收肌，在其外缘取穴。

【**主治**】月经不调，不孕，少腹痛。

【**释义摘录**】

《经穴解》："肝经将入腹矣，廉者，言其

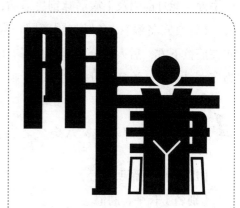

廉，侧边，此处指腹股沟。穴在外阴旁腹股沟中，故名。

隅也，锐也，离股而入腹，有廉之象焉，肝经为阴，故曰阴廉。"

《经穴释义汇解》："穴在羊矢下，去气冲二寸动脉中。羊矢者，在阴旁股内约文（纹）缝中，皮肉间有核如羊矢。侧边曰廉，因穴在阴旁股内侧纹缝中，故名阴廉。"

《针灸穴名释义》："阴，指前阴部。廉，见上、下廉条。穴当前阴部耻骨下方的边缘有棱处，故名。"

《针灸穴名解》："廉，侧也，隅也，又边际也。其处有筋核如羊矢，穴在筋核下方。妇人求子可灸之。月经不调、腿股痛，可以取此。"

12 急脉

【出处】《素问·气府论》。

【别名】羊矢。

【穴义】本穴位于腹股沟股动脉搏动处，犹如湍急的水流，故名"急脉"。

【定位】横平耻骨联合上缘，前正中线旁开 2.5 寸。

【主治】疝气，前阴痛，少腹痛。

穴在腹股沟股动脉搏动处，犹如湍急的水流。

《医经理解》："《气府论》曰：'厥阴毛中急脉各一，盖此穴也。'"

《经穴释义汇解》："穴在阴毛中，阴上两旁相去同身寸之二寸半，行小腹下，引阴丸，寒则为痛，其脉甚急，穴当其处，故名急脉。"

《针灸穴名释义》："急，指拘急，急促。脉，指筋脉，动脉。穴在腹股沟动脉搏动应手处，能舒前阴及下腹筋脉拘急诸病，故名。"

《针灸穴名解》："急脉与阴廉同一穴底，其实则一穴也。急脉穴在筋核上方，阴廉穴在筋核下方，后人强分之耳。核下有脉，其动滑促，因名'急脉'。此乃厥阴之大络，为睾丸之系带，治癫疝可灸之，不可刺，治阴挺、少腹痛。"

13 章门 (脾募穴，八会穴之脏会，足厥阴经、足少阳经交会穴)

【出处】《黄帝明堂经》。

【别名】长平，胁髎。

【穴义】本穴名解有二。其一，章，章服，古称礼服为章服。本穴位于腋中线，第 11 肋游离端，正当古代章服启闭之处，故名。其二，章，通"彰"，显著，引申为气血旺盛；门，指出入要地。本穴为脾之募穴，是脾脏之气血输注于腹部之处；又是八会穴之脏会，是脏气出入之门户，故名"章门"。

【定位】在第 11 肋游离端的下际。

【主治】①疝气，前阴痛，少腹痛，呕吐；②胁痛，痞块，黄疸。

【释义摘录】

《医经理解》："在大横外直季胁端，足少阳厥阴之会，经曰'脏会章门'，盖脏气之会而为章也。"

《经穴解》："草曰本，木曰章，肝阴木，胆阳木也，胁肋正肝胆所治之部分，故曰章门。肝经在腹，只有二穴，皆以门称。以木性曲直，而有启闭之义，故曰门。"

《古法新解会元针灸学》："是五脏之气出入交经之门也，故曰章门。"

《经穴释义汇解》："因穴为脏会，以喻脏气之会而为章，穴主脏病之门户，故名章门。"

《针灸穴名释义》："章，文采貌；山丘上平者亦曰章；又是障的意思。门，为守护与禁要之处。指季胁形如平顶之丘，穴在其下方，为章身之衣与屏障内脏的门户。"

《针灸穴名解》："取之，犹开四障之门，以通痞塞之郁气也，故名章门。"

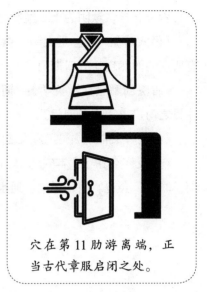

穴在第 11 肋游离端，正当古代章服启闭之处。

14 期门（肝募穴，足厥阴经、足太阴经、阴维脉交会穴）

【出处】《黄帝明堂经》。

【别名】无。

【穴义】期，周期；门，指出入要地。十二经气血的运行，始出手太阴肺经云门穴，终入足厥阴肝经期门穴，如此周而复始。本穴为经气周期运行归入之门户，故名"期门"。

【定位】第 6 肋间隙，前正中线旁开 4 寸。

【主治】①胁下积聚、气喘，呃逆，胸胁胀痛；②呕吐，腹胀，泄泻；③乳痈。

【释义摘录】

《医经理解》："期，周一岁也，岁有十二月，

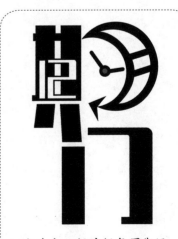

穴为十二经脉经气周期运行归入之门户。

三百六十五日，厥阴为十二经脉之终，期门为三百六十五穴之终，故以期名也。"

《经穴解》："既会足太阴、厥阴、少阴、阳明于府舍，而又会太阴、厥阴于此，若有所期约而然也，故曰期门。"

《古法新解会元针灸学》："期门者，气血出入之终始，贯膈交阳明，出太阴，阴精注目之门户也，故名期门。"

《经穴释义汇解》："穴为人之气血归入之门户，故曰期门。"

《针灸穴名解》："本穴为治血症之要穴，血症以月经为最，月信有期，故名期门。期，时也，会也。门，开也，通也。"

第十四章

督脉穴

1 长强（督脉络穴，督脉、足少阳经、足少阴经交会穴）

【出处】《灵枢·经脉》。

【别名】阴郄，橛骨，穷骨，龟尾，尾翠骨，尾闾骨。

【穴义】人体脊柱从头到尾端，长而强大，且督脉为诸阳之长，阳气最为强盛，本穴位居督脉之首，故名"长强"。

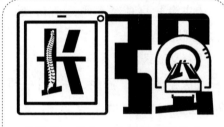

脊柱长而强大，穴在脊柱尾骨端。

【定位】尾骨端与肛门连线的中点处。

【主治】①泄泻，便秘，便血，痔疾，脱肛；②癫狂，小儿惊风；③腰痛，尾骶骨痛。

【释义摘录】

《医经理解》："长强，《灵枢》谓之穷骨，在脊骶骨端，其骨形长而强也。"

《经穴解》："身长之骨，莫长于脊骨，故曰长，而此穴正当其下之最锐处，故曰强。又为足少阴肾、足少阳胆会督脉之处，生痔之根，在于此穴。"

《古法新解会元针灸学》："长强者，长于阳而强于阴，其督脉与任脉之长共九尺。由会阴入胞中四寸而分任督，其生气通于天而化督脉，其质造形而通于地以化任脉。督脉为督催诸阳之经络而长于阳。长强为纯阳初始，使脏中生春阳正气，舒缓各部气器宫，故名长强。"

《针灸穴名释义》："长，长大，旺盛。强，强壮，充实。喻经气与脊柱为人身强大的梁柱与肾气强健的象征。督脉自下而上，强劲端长，为全身之所寄托。杨上善曰：'督脉诸阳脉长，其气强盛，穴居其处，故曰长强也。'如长而不强，则困顿难支，长而过强，则脊强反折，据此以推，则二者皆可取用矣。肾为作强之官，肾强则阳势壮。长强之名，也可与其能治遗精早泄及阳痿等证有关。"

2 腰俞

【出处】《素问·缪刺论》。

【别名】髓空，背解，腰户，腰柱。

【穴义】俞，通"输"，输送。督脉由长强上行越过尾骨至本穴（骶管裂孔处），经气由内输送至外而行于腰背正中，且本穴主治腰部诸疾，凡腰脊强痛、转运不利者均可取之，故名"腰俞"。

【定位】正对骶管裂孔，后正中线上。

【主治】①月经不调；②痔疾；③腰背痛，下肢痿痹。

穴在骶管裂孔，督脉经气由内输送至外而行于腰背正中。

【释义摘录】

《医经理解》："腰俞，在二十一椎节下间宛宛中，一名腰户，一名髓空。盖腰之输气处也。"

《经穴解》："二十一椎之下，椎尽矣。背解者，脊之上通于背者至此而尽，故曰背解。脑为髓海，而脊通之，至此而下输，故曰髓孔。此椎下接于横骨，犹柱之立于壁也，故曰腰柱。风寒湿由此穴而入，遂成腰痛之症，故曰腰户。而图以腰俞名之，尽概上四之名义，故曰至要之穴也。"

《古法新解会元针灸学》："腰俞者，其肾小如赤豆，其腰大如拳，其肾化之精气输入腰，腰之带附脊两旁，络于尾脊，腰肾之精气所过之腧穴，故名腰俞。"

《针灸穴名释义》："腰俞，腰，指腰部，又同要。穴居腰部冲要之地，为腰部经气注输之处也。"

《针灸穴名解》："'俞'为'腧'之简，'腧'为'输'之化。输者，通达传送也。《素问·骨空论》谓：'督脉起于少腹以下骨中央。'本穴乃其外线循行之初步。由长强穴上行，过尾闾，透出荐骨之下，其处为全腰之俞。试将腰部扭转，本穴如户下枢轴。（腰背督脉诸穴，皆具枢动能力。本穴居下，代表全部。）以功能论，本穴能疏解腰部郁滞之气，故名'腰俞'。"

3 腰阳关

【出处】《素问·气府论》王冰注作"阳关",《针灸学简编》始作"腰阳关"。

【别名】背阳关,阳关。

【穴义】关元为腹部元阴元阳相交之处,腰阳关相当于关元穴在背部的投影,背为阳,且督脉为阳脉之海,故名"腰阳关",是治疗腰骶诸疾之要穴。古代中原通往西域有南北两个门户,南边的称之为阳关,"劝君更进一

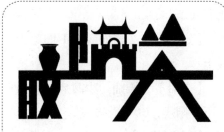

"劝君更进一杯酒,西出阳关无故人"之阳关,与"关元"之阴关相对。

杯酒,西出阳关无故人"中"阳关"指的就是这里;北边的称之为阴关,后更名为玉门关。两道关隘,一南一北,遥相呼应,成为扼守河西走廊的咽喉要道。在人体,任脉的"关元穴"和督脉的"腰阳关"分别对应于阴关和阳关,均为元阴、元阳相交之处,成为人体两相呼应的重要"关隘"。元阴、元阳也叫"真阴""真阳",是人体内最重要的阴阳二气,寄藏于肾。

【定位】第4腰椎棘突下凹陷中,后正中线上。

【主治】①月经不调,遗精,阳痿;②腰骶痛。

【释义摘录】

《医经理解》:"阳关,在十六椎节下间。背为阳,盖阳之关要处也。人身有二阳关:足阳关,少阳之关也;背阳关,太阳之关也。"

《经穴解》:"阳关者,督经之阳气,自腰俞而上行者,已六椎而至此穴,有关之象焉,故曰阳关。"

《古法新解会元针灸学》:"阳关者,阳者气也,关为机关。大肠属气,其输在十六椎两旁,关乎阳气,下通经络,上通命门,相火禀金化气而生三焦,夹脊双关而上,通背化气,助力之用于外,关乎全身之阳强壮力之出入,故名阳关。"

《针灸穴名释义》:"腰,见腰俞条。阳,指下焦之阳气。关。机关,关藏。穴当腰部之要冲,为下焦关藏元气之窟宅与腰部运动之机关。"

4 命门

【出处】《黄帝明堂经》。

【别名】属累。

【穴义】本穴位于两肾之间，为元气之根，生命之本，是关乎生命之重要门户，故名"命门"，是强身健体、治疗虚损性疾病的常用要穴。

【定位】第2腰椎棘突下凹陷中，后正中线上。

【主治】①腰痛，少腹痛，脊强；②赤白带下，阳痿；③下肢痿痹。

【释义摘录】

《医经理解》："命门，在十四椎节下间，当两肾中间，为精道所出，是生之门、死之门也。命门一名属累，言人未有不为此累者也。"

《经穴解》："此穴与脐对，正在内两肾之中间，而足太阳两肾俞穴之内，乃人至命之地，故曰命门。"

《古法新解会元针灸学》："命门者，生命所系初生之门也……男子丹田属精气之海，两肾之间属命门；女子丹田为命门，两肾之间为精血之海，是一而二，二而一，皆主要之部位，皆可曰命门。"

《针灸穴名释义》："命，指生命，重要之意。门，见云门条。指其为生气出入通达与维系生命之处。"

元气之根，关乎生命的重要门户。

5 悬枢

【出处】《黄帝明堂经》。

【别名】无。

【穴义】悬，悬空；枢，指门上的转轴，此处指代腰椎。人仰卧时，腰脊处约有数寸悬空。本穴位于悬空处之上端，且为腰椎转动之处，故名"悬枢"。

【定位】第1腰椎棘突下凹陷中，后正中线上。

【主治】①腹痛，泄泻；②腰脊痛。

【释义摘录】

《医经理解》："悬枢，在十三椎节下间，盖中悬之枢要也。"

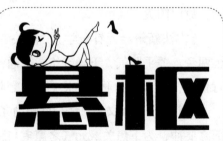

仰卧时本穴位于腰脊悬空处，且为腰椎转动之处。

《经穴解》："枢者，所以司开合之轴也。脊中司俯仰屈伸，亦犹门之阃，在于枢也，此穴在脊中之下，有枢之象焉。曰悬者，以其横悬为俯仰之枢，而非若门之枢，立而司开合者也。"

《古法新解会元针灸学》："悬枢者，悬系枢纽之机关，三焦发源之根基也。"

《针灸释义汇解》："悬，系也，物之有所系属者称悬，这里比喻本穴系属督脉枢要之处，故名悬枢。"

《针灸穴名解》："悬，为托空不着之处；枢，为致动之机。本穴治腰脊强直不得屈伸之症，故名之以枢。"

6 脊中

【出处】《黄帝明堂经》。

【别名】神宗，脊俞。

【穴义】十一椎为脊柱二十一椎[①]全数之折中，本穴在第十一椎之下，临近脊柱正中，故名"脊中"。

【定位】第 11 胸椎棘突下凹陷中，后正中线上。

【主治】①泄泻，黄疸；②癫痫；③腰背痛。

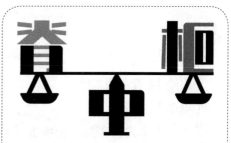

十一椎为脊柱二十一椎全数之折中。脊中穴在第十一椎之下，中枢穴在第十一椎之上。

【释义摘录】

《医经理解》："脊中，在十一椎节下间，背凡二十一节，而此为之中也。"

《经穴解》："脊共二十一椎，上十椎，下十椎，此穴在十一椎之下，区处其中，故为脊中。"

《古法新解会元针灸学》："脊中者，背脊椎，除尾骶骨与葫芦骨外，共计二十一节，其穴居十一椎下，脊之正中，故名脊中。"

7 中枢

【出处】《素问·气府论》王冰注。

【别名】无。

---

①　古人称脊柱为二十一椎，即 12 节胸椎、5 节腰椎、4 节骶椎。

【穴义】枢，指门上的转轴，此处指代脊柱骨。十一椎为脊柱二十一椎全数之折中。本穴在第十一椎之上，临近脊柱正中，故名"中枢"，与"脊中"穴义略同。

【定位】第10胸椎棘突下凹陷中，后正中线上。

【主治】腰背痛。

【释义摘录】

《经穴释义汇解》："枢，中也。凡脊柱有二十一椎，穴在第十椎节与第十一椎节之中间，位临脊柱之中，为督脉之中枢，故以为名。"

《针灸穴名释义》："指穴当脊柱中部枢要之处。"

《针灸穴名解》："本穴在第十一椎之上，亦属脊骨中部枢要处。古书多不记载，后人增之。与脊中、悬枢名义略同，功用亦同。其或取脊中穴之'中'字及悬枢穴之'枢'字，而名之为'中枢'也。"

8 筋缩

【出处】《黄帝明堂经》。

【别名】缩筋。

【穴义】本穴位于第9胸椎下，与足太阳膀胱经肝俞穴齐平，肝主筋，肝病则肌肉挛缩，发生瘛疭、脊强等抽搐筋挛之症，本穴均能治之，故名"筋缩"。

【定位】第9胸椎棘突下凹陷中，后正中线上。

【主治】①小儿惊风，抽搐，癫狂痫，目上视；②脊强。

穴与肝俞相平，肝主筋，可治疗抽搐筋挛之症。

【释义摘录】

《医经理解》："筋缩，在九椎节下间，是背筋伸缩处也。"

《经穴解》："人之俯仰，在乎脊筋之伸缩，伸而不缩，则脊强矣，缩而不伸，则伛偻矣，此穴正在脊中之上，当脊筋伸缩之际，故曰筋缩。"

《古法新解会元针灸学》："筋缩者，因肝俞在九椎下两旁，肝主筋，其短筋总系于腰脊，联筋络肝，故名筋缩。"

《针灸穴名解》："本穴旁平肝俞穴。肝主筋，诸风掉眩皆属于肝。本穴治瘛疭、脊强、天吊，诸般抽搐筋挛之症，因名'筋缩'。又以本穴正当背部大方肌之下角，逐渐狭缩之下，亦'筋缩'命名之一义也。凡治筋缩之症，可以取此。"

9 至阳

【出处】《黄帝明堂经》。

【别名】无。

【穴义】本穴位于第 7 胸椎下，与足太阳膀胱经膈俞穴齐平。人身以背为阳，横膈以下为阳中之阴，横膈以上为阳中之阳。督脉之气上行至此，则由阳中之阴达于阳中之阳，故名"至阳"。

【定位】第 7 胸椎棘突下凹陷中，后正中线上。

【主治】①黄疸；②身重；③腰背痛。

【释义摘录】

《医经理解》："至阳，在七椎节下间。背为阳，三分之而七椎以上为阳中之至阳也。"

《经穴解》："此穴之旁，为足太阳之膈俞穴，膈之上乃纯气之府，血为阴，气为阳，故曰至阳。言督经自下而上行者，至此则入于阳分也。"

《经穴释义汇解》："穴在第七椎节下间。背为阳，心为阳中之阳，穴近心处，故名至阳。"

《针灸穴名解》："至者，达也。又极也，如四时节令，'夏至'为夏之至极；'冬至'为冬之至极。人身以背为阳，而横膈以下为阳中之阴，横膈以上为阳中之阳。阳中之阳，即阳之至极也，故名'至阳'。又可意为督脉之气上行至此，乃由阳中之阴，达于阳中之阳，即背部阴阳交关处也。"

督脉之气上行至此，由阳中之阴达于阳中之阳。

10 灵台

【出处】《素问·气府论》王冰注。

【别名】无。

【穴义】灵台，古代天文台，天子祭祀、朝聘诸侯之所。本穴在第 6 胸椎之下，内应心，心为君主之官，故名"灵台"。

【定位】第 6 胸椎棘突下凹陷中，后正中

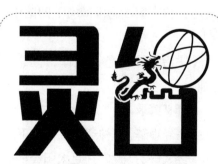

古代天文台，天子祭祀、朝聘诸侯之所。本穴内应心，心为君主之官。

线上。

【**主治**】①咳嗽，气喘；②脊痛，颈项强痛。

【**释义摘录**】

《医经理解》："灵台，在六椎节下间，神道在五椎节下间，心之位，故有神灵之称也。"

《经穴解》："心为人身至灵之官在上，穴在其下，有台之象，状脊之内载其心之象也。"

《古法新解会元针灸学》："灵台者，心灵之台也。上有心俞，下有膈俞，中有黄脂膏垒如台，其两旁为督俞之所系，阳气通其中，心灵居上，故名灵台。"

《经穴释义汇解》："灵台者，心也。穴在第六椎节下间，内应心，喻穴为心灵至尊之处，故名灵台。"

《针灸穴名解》："古代国君有灵台之设，为君主宣德布政之地。即中医学说，心为君主之官，神明出焉。本穴内应神志。《庄子·庚桑楚》注文：'灵台者，心也。'余意凡属有关神志之病，可以取此，俾以加强感通之力，而启性灵之能，故喻本穴为'灵台'。"

11 神道

【**出处**】《黄帝明堂经》。

【**别名**】无。

【**穴义**】本穴在第5胸椎下间，与足太阳膀胱经之心俞穴齐平，内应心。心藏神，穴为心气之通道，主治心脏和神志诸疾，如心痛、惊悸、失眠、健忘等，故名"神道"。

【**定位**】第5胸椎棘突下凹陷中，后正中线上。

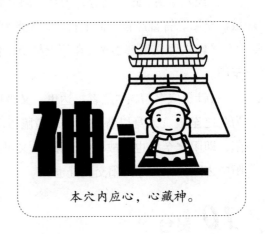

本穴内应心，心藏神。

【**主治**】①悲愁，惊悸，健忘；②寒热，头痛，疟疾；③小儿惊风；④脊痛，脊强。

【**释义摘录**】

《医经理解》："神道在五椎节下间，心之位，故有神灵之称也。"

《经穴解》："此穴在足太阳经两心俞之中，正在心之后，心为主宰之官，神明出焉，故曰神道。"

《古法新解会元针灸学》："神道者，心藏神，心俞在五椎两旁，其统系于脊，心神仗督阳之气，所行之道，故名神道。"

《经穴释义汇解》："穴在第五椎节下间，应心。心藏神，穴主神，为心气之通道，主心疾，故名神道。"

12 身柱

【出处】《黄帝明堂经》。

【别名】无。

【穴义】柱，指承重的柱子。本穴在第3胸椎下，两肩胛的中央，因比喻穴处犹如肩胛荷重的撑柱，故名"身柱"。

【定位】第3胸椎棘突下凹陷中，后正中线上。

【主治】①咳嗽，气喘；②身热，癫狂，惊风，瘛疭；③腰背痛。

穴在两肩胛的中央，比喻穴处犹如肩胛荷重的撑柱。

【释义摘录】

《医经理解》："身柱，言骨柱于上，横接两膊，为一身之柱干也。"

《经穴解》："人之肩所以能负重者，以有身柱也，脊骨为人一身之柱，而此穴近上，犹其用力负重之所，故曰身柱。"

《古法新解会元针灸学》："身柱者，为身之柱骨也。人背脊在第三椎下两旁是肺俞，关系全身之气脉，前对两乳间膻中，宗气之所出，其肺系于第三椎节，其脊髓通下，直上贯于脑。肺气关乎一身之脉，通脑是为主要之台柱，语云'立柱顶千斤'。世俗以千斤骨倒，不出一年即亡。因此为负身之立柱，故名身柱。"

《针灸穴名释义》："身，指全身。柱，梁柱。穴处为全身支柱之意。穴位上接颠顶，下通背腰，平齐两肩，居冲要之地，而又梁柱之用也。"

13 陶道（督脉、足太阳经交会穴）

【出处】《黄帝明堂经》。

【别名】无。

【穴义】陶，指烧制陶瓷的窑洞；道，通道。胸廓中空，有陶之象，此穴在胸廓最高

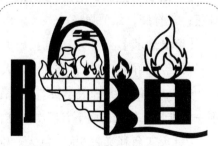

本穴驱散阳热，犹如陶窑火气所出之通道。

处，且主治骨蒸潮热、恶寒发热，驱散阳热，犹如陶窑火气所出之通道，故名"陶道"。

【定位】第1胸椎棘突下凹陷中，后正中线上。

【主治】①寒热，疟疾，骨蒸；②脊强。

【释义摘录】

《医经理解》："陶道，在一椎节下间，陶烧瓦灶也，通窍于上，背凡二十一椎，此为火气所通之道也。"

《经穴解》："陶者，窑也，中虚而能容物之象也。胸与腹在下与前而中虚，此穴在其上之最高处，有陶之象焉，故曰陶道。"

《古法新解会元针灸学》："陶道者，其椎骨较下，而高起如陶丘，导精陶陶然而过其中，合于三焦，上七椎为上焦，下七椎为下焦，中七椎合于中焦。分而为三才，合而为阴阳之天道。（语云）天道阴阳合一，地道相济，人道精神一统全躯，其乐也荣荣，陶陶而过陶丘之下，故名陶道。"

《经穴释义汇解》："丘形上有两丘相重累曰陶，穴在大椎节下间，第二椎节上间。大椎、二椎似两丘相重累，为督脉之气通行之道，故名陶道。"

《针灸穴名释义》："陶，陶丘，陶然；道，道路。指椎体依次高起状如陶丘，且有舒畅情志的陶然之用。"

14 大椎 （督脉、手足三阳经交会穴）

【出处】《黄帝明堂经》。

【别名】百劳。

【穴义】第七颈椎棘突为颈背部最突出的棘突，本穴在此椎骨之下，故因名"大椎"。

【定位】第7颈椎棘突下凹陷中，后正中线上。

【主治】①热病，疟疾，寒热；②咳嗽，气喘，骨蒸；③脊痛，颈项强痛。

【释义摘录】

《医经理解》："大椎，椎骨之最大者也。"

《古法新解会元针灸学》："大椎者，为项后平肩第一大椎骨，从大椎而下，以次类推，故名大椎。"

《针灸穴名释义》："大，巨大。椎，脊椎。第七颈椎为椎体中之最大者，穴在其下，故名。"

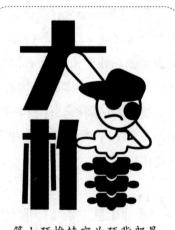

第七颈椎棘突为颈背部最大的棘突，穴在此椎骨之下。

15 哑门（督脉、阳维脉交会穴）

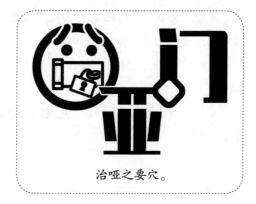

治哑之要穴。

【**出处**】《素问·气穴论》。

【**别名**】舌厌，舌横。

【**穴义**】本穴主治"舌缓，暗不能言"，为治哑之要穴，故名"哑门"。

【**定位**】第2颈椎棘突上际凹陷中，后正中线上。

【**主治**】①暴暗，舌缓，舌强不语，鼻衄；②头痛，脊痛，颈项强痛。

【**释义摘录**】

《医经理解》："哑门，一名舌厌，在项后入发际五分宛宛中，灸之则令人暗，故名也。"

《古法新解会元针灸学》："哑门者，为发音之门，有风寒闭五脏之气出声带入喉，令不得发音而哑，故名哑门。"

《经穴释义汇解》："穴在后发际宛宛中，即在头项正中后发际上五分处，因本穴联系舌根，针之利于发音，为治哑疾之门户，故名哑门。"

《针灸穴名解》："本穴内应舌咽，主治暗症，刺之俾使发音，故称'哑门'。为回阳九针之一。凡诸暗症俱可取此。《针灸大成》谓此穴禁灸，灸之令人哑。以其近于舌咽及脑也，故不宜火攻。"

16 风府（督脉、阳维脉交会穴）

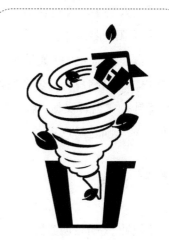

此处易为风邪所侵袭，犹如风邪会聚之处。

【**出处**】《素问·风论》《灵枢·本输》等。

【**别名**】舌本，鬼穴，鬼枕。

【**穴义**】府，有会聚之意；风府，指风邪会聚之处。本穴位于人体头项处，为风邪最易侵袭和蓄积的部位，并主治风疾，故名"风府"。

【**定位**】枕外隆凸直下，两侧斜方肌之间凹陷中。

【**主治**】①咽喉肿痛，鼻衄，暴暗；②头痛，眩晕，癫狂；③中风，舌强不语，半身不遂；④脊痛，颈项强痛。

【释义摘录】

《医经理解》："风府，一名舌本。在项入发际一寸大筋内宛宛中，去脑户一寸五分。盖风所从入之府也，故凡风热病刺此。"

《经穴解》："风自后来者，此穴先受之，故曰风府。凡一切风寒之邪，俱由此穴入，而后及于周身，故有风府之称。"

《经穴释义汇解》："穴在项上入发际一寸，因本穴主治中风舌缓等风疾，故名风府。"

《针灸穴名释义》："风，见风门条。府，见中府条。指其为风邪最易储积与治风所宜取之处。"

17 脑户（督脉、足太阳经交会穴）

【出处】《黄帝明堂经》。

【别名】 匝风，会颅，合颅。

【穴义】 户，指出入通行之处。本穴位于枕外粗隆上缘凹陷处，为督脉入脑之门户，故名"脑户"。

【定位】 枕外隆凸的上缘凹陷处。

【主治】 ①癫狂痫；②眩晕；③脊痛，颈项强痛。

【释义摘录】

《医经理解》："脑户，一名合颅，在枕骨上强间后一寸五分，是脑之户也。"

《经穴解》："穴在枕骨上，本经强间穴后一寸半，足太阳、督脉之会。"

《古法新解会元针灸学》："脑户者，头髓大脑所居之户，故名脑户。又名合颅者，脑后骨之合缝间也。"

《针灸穴名释义》："脑，颅脑；户，可以通过之处。督脉上行之风府，入属于脑，此处犹如入脑之门户。"

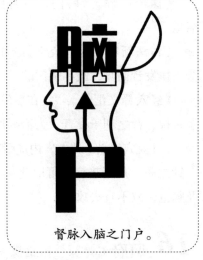

督脉入脑之门户。

18 强间

【出处】《黄帝明堂经》。

【别名】 大羽。

【穴义】 本穴位于脑户之上、后顶之下，近顶骨与枕骨人字缝处，最坚固之所，故名"强间"。

【定位】后发际正中直上4寸。

【主治】①头痛，癫狂痫，瘰疬；②颈项强痛。

【释义摘录】

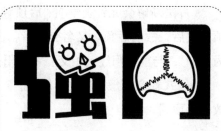

穴在顶骨与枕骨"人字缝"之间，此处骨质强硬。

《医经理解》："强间，在后顶后一寸五分，盖枕骨刚强之间也。"

《经穴解》："穴在脑户之上，后顶之下，最坚固之所，故曰强间。"

《古法新解会元针灸学》："又名大羽者，脑后颅骨，左右两片分为两仪，如鸟之有两翅。上有毛发丛生，又因肾音从阳，从命门贯督脉，其音为羽，护于大脑，故又名大羽。"

《经穴释义汇解》："强间穴在后顶后一寸五分，即顶骨与枕骨人字缝之间，因骨质强硬，穴在其间，故名强间。"

《针灸穴名释义》："强，强硬不和也；间，见二间、三间条，又指中间。穴当顶骨与枕骨结合之间，能治头痛项强诸病。"

19 后顶

【出处】《黄帝明堂经》。

【别名】交冲。

【穴义】顶，颠顶。头部颠顶（百会）前、后1.5寸处各有一穴，本穴位于颠顶之后，故名"后顶"。前顶和后顶均主治头面神志诸症，前顶偏于治额，后顶偏于治项。

【定位】当后发际正中直上5.5寸（脑户上3寸），于百会向后1.5寸处取穴。

【主治】①头痛，眩晕，癫狂痫；②颈项强痛。

穴在颠顶之后。

【释义摘录】

《医经理解》："后顶，枕骨上也。在百会后一寸五分。"

《经穴解》："穴在百会之后，百会为顶也，故曰后顶。一名交冲者，足太阳两脉，既左右交于顶之百会而下，此穴正当左右交冲之中，故曰交冲。"

《古法新解会元针灸学》："后顶者，由百会前一寸半为前顶，后寸半为后顶，穴居顶中之后，故名后顶。又名交冲者，囟骨与颅骨相交，大脑与小脑相接。《经》云'后为太冲'，与前三阳经气相交。背三阳循督脉而至，由是相交而会百会，故又名交冲。"

《经穴释义汇解》："顶，颠也。穴在百会后一寸五分，居颠之后，与前顶相对应，故名后顶。"

20 百会（督脉、足太阳经交会穴）

【出处】《黄帝明堂经》。

【别名】三阳五会，天满，泥丸宫。

【穴义】百会，又名"三阳五会"。头为诸阳之会，本穴居颠顶中央，为督脉与足太阳膀胱经、手足少阳经和足厥阴肝经的交会之处，且临床应用也非常广泛，有"百病皆主"的说法，故名"百会"。

【定位】前发际正中直上 5 寸。

【主治】①头痛，目痛，眩晕，耳鸣，鼻塞；②中风，神昏，癫狂痫，惊风，痴呆；③脱肛，阴挺。

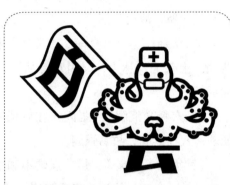

本穴为"诸阳之会"，临床应用广泛，有"百病皆主"的说法。

【释义摘录】

《医经理解》："百会，一名颠上。在前顶后一寸半。顶中央直两耳尖，陷可容指。是督脉、足太阳、手足少阳厥阴之会也。故又名三阳五会。《史记》载扁鹊治虢太子尸厥，针取三阳五会而苏。盖此穴也。"

《古法新解会元针灸学》："百会者，五脏六腑、奇经三阳、百脉之所会，故名百会。"

《经穴释义汇解》："穴在头顶中央。人头者，诸阳之会，穴为手足三阳、督脉之会，百病皆主，故名百会。"

《针灸穴名释义》："百，百脉，百骸。会，朝会。居一身之最高，百脉百骸皆仰望朝会，如天之北辰北极也。"

21 前顶

【出处】《黄帝明堂经》。

【别名】无。

【穴义】顶，颠顶。头部颠顶（百会）前、后1.5寸处各有一穴，本穴位于颠顶之前，故名"前顶"。前顶和后顶均主治头面神志诸症，前顶偏于治额，后顶偏于治项。

【定位】前发际正中直上3.5寸。

【主治】①头痛，眩晕；②面肿，鼻渊；③小儿惊风。

【释义摘录】

《医经理解》："前顶，在囟会后一寸半骨陷中。一云在百会前一寸。盖头之前顶也。"

《经穴解》："百会为顶，此穴在百会之前，故曰前顶。"

《古法新解会元针灸学》："前顶，在囟会之后，正顶之前，故名前顶。"

《经穴释义汇解》："顶，颠也，穴在囟会后一寸五分骨间凹陷处，正是左、右顶骨接合处的骨缝间，因其位在颠之前，与后顶相对应，故名前顶。"

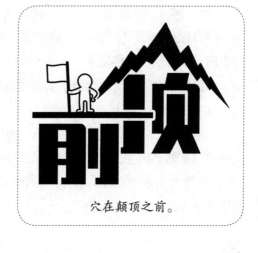

穴在颠顶之前。

22 囟会

【出处】《灵枢·热病》。

【别名】天窗，鬼门，顶门。

【穴义】囟，囟门，胎儿或新生儿颅顶盖各骨间的膜质部；会，聚合。本穴接近前发际，对应"前囟门"①，是颅顶盖各骨的聚合部，故名"囟会"。前囟门大多1至2岁闭合，故婴儿禁刺。

【定位】前发际正中直上2寸。

【主治】①头痛，眩晕，癫狂痫；②鼻塞，鼻衄；③小儿惊风。

【释义摘录】

《医经理解》："囟会，在上星后一寸骨陷中。小儿八岁以下禁针。其囟门未合也。"

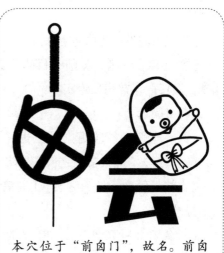

本穴位于"前囟门"，故名。前囟一般一岁半才闭合，故婴儿禁刺。

---

① 婴儿出生时，由于颅骨尚未发育完全，所以骨与骨之间存在缝隙，并在头的顶部和枕后部形成两个没有骨头覆盖的区域，分别称为前囟门和后囟门，闭合后分别形成"十字缝"和"人字缝"。

《经穴解》："囟会者，乃人之囟门，以与督脉会，故曰囟会。"

《古法新解会元针灸学》："囟会者，脑盖骨之穴，在百会前三寸。缘人在母腹中百窍皆闭，唯以脐吸母体之生气，囟会两手相抱，与手心相通，脐与囟换通气脉。任督如一，脑盖骨未合。既生则窍开，鼻息通尾闾气分，而阴阳判开，四象已定，囟门渐渐而合，故名囟会。"

《经穴释义汇解》："穴在上星后一寸骨间凹陷处，此即婴儿时头顶软骨跳动之处，俗称囟门，前名囟会，穴当其处，故以为名。"

《针灸穴名解》："囟，繁体字为顖，从页，从思；思从囟，从心。人当思虑之际，神识会于囟门，故名'囟会'。"

23 上星

【出处】《黄帝明堂经》。

【别名】鬼堂，明堂。

【穴义】本穴位于额顶部，头面上方，如星星悬在上空，可治疗头痛、眩晕、目赤肿痛、目不能视等一切头目不清、上焦阴沉之症，其作用又如黑夜中的一颗明星，故名"上星"。

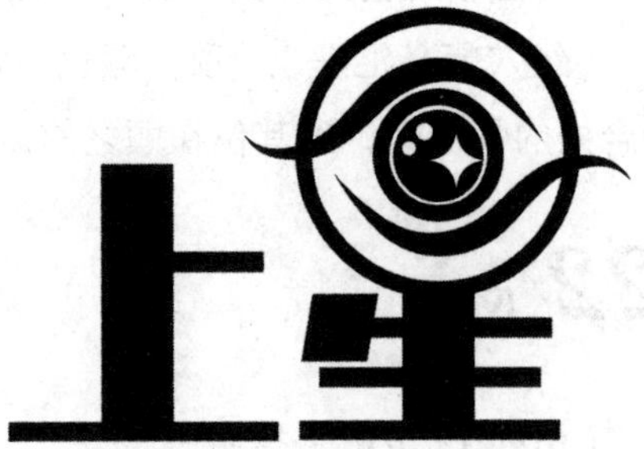

【定位】前发际正中直上 1 寸。

【主治】①鼻渊，鼻衄，目痛；②头痛，眩晕，癫狂；③热病，疟疾。

本穴主治目疾，位在上，犹如黑夜中的一颗明星。

【释义摘录】

《医经理解》："穴如星之居上也。"

《经穴解》："此穴在额之最高处陷中如豆大，如星以悬于天者然，故曰上星。"

《古法新解会元针灸学》："上星者，五脏之精气，上朝头结精于目，居高临上，故名上星。"

《针灸穴名释义》："上，指头部。星，指精气。穴在前头部正中，正为阳精所聚之处。"

24 神庭（督脉、足太阳经、足阳明经交会穴）

【出处】《黄帝明堂经》。

【别名】发际，督脉。

【穴义】庭，指额部中央。因穴居头颅之上近额部，脑在其中，而脑为元神之府，故名。

【定位】前发际正中直上 0.5 寸。

【主治】①鼻渊，鼻衄；②头痛，眩晕，癫狂痫；③呕吐。

穴居头颅之上，脑在其中。脑为元神之府。

【释义摘录】

《医经理解》："神庭，在鼻上入发际五分。头颅之上，人神之所出入也。"

《古法新解会元针灸学》："神庭者，神光所结之庭，目神之光，来原通于六腑六脏神系，是脑府前之庭堂，故名神庭。"

《经穴释义汇解》："庭者，颜也。穴在发际，直鼻，意即指本穴同鼻相垂直而近颜面部。因穴居头颅之上，脑在其中，而脑为元神之府，为人神之所出入处，故名神庭。"

《针灸穴名释义》："神，指脑之元神。庭，宫庭，庭堂。意为此乃脑神所居之高贵处也。"

25 素髎

【出处】《黄帝明堂经》。

【别名】面王。

【穴义】髎，空穴。鼻为肺之窍，五行对应白色，白为素色，且本穴在鼻尖正中，对应鼻柱端的空穴，故名"素髎"。

【定位】鼻尖的正中央。

【主治】鼻塞，鼻渊，鼻衄，鼻息肉，酒糟鼻。

【释义摘录】

《医经理解》："素髎，一名面王，在鼻端。素，始也。人之胚胎，鼻先结形。故谓是太始之骨髎也。"

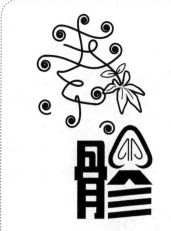

穴在鼻尖正中，鼻五行对应白色（素色）。

《经穴解》："素者，始也；顺也，洁也。人之生也先鼻，有始之义焉，自山根而下，至此而止，有顺之义也，穴在面中最高处，有洁之义焉，故曰素髎。"

《古法新解会元针灸学》："素髎者，肺之原素，其色白，所开之窍，通畅于鼻，穴居鼻头之边正中，故名素髎。又名正面者，鼻之正面也……人面前而立，鼻准端正，故又名正面。"

《经穴释义汇解》："髎，与窌同。窌，空穴也。穴为鼻柱端之空穴，因肺开窍于鼻，其色白素，即白色，故名素髎或素窌。"

26 水沟（督脉、手阳明经、足阳明经交会穴）

【出处】《黄帝明堂经》。

【别名】人中，鬼客厅，鬼宫，鬼市。

【穴义】本穴位于人中沟中，鼻水流注，形如沟渠，故名"水沟"。本穴又名"人中"，天气通于鼻，地气通于口，穴正居口鼻之间，故名。水沟穴为十三鬼穴之一，有醒脑开窍之功，常用于治疗昏迷、癫痫等神志病，为急救要穴。

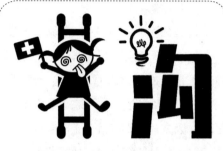

本穴有醒脑开窍之功，重刺激本穴常用于急救。

【定位】人中沟的上 1/3 与中 1/3 交点处。

【主治】①昏迷，晕厥，中风，癫痫；②口眼㖞斜，流涎，口噤，鼻塞，鼻衄；③消渴，水肿；④腰脊强痛。

【释义摘录】

《医经理解》："水沟，一名人中。在鼻下三分人中陷中，形如水沟也。"

《经穴解》："穴名水沟者，以其形有水沟之象，而治水病者，必取此穴以出水，故名水沟以志之。"

《经穴释义汇解》："穴居鼻柱下沟中央，其穴正夹于手足阳明经之中，如经水交合，故名。"

《针灸穴名释义》："水，指水液，涕水；沟，见支沟条。穴在鼻柱下，人中沟中央，近鼻孔处，为鼻水所流注，且能治水病，故名。"

27 兑端

【出处】《黄帝明堂经》。

【别名】无。

【穴义】兑，卦象之一，对应口。端，正，也指事物的尽头。本穴在上唇正中之端，又接近督脉末端，故名"兑端"。

【定位】上唇结节的中点。

【主治】①齿痛，口臭；②癫痫，呕沫，口噤。

【释义摘录】

《医经理解》："兑端，在上唇端。《易》曰：'兑为口也。'"

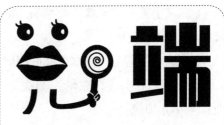

穴在上唇正中，近督经末端。口对应兑卦。

《经穴解》："兑者，口也。穴在唇正中之端，故曰兑端。"

《古法新解会元针灸学》："穴居人中之下，五形之端，有在唇棱锐端，故名兑端。"

《针灸穴名释义》："兑，同锐，又洞穴也，卦也；端，顶端。穴在上唇顶端，口腔这一大洞口之上方，故名。"

28 龈交

【出处】《黄帝明堂经》。

【别名】悬命，鬼禄。

【穴义】龈，牙龈；交，交会。穴在唇内齿上龈缝中，是任、督二脉交会处，亦是齿唇交会之所，故名"龈交"。

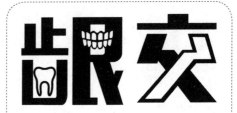

穴在唇内齿上龈缝中，沟通任、督二脉。

【定位】上唇系带与上齿龈的交点。正坐仰头，提起上唇，于上唇系带与齿龈的移行处取穴。

【主治】①牙龈肿痛、出血，鼻塞，鼻息肉；②小儿面部疮癣；③癫狂。

【释义摘录】

《医经理解》："龈交，在唇内上齿龈缝中，是任督之交也。"

《采艾编》："齿唇之际为龈之交。"

《经穴解》："龈者，齿根也，为三阳交会之所，故曰龈交。"

《古法新解会元针灸学》："龈交者，唇与齿相交肉弦断处是穴，故名龈交。"

29 印堂

【出处】《针灸玉龙歌》。

【别名】无。

【穴义】星相学家将额部两眉之间称为"印堂"，穴在其上，故名。

【定位】两眉毛内侧端中间的凹陷中。

【主治】①头痛，眩晕；②失眠；③鼻渊，鼻衄；④小儿惊风。

【释义摘录】

《国际标准针灸穴名简释》："印，泛指图章；堂，庭堂。古代指额部两眉之间为'阙'，星相家称印堂，穴在其上，故名。"

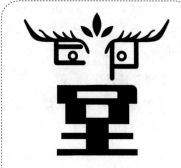

额部两眉之间称为"印堂"，穴在其上。

第十五章
任脉穴

1 会阴

【**出处**】《黄帝明堂经》。

【**别名**】屏翳，金门。

【**穴义**】穴在前后阴之间，故名"会阴"。督脉、任脉、冲脉皆起于胞中，同出于会阴，故可用于治疗子宫、精室、阴器诸疾。

【**定位**】男性在阴囊根部与肛门连线的中点，女性在大阴唇后联合与肛门连线的中点。

【**主治**】①阴中诸病，前后相引痛不得大小便；②阴痛，阴痒，阴肿，遗精，月经不调；③痔疾。

督脉、任脉、冲脉同出于会阴，被称为"一源三岐"。

【**释义摘录**】

《医经理解》："一名屏翳，在前后两阴之间，冲任督三脉之会也。"

《经穴解》："穴名会阴者，以其处在二阴之间，又为冲、任、督相会之所，故曰会阴。"

《古法新解会元针灸学》："会阴者，三阴之气会于阴窍，而至胞中，生一阳，而行督脉。三阴之气并而任脉生。督任合而化冲脉。督脉督诸阳气，强精益肾，助三焦而补脑；任脉统诸阴之血而为经；冲脉贯营而通卫，皆从阴窍出入，又系任脉之络，故名会阴。"

《经穴释义汇解》："穴为任脉别络，夹督脉、冲脉之会，位在前后两阴之间，故名会阴。"

《针灸穴名释义》："穴当下腹最低处前后阴之间，为阴气之所聚会，又为任督冲三脉之会合，故名。"

2 曲骨（任脉、足厥阴经交会穴）

【出处】《黄帝明堂经》。

【别名】尿胞，骨端，屈骨，回骨。

【穴义】曲骨，指耻骨联合部。本穴在耻骨联合部上缘，故名"曲骨"。

【定位】耻骨联合上缘，前正中线上。

【主治】小便不利，遗尿，阴疝，遗精，阳痿，月经不调，带下。

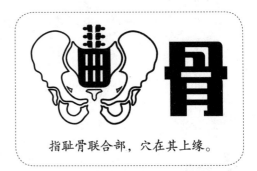

指耻骨联合部，穴在其上缘。

【释义摘录】

《医经理解》："曲骨在横骨上，中极下一寸，毛际陷中动脉，其横骨正曲而向外也。"

《经穴解》："曰曲者，其形弯曲非直也。"

《经穴释义汇解》："穴在横骨上，中极下一寸阴毛部凹陷处，因喻穴位居横骨中央屈曲之处，故名曲骨。"

《针灸穴名释义》："曲骨，古解剖名。穴在曲骨上缘，骨穴同名。"

3 中极（膀胱募穴，任脉、足三阴经交会穴）

【出处】《黄帝明堂经》。

【别名】气原，玉泉，气鱼。

【穴义】中极，星名，居天之中，为众星之主。人体的穴位如满天繁星，而本穴位居人体上下左右的中央，故名"中极"。

【定位】脐中下4寸，前正中线上。

【主治】①月经不调，崩漏，子宫脱垂，阴痒，不孕，恶露不尽，带下；②遗尿，小便不利，疝气，遗精，阳痿。

星名，居天之中。本穴位居人体上下左右的中央。

【释义摘录】

《医经理解》："在脐下四寸，横骨为下极，而此谓之中极。"

《经穴解》："此穴一名玉泉，一名气原，一名中极。名中极者，中指任脉在腹之中也。极者，自承浆而下，此为极处也。"

《古法新解会元针灸学》："中极者，腹脐下四寸中行，胞中内脏，阳经之气落于阴经，入胞中器之，而利阴窍。结灵根而生三奇经，故名中极。"

《经穴释义汇解》："穴应星名，居天之中，因穴在腹部，喻有天体垂布之象，其位居人体上下左右之中央，故名中极。"

《针灸穴名释义》："中，指人身上下之中，根本与内部。极，指方位；又最也，与急通。言穴居人身之中，为元气之根本与最为重要之处，且能治内急不通诸病。"

4 关元 （小肠募穴，任脉、足三阴经交会穴）

【出处】《素问·气穴论》《灵枢·寒热病》。

【别名】次门。

【穴义】本穴位于小腹，为男子藏精、女子蓄血之处，元阴元阳交关之处，故名"关元"。

【定位】脐中下 3 寸，前正中线上。

【主治】①疝气，少腹疼痛；②癃闭，尿频，遗精，阳痿；③月经不调，痛经，带下，子宫脱垂，恶露不尽，不孕；④疝气，小腹疼痛；⑤泄泻；虚劳。

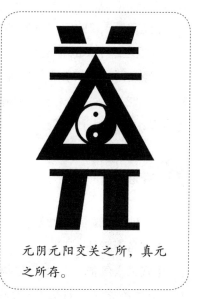

元阴元阳交关之所，真元之所存。

【释义摘录】

《医经理解》："在脐下三寸，男子藏精，女子蓄血之处。人生之关要，真元之所存也。"

《经穴解》："足三阴上行入腹者，必会于此处，有关之象焉，以任脉在中，而三阴共会之，有元之义焉，故曰关元。"

《经穴释义汇解》："穴在脐下三寸，为男子藏精，女子蓄血之处，是人生之关要，真元之所存，元阴元阳交关之所，穴属元气之关隘，故名关元。"

《针灸穴名释义》："关，指关藏，关闭，机关。元，指元气。意为下焦元阴元阳关藏出入之所。"

5 石门 （三焦募穴）

【出处】《黄帝明堂经》。

【别名】利机，精露，丹田，命门。

【穴义】石，同"石女"之石，古人称不育之女为"石女"。古人认为刺灸此穴可致女子不育，故名"石门"。

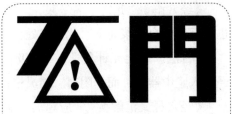

古人称不育之女为"石女"，刺灸致不育之穴曰"石门"。临床当慎刺。

【定位】脐中下 2 寸，前正中线上。

【主治】①疝气，小便不利，遗尿，遗精，阳痿；②月经不调，不孕，恶露不尽，妇人胞中积聚；③腹痛，泄泻，水肿。

【释义摘录】

《医经理解》："石门，在脐下二寸，一名丹田。妇人灸此穴，则终身绝孕。故谓是石门也。"

《经穴解》："此穴之贵要如此，故命曰石门，着其禁也，甚言此穴之不可轻针也。至妇人犯之绝子，的有至验，不可忽也。"

《经穴释义汇解》："穴在脐下二寸。石有坚硬之意。穴主少腹坚痛，历代医家传为妇人禁针之处，犯之无子。所谓女子不通人道者名石女，亦寓此意。穴为任脉之气出入之门户，故名为石门。"

6 气海

【出处】《黄帝明堂经》。

【别名】脖胦，下肓。

【穴义】气海，指生气之海。人身之气生于此处。道家称之为"丹田"，为储存真气的部位，犹如容纳百川之海。且本穴主治"脏气虚惫，真气不足，一切气疾久不瘥"（《针灸资生经·少气》），故名"气海"。

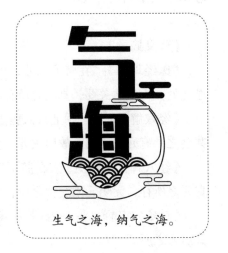

生气之海，纳气之海。

【定位】脐中下 1.5 寸，前正中线上。

【主治】①虚脱，泄泻，腹中绞痛，虚劳羸瘦；②疝气，腹痛；③小便不利，遗尿，遗精，阳痿；④月经不调，带下，子宫脱垂，恶露不尽。

【释义摘录】

《医经理解》："在脐下一寸半宛宛中，肓之原，生气之海也。"

《经穴解》："人身之气生于此穴，而会于膻中，概男女而通言之也。"

《古法新解会元针灸学》:"气海者，化冲气之海，由气海贯两旁通气穴，交于胃气。上至胸膈，入肺管而出于喉间，为气街散入胸中，与卫气相交而行于经，且导卫气入胞中，统阴血，至胞相交于肾。其上之阴交，下之丹田、关元，由气海而分天地，水火由是相交。导气以上，导血以下。故名气海。"

《针灸穴名释义》:"气，指人身元气与各种气病。海，是广大深远之意。穴处为人身生气之海，且能主一身之气疾。"

7 阴交（任脉、冲脉、足少阴经交会穴）

【出处】《黄帝明堂经》。

【别名】少因，横户。

【穴义】本穴为冲脉、任脉和足少阴肾经三条阴经之交会穴，可主治三条经脉在腹部的相关疾病，如绕脐冷痛、泄泻、疝气等，故名"阴交"。

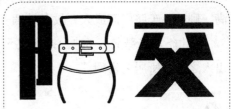

穴在脐中下1寸，为冲、任、足少阴肾经三条阴经之交会穴。

【定位】脐中下1寸，前正中线上。

【主治】①月经不调，带下，不孕，产后诸症，小便不利，疝气；②腹痛；③水肿。

【释义摘录】

《医经理解》:"阴交，在脐下一寸。当膀胱上口，三阴冲任之交会也。"

《经穴解》:"穴名阴交者，以足少阴同冲脉自下而上，共会于此处，故曰阴交。"

《古法新解会元针灸学》:"阴交者，元阳之气相交于阴，癸水之精，合于阴气，上水分合于任水之精，阳气从上而下，与元阴相交注丹田，水火既济，故名阴交。"

《经穴释义汇解》:"穴在脐下一寸，居腹，腹为阴。穴又为任脉、冲脉、少阴交会之处，故名阴交。"

8 神阙

【出处】《黄帝明堂经》作"脐中"，自《铜人腧穴针灸图经》始作"神阙"。

【别名】脐中，气合。

【穴义】神，元神；阙，宫阙，宫城。本穴位于肚脐，十月怀胎时，母体依靠脐带传输营养，孕育胎儿，以培养先天之元神，故

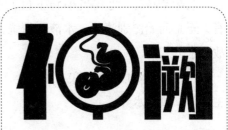

穴在肚脐，为元神之阙庭。

名"神阙"，喻元神之阙庭。

【定位】在脐区，脐中央。

【主治】①脐周痛，腹胀，肠鸣，泄泻；②水肿，小便不利；③中风脱证。

【释义摘录】

《医经理解》："在脐中元神之阙庭也。"

《经穴解》："此穴一名气舍，乃腹之中上下气所舍之地。名神阙者，以任脉上直乎心，心之所藏者神，此穴有隙焉，如王者宫门之有阙，故曰神阙。"

《古法新解会元针灸学》："神阙也，神之所舍其中也，上则天部，下则地部，中为人部……天一生水，而生肾，状如未放莲花，顺五行以相生，赖母气以相传，十月胎满，则神注于脐中而成人，故名神阙。"

《针灸穴名释义》："神，指人之元神与脐神。阙，宫阙，门观；又同缺。意为元神出入之处与所居之宫阙。"

9 水分

【出处】《黄帝明堂经》。

【别名】中守，分水。

【穴义】本穴能够分利腹部水气之清浊，使水液入膀胱、糟粕入大肠，从而主治水肿、泄泻等疾病，故名"水分"。

【定位】脐中上1寸，前正中线上。

【主治】①腹痛，浮满坚硬，腹胀不得食；②水肿，小便不利。

【释义摘录】

《医经理解》："在下脘下一寸，正当小肠。言由此而泌别清浊，水液入膀胱，渣滓入大肠也。"

《经穴解》："此穴当小肠下口，小肠为受盛之官，至是而始泌别清浊，水液入膀胱，滓渣入大肠，故曰水分。"

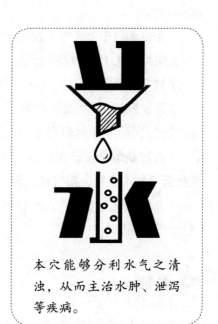

本穴能够分利水气之清浊，从而主治水肿、泄泻等疾病。

《经穴释义汇解》："穴在下脘下一寸，脐上一寸，因此穴能分利腹部水气之清浊，主水病，故名水分。"

10 下脘（任脉、足太阴经交会穴）

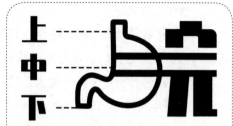

【出处】《黄帝明堂经》。

【别名】下管。

【穴义】脘，指胃脘。本穴对应胃之下口，故名"下脘"。

【定位】脐中上2寸，前正中线上。

【主治】①呕吐，食入即出；②腹满，腹硬，腹中包块，不思饮食，消瘦。

下脘穴对应胃之下口；中脘穴对应胃脘中部，近于胃小弯；上脘穴对应贲门，即胃上口。

【释义摘录】

《医经理解》："脘，胃府也。下脘，在建里下一寸，脐上三寸，是胃之下口也。"

《经穴解》："胃有三脘，此穴正当其内下脘，迂曲于肠之下，上小而中大，下脘仍微小于中，下口则愈小，以交于小肠，水谷至此，已为脾之真火磨化已融，方下入小肠，而分清浊，故曰下脘。"

《古法新解会元针灸学》："下脘者，脘是胃脘，分上中下三部，胃之上口，偏斜当右，胃之中弯向左，胃之下当中。上中下分三弯，当下弯者，胃之下口也，故名下脘。"

《经穴释义汇解》："脘，胃府也，又通管。穴在建里下一寸，脐上二寸。当胃之下口，故名下脘。"

11 建里

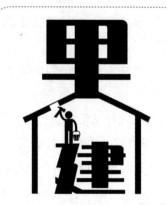

【出处】《黄帝明堂经》。

【别名】无。

【穴义】建，通"健"，强健；里，指居住。脾胃为"后天之本"，化生精微而滋养五脏六腑。凡属胃中不安之症、胃病康复期，刺激本穴皆可理中和胃，强健后天之本，而使五脏能够"安居乐业"，故名"建里"。

【定位】脐中上3寸，前正中线上。

【主治】胃痛，呕吐，食欲不振，腹痛，肠鸣，腹胀，腹肿。

本穴可理中和胃，强健后天之本，而使五脏"安居乐业"。

【释义摘录】

《医经理解》："建里在中脘下一寸，脐上三寸，言建立于里道之中也。"

《经穴解》："里者，土也；建者，厚之之意。以内所当者，正在胃中脘之下，恐其弱也，故命曰建里。"

《针灸穴名释义》："建，建立，建树，强健。又顺流而下亦谓之建。里与裡通。言其可以建立中焦之裡气，水谷亦由此流入腹里也。"

《针灸穴名解》："建者，筑也，置也。里者，居也，止也……本穴治胃痛呃逆、不欲食、胸中苦闷等症。后人演得经验，兼取内关穴，用以安定闾里，通彻门户，而和中也。不愈，则检取他穴，促使吐泻，以逐外邪。但愈后仍须补此。即安内重在善后也。凡属胃中不安之症，本穴皆可为力，俾以奠定闾里，而人得安居也，故曰'建里'。"

12 中脘（胃募穴，八会穴之腑会，任脉、手太阳经、手少阳经、足阳明经交会穴）

【出处】《黄帝明堂经》。

【别名】 太仓，胃管，中管。

【穴义】 脘，胃脘。本穴对应胃脘中部，近于胃小弯，相对于上脘及下脘而言，故名"中脘"。

【定位】 脐中上4寸，前正中线上。

【主治】 ①胃脘痛，腹胀，腹中包块，泄泻，便秘，不思饮食，呕吐；②黄疸。

【释义摘录】

《医经理解》："在上脘下一寸，脐上四寸，居歧骨与脐之中正胃府之中也。"

《经穴解》："穴正在任之中行，而实为在内胃之中脘，乃胃气所结之地，故曰胃募。"

《古法新解会元针灸学》："脾胃居肺肝心肾之中，当于上中下，胃脘之中，故名中脘。"

《经穴释义汇解》："脘，胃府也；通管。穴在上脘（管）下一寸，居心蔽骨与脐之中，正当胃之中，故名中脘。"

《针灸穴名释义》："指穴当胃体的中部，相对于上脘及下脘而言。"

13 上脘（任脉、手太阳经、足阳明经交会穴）

【出处】《黄帝明堂经》。

【别名】上管，胃管，胃脘。

【穴义】脘，胃脘。本穴对应贲门，即胃上口，故名"上脘"。

【定位】脐中上 5 寸，前正中线上。

【主治】①胃痛，呕吐，呕血，呃逆，食欲不振，腹胀，腹中积聚；②癫痫。

【释义摘录】

《医经理解》："上脘，在巨阙下一寸五分，去蔽骨三寸，脐上五寸，是胃上口也。"

《经穴解》："此穴在内为饮食初入于胃之所，故曰上脘。"

《古法新解会元针灸学》："穴当胃脘之上口，故名上脘。脘主胃之膏油，当胃弯之上，故又名胃脘也。"

《针灸穴名解》："本穴内应贲门。贲门，即胃上口也。故曰'上脘'。"

14 巨阙（心募穴）

【出处】《黄帝明堂经》。

【别名】无。

【穴义】本穴名解有二。其一，巨阙，古代最有名的宝剑剑号①。本穴在胸骨剑突之下，主治惊悸、癫狂、心痛、心烦等清浊相干、心神不宁之证，犹如仗剑立朝，除暴戡乱，故名"巨阙"。其二，穴在肋下，两肋如门之两阙，故名。

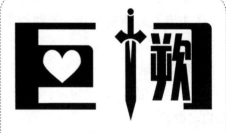

巨阙，为宝剑剑号。本穴在脐中上 6 寸，胸骨剑突下。

【定位】脐中上 6 寸，前正中线上。

【主治】①心悸，心烦，心痛，胸痛，气喘；②癫狂痫。

【释义摘录】

《医经理解》："阙者，至尊之门，巨阙在鸠尾下一寸，为心之幕。言是心君之门魏阙之地也。"

《经穴解》："穴名为巨阙者，心为一身之主，在乎上之内，此穴在胸之下，两胁在其旁，有阙象焉，故曰巨阙。巨者，大也，尊称也。"

---

① "巨阙"剑相传为春秋时期铸剑名师欧冶子所铸，与干将、莫邪、辟闾号称古代"四大剑"。传说巨阙剑初成时，宫中有一马车失控，横冲直撞。于是越王勾践立刻拔出此剑，指向马车，欲命勇士上前制止，但却在这拔剑一指时将马车砍为了两节。于是越王又命人取来一个大铁锅，用此剑轻轻一刺，便将铁锅刺出了一个大缺口。越王以其威力强大，能"穿铜釜，绝铁䍦，胥中决如粢米"，便将此剑命名为"巨阙"。

《古法新解会元针灸学》："巨阙者，在胸坎肋下如门之两阙，齐蔽骨下一寸，蔽骨系黄庭方寸之地，巨长只寸许，心气所依注之穴，故名巨阙。"

《针灸穴名解》："古者剑号'巨阙'。剑为除暴戡乱之器。本穴在胸骨剑突之下，其所治证为胸满、癥疚、霍乱、吐逆、痰饮、心痛等证。凡属清浊相干，不得宁静者，本穴均可治之。犹仗剑立朝，清除君侧，而戡定变乱也。因名'巨阙'。"

15 鸠尾（任脉络穴）

【**出处**】《灵枢·九针十二原》。

【**别名**】尾翳，𩨗骬。

【**穴义**】剑突中垂，犹如鸠鸟之尾；而两侧肋骨，犹如两翼横张。因本穴位于胸骨剑突下，故名"鸠尾"。

【**定位**】胸剑结合下 1 寸，前正中线上。

【**主治**】①胸痛引背，气喘；②腹胀，呃逆；③癫狂痫。

【**释义摘录**】

《医经理解》："鸠鸟短尾，蔽骨之下垂者象之，故以名也。"

《经穴解》："穴名鸠尾者，以其骨之下垂如鸠尾也。"

剑突中垂犹如鸠鸟之尾，穴在胸骨剑突下。

《经穴释义汇解》："穴在𦜝前蔽骨下五分。蔽骨，即蔽心骨，又名鸠尾骨。即穴处胸前鸠尾骨之下，因其骨垂形如鸠尾，故以为名。"

16 中庭

【**出处**】《黄帝明堂经》。

【**别名**】无。

【**穴义**】庭，庭院。本穴在胸剑结合之凹隙处，胸骨犹如屏门，本穴两旁为足少阴经之步廊穴，穴处犹如屏门之内、走廊之间的庭院，故名"中庭"。

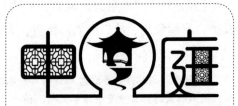

穴在胸剑结合之凹隙处，穴处犹如屏门之内、走廊之间的庭院。

【**定位**】剑胸结合终点处，前正中线上。

【主治】①胸胁胀满；②噎膈，呕吐。

【释义摘录】

《医经理解》："中庭，在膻中下一寸六分陷中，心居中而处尊，故谓是至中之殿庭也。"

《采艾编》："中央之前庭也。"

《经穴解》："中庭者，为心之庭也，心在内，而此穴为外见之庭。"

《古法新解会元针灸学》："中庭者，在心上肺下陷中，不出心之宫庭，在上膈，如月当天之中，故名中庭。"

《针灸穴名解》："穴在蔽骨之凹隙处。蔽骨犹屏门，'中庭'则庭除也。又屋之正室为庭。本穴两旁为足少阴之步廊穴，犹主室之旁，房廊相对也。如此者，则形成空庭院落。不然，'步廊'二字，在人体有何取意。盖古人所譬，心为主人，则胸廓为其庭院，再进则升堂入室矣。故喻本穴为'中庭'"。

17 膻中（心包募穴，八会穴之气会，任脉、足太阴经、足少阴经、手太阳经、手少阳经交会穴）

【出处】《黄帝明堂经》。

【别名】元儿，胸堂，上气海。

【穴义】膻，同"袒"，袒胸露乳。本穴在两乳间胸脯中央，故名。

【定位】横平第4肋间隙，前正中线上。

【主治】①胸闷，心痛；②咳嗽，气喘；③噎膈；④产后缺乳。

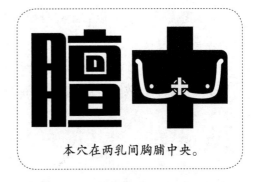

本穴在两乳间胸脯中央。

【释义摘录】

《医经理解》："两乳之中，气所回旋处也，故又名上气海。本经有二气海，下气海生气之海也，上气海宗气之海也。"

《古法新解会元针灸学》："膻中者，为心主臣使之官，属心包也。心内系上通于肺，故脉搏出于心，心跳则膻中颤动，故名膻中。"

《经穴释义汇解》："胸中两乳间曰膻。穴在两乳间陷中，故名膻中。"

《针灸穴名释义》："膻，同袒。中，指胸中。膻中，心包络名。袒胸露乳，此处又正当其中。"

18 玉堂

【出处】《黄帝明堂经》。

【别名】玉英。

【穴义】玉堂，宫殿的美称，此处指君主之居处。心为君主之官，本穴在中庭之上，主人过庭院后即登堂入室[①]，故名"玉堂"。

【定位】横平第3肋间隙，前正中线上。

【主治】①咳嗽，气喘，胸闷，胸痛；②乳房胀痛；③呕吐。

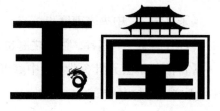

本穴内应心，心为君主之官，喻穴处为心之居所。

【释义摘录】

《医经理解》："玉堂紫宫，皆至尊之居也。"

《采艾编》："清净之座。"

《经穴解》："玉堂者，心之堂也，心在内，而此其堂也。"

《古法新解会元针灸学》："玉堂者，心之德有五：温仁、中义、通理、达智、信在其中。其恩施于外，是以君子守身如执玉，居心之上，为五脏六腑经络精气来朝之堂，故名玉堂。"

《经穴释义汇解》："穴在紫宫下一寸六分凹陷处，正居心位，心者，君主之官，因古以玉堂作殿名，故喻本穴似君主之居处，而名玉堂。"

19 紫宫

【出处】《黄帝明堂经》。

【别名】无。

【穴义】紫宫，星名，紫微[②]的别称。紫微垣十五星，紫微为诸星之首，号称"帝星"，属帝王之所居。本穴对应心，犹如君主

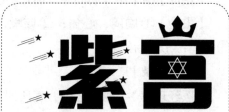

紫宫，紫微别称，为诸星之首，号称"帝星"。本穴内应心，心为君主之官，喻穴处为心之居室。

---

① 战国辞赋家宋玉的《风赋》中有："然后徜徉中庭，北上玉堂，跻于罗幢，经于洞房，乃得为大王之风也。"

② 在中国古典天文学中，"垣"是划分满天星斗的一个单位。中国古人把天上的恒星分为很多星官（相当于西方天文学中的"星座"），其中有三个星官被称为"三垣"，分别是"紫微垣""太微垣""天市垣"。

的居室，故名"紫宫"。

【定位】横平第2肋间隙，前正中线上。

【主治】①胸痛；②咳嗽，气喘。

【释义摘录】

《医经理解》："玉堂、紫宫，皆至尊之居也。"

《经穴解》："紫宫者，紫微之宫也，心正在内，此穴为宫。"

《经穴释义汇解》："紫宫，星名。乃紫微垣之异名。紫微垣十五星，一曰紫微，天帝之座也，天子之所居……穴在华盖下一寸六分凹陷处，正心位，心者，君主之官，喻穴之君主之居，又应紫宫星名，故名紫宫。"

20 华盖

【出处】《黄帝明堂经》。

【别名】无。

【穴义】华盖，指古代帝王车上的伞盖，中医称肺为"华盖"。本穴平第1肋间隙，几近肺之上缘，主治咳嗽、气喘、胸痛等胸肺之症，故名"华盖"。

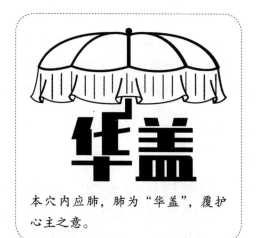

本穴内应肺，肺为"华盖"，覆护心主之意。

【定位】横平第1肋间隙，前正中线上。

【主治】胸痛，咳嗽，气喘。

【释义摘录】

《医经理解》："华盖在璇玑下一寸陷中，肺叶垂布，为五脏之华盖也。"

《采艾编》："华盖而拥紫宫，在天成象也。"

《经穴解》："此穴则在心之上，故谓华盖，如盖之覆乎人顶也。"

《古法新解会元针灸学》："华盖者，五脏六腑之精华，上朝于肺，肺居在高位，名为上腑，上系吭嗌，缘布于胸，故名华盖。"

《经穴释义汇解》："穴在璇玑下一寸凹陷处，主肺疾，肺之为脏，有称五脏之华盖；又因华盖为天上九星之星名，以喻天象，故名华盖。"

21 璇玑

【出处】《黄帝明堂经》。

【别名】旋机。

【穴义】璇玑，有转动之意①，古人常用于形容圆润光滑之物。本穴功用在于滋润滑利，主治喉部干涩枯燥之症，如喉痹、咽肿、涩痛等，故名"璇玑"。

【定位】胸骨上窝下 1 寸，前正中线上。

【主治】胸痛，咳嗽，气喘；咽喉肿痛。

【释义摘录】

《医经理解》："璇玑，浑天仪也，以象天机之运旋。肺金上浮，天象也，其系上悬，为转运之机，故以象之。穴在天突下一寸也。"

《采艾编》："胸中之行街也。"

《经穴解》："璇玑者，乃紫微垣之星，在华盖之上，此穴亦在华盖之上，故名。"

《针灸穴名解》："养生家以璇玑为喉骨环圆动转之象，文学家以璇玑为珠玉之别称，均喻其圆润光滑也……再考其所治诸症，为喉痹、咽肿、胸满涩痛等等，是其功能富于滋润滑利，有通滞去瘀消肿之能，以治干涩枯燥之症。"

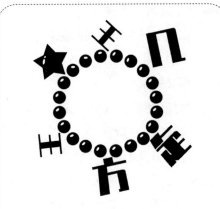

形容圆润光滑之物。本穴功在滋润滑利，主治喉部干涩之症。

22 天突

【出处】《素问·气穴论》《灵枢·本输》。

【别名】玉户，五户。

【穴义】天，人体上部，此处指胸腔；突，突出，灶突，即烟囱。天气通于肺，穴处犹如肺气出入之灶突，故名"天突"。

【定位】在颈前区，胸骨上窝中央，前正中线上。

【主治】①咳嗽，气喘，胸痛，咳血；②咽喉肿痛，失音；③瘰疬；④噎膈。

【释义摘录】

《医经理解》："在结喉下三寸宛宛中，言气之突起于天部也。"

《经穴解》："天者，言其高出也，任脉入胸穴者

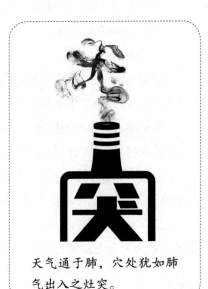

天气通于肺，穴处犹如肺气出入之灶突。

---

① 北斗七星，第二星为璇，第三星为玑，北斗自转，璇、玑随之。

在于骨，至此穴乃为空隙之处，而所在又甚高，故名天突。"

《古法新解会元针灸学》："天突者，人之呼吸，通乎天，从上而降下，则突然而动，故名天突。"

《经穴释义汇解》："因喻穴处之脉气突起于天部，故名天突。"

《针灸穴名释义》："天，指天气及人身之上部。突，指灶突。天气通于肺，穴处犹如肺气出入之灶突也。"

23 廉泉（任脉、阴维脉交会穴）

【出处】《黄帝明堂经》。

【别名】本池。

【穴义】廉，棱角。喉结突起，形如棱角，穴在结喉上方凹陷中，且穴下为舌下腺体，刺激本穴则津液分泌犹如泉水涌出，故名"廉泉"。

【定位】在颈前区，结喉上方，舌骨上缘凹陷中，前正中线上。

【主治】①中风失语，吞咽困难，舌缓，流涎；②舌下肿痛，咽喉肿痛。

【释义摘录】

《经穴解》："穴名廉泉者，乃舌下生津液之本也，舌下津液，由此而生，乃任脉自下行者，入交于舌之下，而生津液，有泉之象焉。"

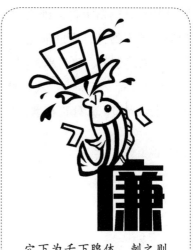

穴下为舌下腺体，刺之则
津液分泌犹如泉水涌出。

《古法新解会元针灸学》："廉泉者，言其通金津玉液，廉洁之甘泉也，故名廉泉。"

《经穴释义汇解》："廉，这里作棱形解，因喉头结节如棱，且舌根下伴有舌下腺体，津液所出犹如清泉，故名廉泉。"

《针灸穴名释义》："廉泉，水名。穴当喉结上缘有棱之处，有如吐液之泉源。"

24 承浆（任脉、足阳明经交会穴）

【出处】《黄帝明堂经》。

【别名】天池，鬼市，悬浆。

【穴义】承，受纳；浆，指唾液，古人称唾液为琼浆玉液，称口为天池。本穴位于口唇下，正对存储琼浆玉液之天池，故名为"承浆"。

【**定位**】在面部，颏唇沟的正中凹陷处。

【**主治**】①口眼㖞斜，口噤，齿龈肿痛；②失音；③癫，狂，痫；④消渴多饮；⑤头项强痛。

【**释义摘录**】

《医经理解》："在下唇下陷中，盖水浆入口，则下唇相承也。"

《经穴解》："穴名承浆者，口中饮食所余而在外者，此穴其承之之地，故曰承浆。"

《古法新解会元针灸学》："承浆者，因肾水从督脉升顶降甘露落上池，则任脉上华面，由上下牙齿相通，牙生酸汁，而助消化，与甘露相合为浆，承于上，而落于下，故名承浆。"

《经穴释义汇解》："穴在颐前下唇棱下凹陷处，因喻水浆入口，穴处正相承，故名承浆。"

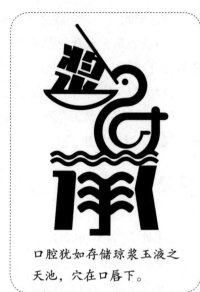

口腔犹如存储琼浆玉液之天池，穴在口唇下。

258

Chapter 1

Introduction

1 The origin and development of acupoint names

In ancient times, human beings instinctively found that when some pain spots were stimulated by pressing, tapping, etc., there would be the phenomenon of "pressing and the person feels comfortable" and "pressing and pain relief". These spots were generally referred to as "Places for Bian-stone and moxibustion", thus the earliest prototype of acupoints-"acupoint is where pain is" was formed.

With the accumulation of practical experience, people gradually realized the specific therapeutic functions of some acupoints, and the location of acupoints became more solidified. In the medical slips unearthed from the Han tomb in Laoguanshan, the acupoints were mainly named after the phrase of body parts plus yin-yang attribute. For example, "Xiang Juyang", "Xiang" indicates a specific body part of the neck; "Juyang" is the yin-yang attribute, indicating the vertical pathway. Although this kind of location was not precisely explained, in the age when anatomy and physiology were not developed, the ancients used their own subtle expressions to start the most primitive naming of acupoints.

The earliest ancient book with acupoint names recorded is *The Yellow Emperor's Inner Classic* (*Huáng Dì Nèi Jīng*, 黄帝内经), which was written during Warring States Period to Qin-Han period. The book included 173 acupoints, of which there were as many as 148 acupoints with clear names and still in use today. Since then, acupoint names have achieved the historical evolution from imprecise area to exact point. The names of these acupoints have a wide range of meanings, containing ancient Chinese astronomy, meteorology, geography, somatology, personal affairs and other aspects.

The Yellow Emperor's Mingtang Classic (*Huáng Dì Míng Táng Jīng*, 黄帝明堂经), which was finished between the end of the Western Han Dynasty and the Yanping period of the Eastern Han Dynasty, is regarded as the first monograph on acupoints in China. This book provided a comprehensive summary of the acupoints in different medical books prior to the Han Dynasty, including their names, locations, indications and needling and moxibustion methods, etc. The original book of *Huáng Dì Míng Táng Jīng* has been lost. Fortunately, its content has been compiled and preserved through later literatures. The earliest citation of *Huáng Dì Míng Táng Jīng* was Huangfu Mi's *The Systematic Classic of Acupuncture and Moxibustion* (*Zhēn Jiǔ Jiǎ Yǐ Jīng*, 针灸甲乙经), which is the earliest extant monograph on acupuncture and moxibustion in China. The book included 349 meridian points, marking the improvement of the arrangement of acupoints. Since then, the number of acupoints has rarely changed. In the Qing Dynasty, presented in Li Xuechuan's book *The Source of Acupuncture and Moxibustion* (*Zhēn Jiǔ Féng Yuán*, 针灸逢源), the number of meridian points increased to 361. The names and number of acupoints in this book have been used in modern times. The national standard *Names and Locations of Acupuncture points* (GB/T 12346–2021), issued in 2006, absorbed the extra–point "Yintang" in Governor Vessel. So far, the number of meridian points has become 362.

It can be seen that the naming of acupoints was not done by one person at a time, and it is an evolutionary process of from zero to one, from area to point, and from less to more. It was doctors of past dynasties that have brought out the names after thousands of years' accumulation under the historical conditions at the time, based on the understanding of nature, astronomy and geography, general outline of yin and yang and the five elements, theories about the viscera and meridians, and functions of acupoints.

2 The origin and the development of explanations of acupoint names

During the Sui and Tang Dynasties, Yang Shangshan was the first to start explaining acupoints and their names. Yang Shangshan annotated the names of the fifteen connecting points in the ninth volume of the *The souce of Yellow Emperor's Inner Classic* (*Huáng Dì Nèi Jīng Tài Sù*, 黄帝内经太素), the Chapter of *Fifteen collateral vessels*. In addition, in *Huáng Dì Míng Táng Jīng*, he also commented on the fourteen meridian points. Unfortunately, the only preserved content of this book is the Hand Taiyin volume which contains 10 acupoints

(Missing the acupoint YunMen LU–2), and the rest have been lost.

In the Song, Jin, Yuan and Ming dynasties, there were only a few books on the interpretation of acupoints. Zhang Jiebin's *The Classified Classic* (*Lèi Jīng*, 类经) in the Ming Dynasty made a comprehensive overview of the meaning of acupoint names. For example, it is pointed out in *Lèi Jīng*: "Among all the acupoints in meridians, some are named after stars or the heaven, which correspond to the sky. Some are named after mountains, hills, streams, valleys, deeps, seas, springs, marshes, capitals or residential areas, which correspond to the ground. Those who are called houses or palaces are gathering spots for the spirit. Those who are called portals are for the entry and exit of the spirit. Those who are called residences or bedrooms are for the spirit to live. Those are called terraces are for the parade of the spirit. There is a reason for naming, and by analogy, it can be seen from the common things." Although there was no detailed explanation of acupoints, the thinking and summary of the interpretation of acupoint names provided a basic idea for later generations of doctors to further understand acupoints.

The development of study on acupoints came to its peak in the Qing Dynasty when many books that fully interpret the acupoint names of the meridians appeared. Those interpretations were rich in content and different from each other.

Comprehension of Medical Classics (*Yī Jīng Lǐ Jiě*, 医经理解) was written by Cheng Zhi in the Qing Dynasty. Volume 3 of the book was set as "Explanation of Acupoint Names", which interpreted the names of acupoints in the Fourteen channels. Cheng said that "I wish that scholars in the world can understand the meaning of acupoint names, thus they will understand the acupoints and master and seek these acupoints more easily." By saying these words, he pointed out the most direct reason for annotating the names of acupoints and exploring their meanings.

Harvesting Mugwort Collection (*Cǎi Ài Biān*, 采艾编) written by Ye Guangzuo in the Qing Dynasty was the representation of the culture of Lingnan (the south of the Five Ridges). The book consisted of four volumes, in which the second volume gave a very brief comment on the acupoint names of the twelve channels. For example, according to the book, "MeiChong BL–3 is located directly above the inner corner of the eyebrow, between ShenTing GV–24 and QuCha BL–4. It is right above the eyebrow close to the midline." "TongTian BL–7 is so named because it is located below the brain and upon the nose, which means it helps qi go up."

A doctor named Yue Hanzhen, from Shandong Province in the Qing Dynasty, had comprehensively introduced the locations and indications, the contraindication of acupuncture, and the meaning of the fourteen meridian points names in his book *Interpretation of Meridians and Acupoints* (*Jīng Xué Jiě*, 经穴解). When annotating acupoints, Yue did a great job on explaining the origin of acupoint names based on human anatomy and meridian theories by using linguistics. For example, the book says: " 承 Cheng is the scene of the lower supporting the upper. 光 Guang refers to BaiHui GV-20, which locates on the top of the head, acting as a monarch of acupoints. ChengGuang BL-6 is below the both sides of BaiHui GV-20, which is a figure of ministers serving the monarch by its side, hence its name." As for NeiGuan PC-6, the book says: " 内 Nei is the contrary word to 外 Wai. The former means inner and the latter means outer. Both NeiGuan PC-6 and WaiGuan TE-5 go far away from the elbow to the wrist and locate in the place where the meridians meet between bones, showing the image of a gateway. Hence the name."

In addition, the author also ingeniously made a comparison and a discussion between acupoints which had similar names, meanings or locations in the book, to help readers differentiate them. For example, to distinguish ChongMen SP-12 from other acupoints located around the groin, the book says that "This acupoint is the entry for the Spleen channel to go into the abdomen. The three yin meridians of foot and the Foot Yangming channel enter the abdomen from the thigh and arrange horizontally. The Kidney channel of Foot Shaoyin is on the medial side, which has HengGu KI-11 as its first acupoint to enter the abdomen, 1 cun to the midline. The second is the Stomach channel of Foot Yangming, which has QiChong ST-30 as its entry to the abdomen, 2 cun to the midline. Next, the Liver channel of Foot Jueyin enters the abdomen by YinLian LR-11, 2 cun inferior to QiChong ST-30. Then comes the Spleen channel of Foot Taiyin with ChongMen SP-12 as its entry to the abdomen. While QiChong ST-30 is 2 cun to the midline and ChongMen SP-12 is farther to the midline with 4.5 cun, ChongMen SP-12 is so named because it is close to QiChong on the Stomach channel."

There was an academic wave of Western learning spreading to the east during the early period of the Republic of China. In this context, the book named *(Ancient Method New Interpretation) Huiyuan Acupuncture and Moxibustion* [*(Gǔ Fǎ Xīn Jiě) Huì Yuán Zhēn Jiǔ Xué*,（古法新解）会元针灸学] had strong characteristics of the times. Jiao Huiyuan, the author, tried to explain the names of acupoints in a way of integrating Chinese and Western culture in this book. For example, WeiDao GB-28 was described to be "upper connecting the uterine belt, lower connecting ligament and Sanjiao". As for ChengGuang BL-6, the book says, "the eye pupil is like water essence, the spleen is like grinding motor, the kidney and life gate are like generators, the cerebrum and cerebellum are like engines receiving electric, the occipital bone is like a flat mirror which can send back light, and the yang of the brain gathers in the forebrain, which is used for application." Although these explanations seem far-fetched now, they can reflect the author's awareness of using modern knowledge to interpret Chinese Traditional Medicine and his desire to make it scientific.

After the founding of the People's Republic of China, acupuncture and moxibustion have been developing day by day. In the early 1980s, a number of influential monographs emerged on the interpretation of acupoint names. *Explanation of the Names of Acupuncture Points* (*Zhēn Jiǔ Xué Míng Jiě*, 针灸穴名解) written by Gao Shiguo and *Interpretation of Acupuncture Points* (*Zhēn Jiǔ Xué Míng Shì Yì*, 针灸穴名释义) written by Zhou Meisheng probed and interpreted the names of acupoints of the fourteen meridians one by one in a similar style. The former paid great attention to ancient culture and combined the author's own experience in clinical treatment. The latter cited ancient classics such as *Book of Songs* (*Shī Jīng*, 诗经), *Records of the Grand Historian* (*Shǐ Jì*, 史记), *Elucidations of Script and Explications of Characters* (*Shuō Wén Jiě Zì*, 说文解字) in order to first decipher words and then phrases. Thus the "Exegesis" research system of acupoint names formed. *Interpretation of Meridian Points* (*Jīng Xué Shì Yì Huì Jiě*, 经穴释义汇解) written by Zhang ShengXing and Qi Gan was a combination of the essence of dozens of ancient and modern theories and the authors' own opinions. It was characterized by short and pithy explanations and quoting documents precisely and meticulously. There were text notes about aliases and English translations of the acupoints in this book. The translation adopted the method of literal translation to retain the rich cultural connotations of the acupoint names. What also worth mentioning is *Categorized collection of literatures on Chinese acupoints* (*first edition in 1994*)(*Zhōng Guó Zhēn Jiǔ Xué Wèi Tōng Jiàn*, 中国针灸穴位通鉴) edited by Wang Deshen. The "Interpretation of Acupoint Names" part of the book comprehensively collected the annotations of each acupoint from ancient times to the present. So, it could be called the generalization of interpretations of acupoint names, which was of great reference value for the research on acupoint names.

3 Naming and Classification of Acupoints

"Names are used to identify the difference. From ancient times to the present, it has been used properly to succeed and improperly to fail." (*Yǐn Wén Zǐ · Dà Dào Shàng*, 尹文子·大道上). Chinese culture has attached great importance to the naming of objects since ancient times, and this is particularly true of the acupuncture–moxibustion culture it has spawned, where each name of an acupoint has its own special meaning. As Sun Simiao says in *Supplement to 'Important Formulas Worth a Thousand Gold Pieces'* (*Qiān Jīn Yì Fāng*, 千金翼方), "All acupoints, where the name is not in vain, have profound implications."

3.1 Thinking methods of naming acupoints

There are mainly two thinking methods about naming acupoints, that is, the analogical method of taking images and the realistic recording method.

Most acupoints are named with the analogical method of taking images, which means that the acupoints are named according to their anatomical location, the five elements and yin–yang theories, the flow of qi and blood, and their functions combining with a rich imagination to find things that are similar to them in astronomy, geography, flora and fauna, buildings and artifacts. It is said in *Plain Questions* (*Sù Wèn*, 素问): "Man is born of the qi of heaven and earth." The human body is a small universe, and its functions are the manifestation of the traffic between the qi of yin–yang of heaven and earth. This is the philosophical basis for the naming method of analogical method of taking images. Here is an evident from the summary of the interpretation of the acupoint names in *Comprehension of Medical Classics* (*Yī Jīng Lǐ Jiě*, 医经理解): " 海 Hai means to which it belongs. 渊 Yuan and 泉 Quan, which means that they are deep. 沟 Gou and 渎 Du represent narrowness. 池 Chi and 渚 Zhu represent shallow. 市 Shi and 府 Fu means gathering. 里 Li and 道 Dao refer to the origin. 室 Shi and 舍 She refer to the place of residence. 门 Men and 户 Hu, refer to the place where one enters and exits. 阙 Que and 堂 Tang refer to somewhere noble. 关 Guan and 梁 Liang refer to important meeting places. 丘 Qiu and 陵 Ling refer to the protrusion of flesh and bone. 髎 Liao means the hollow area of the bone. 俞 Shu means the transmission of qi. 天 Tian, in place of the upper part. 地 Di, standing for the lower part." Due to this, the names of acupoints are rich in meaning and connotation. Understanding the meaning of the names of acupoints is beneficial to understanding the philosophical thinking of the ancients and is important for gaining an in-depth understanding of the distribution characteristics, clinical applications, and flow of qi and blood in acupoints.

The realistic recording method, which means that the characteristics of the acupoints in terms of their location and function are recorded in reality. For example, JuGu(LI–16), WanGu(LI–1), JingGu(BL–64), RuZhong(ST–16) and DaZhui(GV–14) are named for their locations. JingMing(BL–1), YangLao(SI–6), Ying Xiang(LI–20), GuangMing(GB–37) and

FeiYang(BL–58) are named for their functions.

The two methods can be used separately or often combined, such as XueHai(SP–10), TingGong(SI–19), FengShi(GB–31), NeiGuan(PC–6) and YaMen(GV–15).

3.2　Classification of acupoints naming

The ancients named acupoints from astronomy, geography, life, and anything that could be obtained by observing and imitating the phenomena around them. Therefore, the following is a summary of the idea of naming acupoints with the Sancai principle of "imitating the sky", "imitating the earth" and "imitating people".

3.2.1　Imitating the sky

" 天 sky" represents two meanings. Firstly, " 天 sky" stands for astronomy and meteorology. In ancient China, astronomy and meteorology began to emerge from primitive society. The "Jiangjunya petroglyphs" found in Jiangsu province clearly depicting the sun and the banded nebulae are about 4,000 years old at least, probably the world's oldest retained star charts. The oracle bone inscriptions from the Yin Ruins excavated in Anyang, Henan province, also contain rich meteorological records of wind, clouds, rain and thunder. Ancient people were diligent in observing the positions of the sun, moon and stars and their changes, so that they could learn the rules and use them to compile calendars and to serve their production and livelihood. Thus, ancient astronomy and meteorology had a profound impact on Chinese culture and medicine. Besides, " 天 sky" also refers to the gods of heaven, those who rule the universe, the sun, the moon, the stars, the wind and rain, and so on.

3.2.1.1　Astrometeorology

Acupoints named after astronomical terms such as sun, moon and stars include ZiGong(CV–19), HuaGai(CV–20), XuanJi(CV–21), TianShu(ST–25), QuYuan(SI–12), ShangXing(GV–23), RiYue(GB–24), TaiYi(KI–3), TianZong(SI–11), TianXi(SP–18), JiMen(SP–11) and TaiBai(SP–3). Acupoints named after meteorological terms include YunMen(LU–2), LieQue(LU–7) and FengLong(ST–40). These acupoints are mostly distributed above the waist, including the head, neck and chest, and metaphorically represent the channel qi flowing through the heaven. Among them, acupoints named after the stars, such as ZiGong(CV–19), HuaGai(CV–20), XuanJi(CV–21), QuYuan(SI–12) and TianZong(SI–11), are mostly located in the chest and upper back. Ancient Chinese astronomers divided the stars into three enclosures, Supreme Palace Enclosure in the upper enclosure, Purple Forbidden Enclosure in the middle enclosure and Heavenly Market Enclosure in the lower enclosure.

The names of the above stars belong to the Purple Forbidden Enclosure, which is also called Purple Forbidden Palace with the meaning of the imperial palace, where the Emperor of Heaven resides. This is why the names of these stars are assigned to the heart and chest of the human body, to compare the heart as the organ similar to the emperor and the lungs as the organ similar to the prime minister. It is interesting to know that the first record of the Purple Forbidden Enclosure as a star is in *Gan and Shi's Canon of Star* (*Gān Shí Xīng Jīng*, 甘石星经), a book that was written roughly during the Warring States Period, which also happens to be the period when *The Yellow Emperor's Inner Classic* (*Huáng Dì Nèi Jīng*, 黄帝内经) was written.

3.2.1.2 Deity

There is a Chinese common saying that "there is a god at three feet above the head", which originated from people's rituals. During early human civilization, people were mystified and frightened by many natural phenomena, so the idea of "gods" was formed, believing that 'gods' were omniscient and omnipotent creators and masters of everything in the world, thus giving rise to the worship of deities. There are many acupoints named after deities. Some of the acupoints related to " 神 God" include ShenMen(HE–7), ShenTang(BL–44), BenShen(GB–13), ShenCang(KI–25), ShenFeng(KI–23), ShenDao(GV–11) and ShenQue(CV–8), etc. Acupoints related to " 灵 Spirit" include LingDao(HE–4), QingLing(HE–2), ChengLing(GB–18), LingXu (KI–24), LingTai(GV–10), etc. According to Traditional Chinese Medicine, "The heart is the organ similar to the monarch and is responsible for spirit and mental activity." (*Plain Questions*, 素问). Most of these acupoints are therefore located in the chest and upper back or are related to the physiological functions and indications based on the phrase "heart stores spirit", as a metaphor for the place where the heart qi is stored and gathered, or the passage through which it enters and exits.

3.2.2 Imitating the earth

The ancients observed geography and found that the surface of the earth rose and fell, creating topographical features such as mountains, plains, river valleys, dunes and rivers. Channels and acupoints of the human body have many similarities to these landscapes, so they are described in geographical terms. For example, in *The·Spiritual·Pivot: River Channels* (*Líng Shū · Jīng shuǐ*, 灵枢·经水), the size and depth of the twelve rivers on the ancient map of Qing, Wei, Hai, Hu, Ru, Mian, Huai, Luo, Jiang, He, Ji and Zhang are used as a metaphor for the flow of qi and blood of the twelve channels. The saying in *Plain Questions·On Qi Acupoints* (*Sù Wèn · Qì Xué Lùn*, 素问·气穴论), "the big depression between muscles is called 谷 valley, and the small gap between muscles is called 溪 stream. Between the muscles, the part where 溪 streams and 谷 valleys meet can pass through the *Ying*-nutrient qi and *Wei*-defensive qi, and unite the *Zong*-pectoral qi.", is an explanation of the concept of qi points in terms of " 溪 stream" and " 谷 valley". In naming acupoints, the ancients also drew on a large number of geographical and topographical terms to describe the anatomical features of the body part where acupoints are located, such as 山 mountain, 谷 valley, 丘 hill, 陵 mound, 海 sea, 溪 stream, 池 pond and 泽 marsh. According to statistics, of the 148 acupoints with names appearing in *The Yellow Emperor's Inner Classic* (*Huáng Dì Nèi Jīng*, 黄帝内经), the most are named after mountains and waterways, with 37 points. In addition, plants and animals on the ground are also important materials for naming acupoints.

3.2.2.1 Valleys and hills

For example, QiuXu(GB-40) is anterior and inferior to the external malleolus, which protrudes like a hill, hence the name. DaLing(PC-7) is in the depression between the palmaris longus tendon and the flexor carpi radialis tendon. This is a place visibly undulating because the palm bone is high and protruding like a mountain. Hence the name. XianGu(ST-43) is located in front of the union of the second and third metatarsal bones and is depressed like a valley. Others include WaiLing(ST-26), LiangQiu(ST-34), ShangQiu(SP-5), WaiQiu(GB-36), HeGu(LI-4), QianGu(SI-2), RanGu(KI-2), YangGu(SI-5), ShuaiGu(GB-8), ChengShan(BL-57), KunLun(BL-60), etc. Most of these acupoints are located on the limbs of the body near the bones.

3.2.2.2 Rivers and lakes

" 海 Hai means to which it belongs. 渊 Yuan and 泉 Quan, which means that they are deep. 沟 Gou and 渎 Du represent narrowness. 池 Chi and 渚 Zhu represent shallow." (*Comprehension of Medical Classics*, 医经理解) For example, XueHai(SP-10) has the capability of guiding the flow of blood, a metaphor for its capability as if guiding a torrent into the sea. JiQuan(HT-1) is located at the highest point of the Heart Channel of Hand Shaoyin, which is a metaphor for the channel qi flowing down from a very high spring. QingLingYuan(SJ-11) is a metaphor for the flow of qi and blood from the Sanjiao Channel of Hand Shaoyang into this point, like water injecting into a deep pool. Similar acupoints include XiaoHai(SI-8), ShaoHai(HT-3), ZhaoHai(KI-6), QiHai(CV-6), ChiZe(LU-5), ShaoZe(SI-1), YangChi(SJ-4), TianChi(PC-1), QuChi(LI-11), YangXi(LI-5), TaiXi(KI-3), HouXi(SI-3), TaiYuan(LU-9), YongQuan(KI-1), QuQuan(LR-8), ShuiQuan(KI-5), TianQuan(PC-2), LianQuan(CV-23), SiDu(SJ-9), etc. Most of these acupoints are located on the limbs, including many of the five transport points. Some acupoints are named after waterways to describe the flow of channel qi, such as 海 Hai,

泽 Ze, 池 Chi, 溪 Xi, 渊 Yuan, 泉 Quan, 冲 Chong. Meanwhile, degree–terms such as "大 big", "小 small" are often used in the acupoint names to describe the strength of qi and blood, such as XiaoHai(SI–8), ShaoHai(HT–3), ShaoZe(SI–1), TaiYuan(LU–9), TaiChong(LR–3), etc.

3.2.2.3 Animals and plants

Animals and plants are an important part of the nature. The ancients used the analogical method of taking images to name acupoints with similar characteristics after common animals and plants, demonstrating their rich imagination. Take JiuWei(CV–15) for an example, 鸠 Jiu is an alias for the cuckoo, whose tail often hangs down to shelter itself, so here it is used as an analogy for the sternum. YuJi(LU–10) is located proximal to the radial side of the palmar muscle, where the muscle is thick and shaped like a fish belly. Similar acupoints include FuTu(ST–32), DuBi(ST–35), Cuanzhu(BL–2), HeLiao(LI–19), etc.

3.2.3 Imitating people

"The sages of ancient times studied the form of the human body, discerned the internal organs, and learned about the distribution of the channels. The twelve channels merge and converge. Each acupoint has its own location and name." (*Sù Wèn·Yīn Yáng Yìng Xiàng Dà Lùn*, 素问·阴阳应象大论) Thus, the method of "imitating people" first names the acupoints according to their anatomical location in the human body, related internal organs, main therapeutic effects, properties of the five elements and yin–yang. Besides, "imitating people" also includes people's household goods, residences, etc.

3.2.3.1 Anatomical position

For example, JuGu(LI–16), WanGu(SI–4), JingGu(BL–64) and DaZhui(GV–14) are named directly after bones. TaiChong(LR–3), RenYing(ST–8), DaiMai(GB–26) and JiMai(LR–12) are named directly after meridians or blood vessels. ShangWan(CV–13), ZhongWan(CV–12), XiaWan(CV–10), as well as the back–shu points such as FeiShu(BL–13), XinShu(BL–15), GanShu(BL–18), PiShu(BL–20), ShenShu(BL–23) are named directly after internal organs. Acupoints in the holes of bone surfaces or in the depressions at the edges of bones are often named with the Chinese character " 髎 Liao". For example, BaLiao(BL–31, BL–32, BL–33, BL–34) is in the space at the back of the sacrum. JianLiao(SJ–14) is in the depression posterior to the acromion. TianLiao(SJ–15) is in the depression at the edge of superior angle of scapula. QuanLiao(SI–18) is in the depression at the lower edge of the cheekbones.

" 上 Shang and 下 Xia", " 头 Tou and 足 Zu", " 手 Shou and 足 Zu", " 前 Qian and 后

Hou" and other even–words are also often used in names of acupoints to describe the location of the acupoints. For example, ShangGuan(GB–3) and XiaGuan(ST–7), TouQiaoYin(GB–11) and ZuQiaoYin(GB–44), TouLinQi(GB–15) and ZuLinQi(GB–41), ShouSanLi(LI–10) and ZuSanLi(ST–36), QianDing(CV–21) and HouDing(CV–19), QianGu(SI–2) and HouXi(SI–3), etc.

3.2.3.2 Capability of acupoints

GuangMing(GB–37) is mainly used to treat eye diseases. YaMen(CV–15) is an important acupoint for treating dumbness. YingXiang(LI–20) can treat nasal congestion and inability to smell. ZhouRong(SP–20) can promote the flow of qi and blood throughout the body so that to nourish the body. Similar acupoints include ChengJang(CV–24), ChengGuang(BL–5), FeiYang(BL–60), JingMing(BL–1) and YangLao(SI–6). Most of the acupoints for the treatment of pain caused by wind evil are named after " 风 Feng". For example, FengFu(GV–16), FengChi(GB–20) and YiFeng(SJ–17) can treat long–lasting headache. FengMen(BL–12) and BingFeng(SI–12) can treat pain of shoulder and back. FengShi(GB–31) can treat pain of lower limb. There are also acupoints related to " 水 Shui", such as ShuiDao(ST–28), ShuiFen(CV–9) and ShuiQuan(KI–5). ShuiDao(ST–28), with the small intestine deep inside, close to the bladder, is used for treating symptoms such as difficult urination. ShuiFen(CV–9) is used to divide the fluid into the bladder and the dregs into the large intestine. ShuiQuan(KI–5) is the *Xi*–Cleft point of the Kidney Channel of Foot Shaoyin and is used to treat irregular menstruation and difficult urination. It is easy to conclude that most of the above " 水 Shui" acupoints are related to their capabilities in regulating water metabolism.

3.2.3.3 Yin–yang and five elements

"Yin–yang theory" and "Five elements theory" are important philosophical foundations and thinking methods in Traditional Chinese Medicine, and those thinking methods are fully reflected in the naming of acupoints.

"Yin–yang" is a generalization of the properties of the two opposing sides of interrelated things or phenomena in the universe, and the human body is also an organic whole made up of a combination of yin and yang. Acupoints named after " 阳 Yang" are therefore mostly attributed to the yang channels, such as ZhiYang(GV–9), HuiYang(BL–35), YangJiao(GB–35), SanYangLuo(SJ–8), YangLingQuan(GB–34) and YangGu(SI–4). Acupoints named after " 阴 Yin" are mostly attributed to or associated with the yin channels, such as HuiYin(CV–1), YinJiao(CV–7), SanYinJiao(SP–6), YinLingQuan(SP–9), YinGu(KI–10), ZhiYin(BL–67).

"Five elements" are the five substances of wood, fire, earth, gold and water, and their movements and changes. Through the analogical method of taking images and deduction, the five elements link the organs of the human body to all things in nature. According to the "Five elements theory", the lung stores corporeal soul (魄 Po) , the heart stores spirit (神 Shen), the liver stores the ethereal soul (魂 Hun), the spleen stores thought(意 Yi), and the kidney stores will(志 Zhi) . Therefore, the points PoHu(BL-42), ShenTang(BL-44), HunMen(BL-47), YiShe(BL-49), ZhiShi(BL-52) are level with FeiShu(BL-13), XinShu(BL-15), GanShu(BL-18), PiShu(BL-20) and ShenShu(BL-23) respectively. For another example, the lung belongs to "gold" according to the "Five elements theory", and corresponds to "white" in colors and corresponds to " 商 Shang" in tones, so there are the points named of XiaBai(LU-4) and ShaoShan(LU-11) in the lung meridian.

3.2.3.4 Circulation of channels

The channels flow like a four-way road, with straight lines and bifurcations, and sometimes they meet each other. Some of the acupoints are named to reflect the running route of the channel, for example, QuCha(BL-4) reflects the zigzagging and uneven course here of the Bladder Channel of Foot Taiyang. FuLiu(KI-7) reflects the Kidney Channel of Foot Shaoyin travels diagonally from the center of the foot towards the medial malleolus, and then resuming its positive direction after travelling diagonally to this acupoint. Some acupoint names reflect the branching of the channel. For example, ZhiZheng(SI-7) is the *Luo-* Connecting point of the Small Intestine Channel of Hand Taiyang, from which the collaterals of small intestine channel runs separately from the main channel. FuFen(BL-41) reflects the second lateral line of the Bladder Channel of Foot Taiyang starts from this acupoint and is attached to the first lateral line, becoming a branch of this channel. Some acupoints are named after " 交 Jiao" or " 会 Hui", reflecting the rendezvous of two or more channels. For example, SanYinJiao(SP-6) is the meeting of the Spleen Channel of Foot Taiyin, the Kidney Channel of Foot Shaoyin and the Liver Channel of Foot Jueyin. YangJiao(GB-35) is the meeting of the Gallbladder Channel of Foot Shaoyang and Yang Linking vessel. JiaoXin(KI-8) is the meeting of the Kidney Channel of Foot Shaoyin and Yin heel vessel. HuiYin(CV-1) is the meeting of Conception vessel, Governor vessel and Thoroughfare vessel.

3.2.3.5 Architecture and accommodation

Architecture and accommodation, ranging from the administrative zoning to the doors and windows of houses, are the products of human activity and provide places for human activity. "The meridian sinews are like mountains, the channels are like rivers, and the acupoints are like towns spread along the banks of the river." (*Explanation of the Names of Acupuncture Points*, 针灸穴名解). In life there are pavilions, so as in the human body. There are many acupoints named after architecture and accommodation, including 22 names that contain the Chinese character " 门 Men", as well as DaDu(SP-2), ZhongDu(LR-6), YinDu (KI-19), XiongXiang(SP-19), QiJie(ST-30), FuShe(SP-13), ZhongFu(LU-1), TianFu(LU-3), LingTai(GV-10), BuLang(KI-22), ShenTang(BL-44), YuTang(CV-18), ZiGong(CV-19), KuFang(ST-14), YingChuang(ST-16), and so on. Most of the acupoints named after buildings, such as " 宫 Gong", " 府 Fu", " 堂 Tang", " 庭 Ting" and " 廊 Lang" are located in the thoracic region.What is more interesting is that they are distributed very regularly. For example, following the direction of the Conception vessel is like going deeper into a palace. When you open the door of "JuQue(CV-14)", "ZhongTing(CV-16)" in front of the hall comes into view, then you pass through "Yutang(CV-18)" where guests meet and deliberate, and finally you enter "ZiGong(CV-19)" where the king lives. On both sides of the hall is "BuLang(KI-22)" that resembles aisle. This is typical of ancient Chinese courtyard architecture, and the layout not only embodies the ancient art of architecture, but also reflects the patriarchal and feudal ethical code system of the society of the time. The thorax contains the heart and lungs. The heart is the organ similar to the monarch and the lung is the organ similar to the prime minister, so the thorax is like a residence for the heart and lungs. Therefore, the acupoints are named after palaces and buildings, in keeping with the rituals of the ruler.

3.2.3.6 Household goods

In the naming of acupoints, there are also " 钟 Zhong", " 枕 Zhen", " 箕 Ji", " 鼎 Ding" and " 盆 Pen", which are used in people's daily lives and are mostly named by the analogical method of taking images. For example, the Chinese character " 箕 Ji" of JiMen(SP-11) is analogous to the shape of two legs spread apart. The Chinese character " 鼎 Ding" of TianDing(LI-17) is analogous to the medial end of the clavicle, the protrusion of the throat and the two ears, which form the shape of three feet and two ears. The Chinese character " 盆 Pen" of QuePen(ST-12) is analogous to the shape of the supraclavicular fossa.

Chapter 2
The Lung Channel Points of Hand Taiyin

1 中府 **ZhongFu LU–1** (Front–*Mu* point of the Lung, Meeting point of the Lung and Spleen channels)

【Source】《黄帝明堂经》 *Huangdi Mingtang Jing*

【Annotation】中 Zhong means middle–jiao. 府 Fu means gathering. The Lung channel of Hand Taiyin originates in the middle–jiao, and its qi and blood are derived from the essence of water and grain produced by the spleen and the stomach. Being the Front–*Mu* point of the lung, this acupoint is a palace where the qi of the lung gathers and concentrates, hence it is named 中府 ZhongFu.

【Location】On the chest, at the same level as the first intercostal space, lateral to the infraclavicular fossa, 6 cun lateral to the anterior midline.

【Indications】Cough, dyspnea, chest pain, fullness of the chest, heat in the chest; pain of the shoulder and back.

2 云门 **YunMen LU–2**

【Source】《素问·水热穴论》 *Suwen: Shui Re Xue Lun*

【Annotation】云 Yun refers to clouds, a metaphor for channel qi. 门 Men, is a gateway for entrance and exit. This acupoint is the highest point to which the qi of the Lung channel goes up and then leaves the chest and enters the arm like clouds. Therefore, it has the function of relieving depression and can be used to diffuse the lung to suppress cough, resolve phlegm, and dissipate binds, like a gateway for cloud and mist to ascend, hence it is named 云 门 YunMen.

【Location】Above the coracoid process of the scapula, in the depression of the infraclavicular fossa, 6 cun lateral to the anterior midline.

【Indications】Cough, dyspnea, heart pain, fullness of the chest; pain of the shoulder and back.

3 天府 TianFu LU-3

【Source】《素问·气穴论》 *Suwen: Qixue Lun*

【Annotation】天 Tian refers to the upper part of the body. 府 Fu means a treasury. This acupoint is the highest point of the Lung channel at the arm. Its channel flows from the chest into the arm through this point, unifying the channel qi from the upper arm down to the elbow and infusing it into other points of this meridian, hence this acupoint is named 天府 TianFu. Compared to a treasury (府 Fu), this point can concentrate the dissipated qi in the thorax to treat cough and dyspnea caused by qi deficiency when tonifying methods are applied.

【Location】On the inner side of the arm, lateral to the border of the biceps brachii muscle, 3 cun inferior to the anterior axillary fold.

【Indications】①Nosebleed, cough, dyspnea; ②goiter; ③pain of impediment.

4 侠白 XiaBai LU-4

【Source】《黄帝明堂经》 *Huangdi Mingtang Jing*

【Annotation】侠 Xia, an interchangeable word of 夹 Jia, means between. 白 Bai means white, which is the corresponding color of the lung according to the five phases theory. This acupoint belongs to the Lung channel and is located on the inner side of the upper arm, between the lateral border of the biceps brachii muscle and the shaft of the humerus, hence it is named 侠白 XiaBai.

【Location】On the inner side of the arm, lateral to the border of the biceps brachii muscle, 4 cun inferior to the anterior axillary fold, or 5 cun superior to the cubital crease.

【Indications】①Heart pain, cough, dyspnea, agitation and fullness; ②retching; ③pain of the arm.

5 尺泽 ChiZe LU–5 (*He*–Sea point)

【Source】《灵枢·本输》*Lingshu: Benshu*

【Annotation】The location of this acupoint is related to 尺 Chi, a unit of length in ancient China (about a one–third meter). The point is located on the cubital crease, which is about one Chi distance from the wrist pulse. Meanwhile, the function of this acupoint is related to 泽 Ze, a marshland where water gathers and retains. As a *He*–Sea and Water point, the qi of the Lung channel gathers and retains here as water flows to a marshland, hence it is named 尺 泽 ChiZe.

【Location】At the elbow, on the cubital crease, in the depression lateral to the biceps brachii tendon.

【Indications】①Cough, dyspnea, fullness of the chest, hemoptysis, swelling and pain of the throat, pain of the elbow and arm; ②infantile convulsion; ③retching, diarrhea.

6 孔最 KongZui LU–6 (*Xi*–Cleft point)

【Source】《黄帝明堂经》*Huangdi Mingtang Jing*

【Annotation】孔 Kong means clefts. As the *Xi*–Cleft point of the Lung channel, this acupoint is a cleft where the channel qi and blood accumulate deeply. According to *Shuo Wen Jie Zi*, 孔 Kong also means opening the orifices. 最 Zui means extreme. Putting these two Chinese characters together indicates that this acupoint is vital to open the orifices and regulate the blood. Therefore, it is named 孔　最 KongZui and is usually used to treat hemoptysis, nosebleed, and febrile disease without sweating.

【Location】On the forearm, 7 cun superior to the palmar wrist crease, on the line connecting ChiZe (LU–5) with TaiYuan (LU–9).

【Indications】①Febrile disease without sweating; ②cough, dyspnea, hemoptysis, swelling and pain of the throat; ③pain of the elbow and arm.

7 列缺 LieQue LU–7 (*Luo*–Connecting point, Confluent point of the Conception vessel)

【Source】《灵枢·经脉》*Lingshu: Jingmai*

【Annotation】The god of thunder and lightning was known as 列缺 LieQue in ancient China. Firstly, the qi of the Lung channel flows from this acupoint to the Large Intestine channel through a collateral vessel, just like the shape of lightning. Secondly, thunder and lightning in the atmosphere can pass through the upper and lower. As the saying goes, use LieQue to treat headache. Stimulating this acupoint can refresh the head and eyes as if a thunderbolt dissipates the haze and clears the sky, thus it is named 列缺 LieQue.

【Location】On the forearm, 1.5 cun superior to the palmar wrist crease, between the tendons of the extensor pollicis brevis and the abductor pollicis longus, in the groove of the abductor pollicis longus tendon.

【Indications】①Cough, dyspnea; ②toothache, swelling and pain of the throat, deviated eye and mouth; ③headache, pain and stiffness of the neck and nape; ④hemiplegia, weakness or pain of the wrist.

8 经渠 JingQu LU–8 (*Jing*–River point)

【Source】《灵枢·本输》*Lingshu: Benshu*

【Annotation】经 Jing means going through without staying. 渠 Qu means a ditch. As the *Jing*–River point of the Lung channel, this acupoint is like a ditch where the channel qi constantly flows as water. Besides, it can dissipate stasis and purge heat to regulate lung qi, as if the function of diverting the flood for irrigation of a ditch. Hence it is named 经渠 JingQu.

【Location】On the radial side of the forearm, between the radial styloid process and the radial artery, 1 cun superior to the palmar wrist crease.

【Indications】① Cough, dyspnea, chest pain, swelling and pain of the throat; ②weakness or pain of the wrist.

9 太渊 TaiYuan LU–9 (*Shu*–Stream and *Yuan*–Source point, *Hui*–Meeting point of the Vessel)

【Source】《灵枢·九针十二原》《灵枢·本输》*Lingshu: Jiuzhen Shieryuan, Lingshu: Benshu*

【Annotation】太 Tai refers to vast and extreme. 渊 Yuan refers to a deep ravine. This acupoint is the *Hui*–Meeting point of the vessel as if a vast and deep ravine where water gathers and concentrates, hence it is named 太渊 TaiYuan.

【Location】At the wrist joint, between the radial styloid process and the scaphoid bone, in the depression ulnar to the abductor pollicis longus tendon.

【Indications】① Cough, dyspnea, hemoptysis, swelling and pain of the throat; ② pulseless syndrome; ③ weakness or pain of the wrist.

10 鱼际 YuJi LU-10 (*Ying*-Spring point)

【Source】《灵枢·本输》 *Lingshu: Benshu*

【Annotation】际 Ji means border. The acupoint is located at the border between the red and white flesh on the radial side of the thumb, where the muscles are thick with the shape of a fish belly, hence it is named 鱼际 YuJi.

【Location】On the lateral side of the hand, at the border between the red and white flesh, radial to the midpoint of the first metacarpal bone.

【Indications】① Cough, hemoptysis, dry throat, swelling and pain of the throat; ② fever, heat in the palms, headache; ③ infantile malnutrition with accumulation.

11 少商 ShaoShang LU-11 (*Jing*-Well point)

【Source】《灵枢·本输》 *Lingshu: Benshu*

【Annotation】少 Shao means small. 商 Shang, is one of the five notes of the ancient Chinese pentatonic scale, corresponding to the lung according to the five phases theory. As the *Jing*-Well point of the Lung channel, this acupoint works as a well where channel qi of the lung origins like a small shallow stream, hence it is named 少商 ShaoShang.

【Location】On the thumb, radial to the distal phalanx, 0.1 cun proximal-lateral to the radial corner of the thumbnail.

【Indications】① Swelling and pain of the throat, nosebleed, cough, dyspnea; ② infantile convulsion; ③ spasm and pain of the fingers.

Chapter 3
The Large Intestine Channel Points of Hand Yangming

1 商阳 ShangYang LI-1 (*Jing*-Well point)

【Source】《灵枢·本输》*Lingshu: Benshu*

【Annotation】商 Shang, is one of the five ancient Chinese pentatonic scale notes. The large intestine is related to the lung. According to the five phases theory, both are subsumed to metal, which corresponds to 商 Shang as well. This acupoint is the *Jing*-Well point of the Large Intestine channel, undertaking the purifying qi from the lung and transforming yin into yang, hence it is named 商阳 ShangYang.

【Location】On the index finger, radial to the distal phalanx, 0.1 cun proximal-lateral to the radial corner of the index fingernail.

【Indications】① Swelling and pain of the throat, toothache, swelling of the cheek, tinnitus, deafness, bluish blindness; ② febrile disease without sweating, loss of consciousness; ③ numbness, swelling and pain of the fingers.

2 二间 ErJian LI-2 (*Ying*-Spring point)

【Source】《灵枢·本输》*Lingshu: Benshu*

【Annotation】二 Er means two. 间 Jian refers to an interosseous space. This acupoint locates in a depression distal and radial to the second metacarpophalangeal joint and is the second acupoint of the Large Intestine channel, hence it is named 二间 ErJian.

【Location】Distal to the radial side of the second metacarpophalangeal joint, at the border between the red and white flesh.

【Indications】①Swelling and pain of the throat, toothache, cloudy vision, nosebleed, deviation of the mouth and eye; ②febrile disease.

3 三间 SanJian LI-3 (*Shu*-Stream point)

【Source】《灵枢·本输》*Lingshu: Benshu*

【Annotation】三 San means three. 间 Jian refers to an interosseous space. This acupoint locates in a depression proximal and radial to the second metacarpophalangeal joint and is the third acupoint of the Large Intestine channel, hence it is named 三间 SanJian.

【Location】On the index finger, in the depression proximal and radial to the second metacarpophalangeal joint.

【Indications】①Swelling and pain of the throat, toothache, eye pain; ②fullness of the chest, fever with panting; ③borborygmus; ④swelling and pain of the dorsum of hand and the fingers.

4 合谷 HeGu LI-4 (*Yuan*-Source point)

【Source】《灵枢·本输》*Lingshu: Benshu*

【Annotation】合 He refers to the action of opening and closing. 谷 Gu represents a valley-like shape, a metaphor for the big gap or depression between the tendons and muscles. This acupoint is located between the first and second metacarpal bones. When the two bones split, the area between them will be slightly sunken, just like a valley, hence the name 合谷 HeGu.

【Location】On the dorsum of the hand, radial to the midpoint of the second metacarpal bone.

【Indications】①Swelling and pain of the throat, toothache, headache, redness, swelling and pain of the eyes, nosebleed, deafness, deviation of the mouth and eye, lockjaw; ②aversion to cold with fever, absence of sweating, copious sweating; ③prolonged labor, amenorrhea, dysmenorrhea; ④rigid tongue after stroke, paralysis of the upper limbs.

5 阳溪 YangXi LI-5 (*Jing*-River point)

【Source】《灵枢·本输》*Lingshu: Benshu*

【Annotation】阳 Yang means a yang position, which refers to the dorsum of the hand here. 溪 Xi means a stream. As said in *Nei Jing*, it also refers to the small gap or depression between the tendons and muscles. This acupoint is located in the depression between the tendons of the extensor pollicis longus and brevis, as if it is located in a stream, hence it is named 阳溪 YangXi.

【Location】At the wrist joint, on the radial side of the dorsal wrist crease, distal to the radial styloid process, in the depression of the anatomical snuffbox.

【Indications】①Redness, swelling and pain of the eyes, toothache, swelling and pain of the throat, headache; ②swelling, pain, and weakness of the wrist.

6 偏历 PianLi LI-6 (*Luo*-Connecting point)

【Source】《灵枢·根结》*Lingshu: Genjie*

【Annotation】偏 Pian means to deviate. 历 Li means to go through. As the *Luo*-Connecting point of the Large Intestine channel, this acupoint is where the collateral vessel of this channel deviates from the main stem and contacts the Lung channel, hence it is named 偏 历 PianLi, that's why it can treat lesions of both the Large Intestine channel and the Lung channel.

【Location】On the forearm, 3 cun superior to the dorsal wrist crease, on the line connecting YangXi (LI-5) with QuChi (LI-11).

【Indications】①Toothache, nosebleed, swelling and pain of the throat, tinnitus, deafness; ②edema, difficult urination; ③aching pain and weakness of the arm.

7 温溜 WenLiu LI-7 (*Xi*-Cleft point)

【Source】《黄帝明堂经》*Huangdi Mingtang Jing*

【Annotation】温 Wen means to warm up. 溜 Liu means to flow. This acupoint can treat syndromes of internal obstruction of cold-dampness, including cold pain of the elbow and arm and headache caused by cold. With the ability to unblock, it can also treat abdominal pain and hyperactive borborygmus. Therefore, the name 温溜 WenLiu means that this acupoint is where the channel qi flows through like a warm stream, warming the meridian to dissipate cold and to unblock.

【Location】5 cun superior to the dorsal wrist crease, on the line connecting YangXi (LI–5) with QuChi (LI–11).

【Indications】①Headache, swelling of the face, swelling and pain of the throat ②abdominal pain, hyperactive borborygmus; ③febrile disease; ④aching pain of the shoulder and back, deep–rooted sores.

8 下廉 XiaLian LI–8

【Source】《黄帝明堂经》*Huangdi Mingtang Jing*

【Annotation】上 Shang and 下 Xia respectively refer to high and low, front and back. 廉 Lian refers to the side, edge, or border. The ancient name for the side of a central room in Chinese culture is 廉 Lian. ShangLian (LI–9) and XiaLian(LI–8) are located on the radial border of the forearm. The lower one is XiaLian(LI–8), and the upper one is ShangLian(LI–9). They are both named after their locations.

【Location】4 cun inferior to the cubital crease, on the line connecting YangXi (LI–5) with QuChi (LI–11).

【Indications】①Dizziness, pain of the eye; ②swelling, spasm and pain of the elbow and arm.

9 上廉 ShangLian LI–9

【Source】《黄帝明堂经》*Huangdi Mingtang Jing*

【Annotation】上 Shang and 下 Xia respectively refer to high and low, front and back. 廉 Lian refers to the side, edge, or border. The ancient name for the side of a central room in Chinese culture is 廉 Lian. ShangLian (LI–9) and XiaLian(LI–8) are located on the radial border of the forearm. The lower one is XiaLian(LI–8), and the upper one is ShangLian(LI–9). They are both named after their locations.

【Location】3 cun inferior to the cubital crease, on the line connecting YangXi (LI–5) with QuChi (LI–11).

【Indications】①Headache; ②abdominal pain, hyperactive borborygmus; ③aching pain and numbness of the shoulder and arm.

10 手三里 ShouSanLi LI-10

【Source 】Presented as 三里 SanLi in《黄帝明堂经》*Huangdi Mingtang Jing* and as 手三里 ShouSanLi in《针灸甲乙经》*Zhenjiu Jiayi Jing*.

【Annotation 】里 Li means cun. When the elbow is flexed, this acupoint is 3 cun away from the tip of the elbow, hence it is named 三里 SanLi. As it locates on the upper limbs, it is named 手三里 ShouSanLi in order to distinguish it from 足三里 ZuSanLi (ST-36). (手 Shou means hand and 足 Zu means foot.)

【Location 】On the forearm, 2 cun inferior to the cubital crease, on the line connecting YangXi (LI-5) with QuChi (LI-11).

【Indications 】①Toothache, swelling of the cheek; ②pain and motor impairment of the elbow and arm, pain of the shoulder and back, lumbar pain.

11 曲池 QuChi LI-11 (*He*–Sea point)

【Source 】《灵枢·本输》*Lingshu: Benshu*

【Annotation 】 曲 Qu means to bend. 池 Chi means a pond. When the arm is flexed, this acupoint is in the depression at the lateral end of the cubital crease, which looks like a shallow pond. Meanwhile, it is the *He*–Sea point of the Large Intestine channel, where the channel qi flows as water pours into a pond, hence the name 曲池 QuChi.

【Location 】At the lateral end of the cubital crease, the midpoint of the line connecting ChiZe (LU-5) with the lateral epicondyle of the humerus.

【Indications 】①Swelling and pain of the throat, toothache, eye disease; ②urticaria, eczema, scrofula; ③febrile disease, fright epilepsy; ④swelling and pain of the arm, paralysis of the upper limbs.

12 肘髎 ZhouLiao LI-12

【Source 】《黄帝明堂经》*Huangdi Mingtang Jing*

【Annotation 】肘 Zhou means the elbow. 髎 Liao means interosseous space. This acupoint is located in the depression lateral to the elbow, hence it is named 肘髎 ZhouLiao.

【Location 】Flex the elbow, 1 cun proximal and lateral to QuChi (LI-11), on the border of the humerus.

【Indications】Aching pain, numbness, and spasm of the elbow and arm.

13 手五里 ShouWuLi LI-13

【Source】《黄帝明堂经》 *Huangdi Mingtang Jing*

【Annotation】五 Wu means five, and 里 Li is a measuring unit that equals to cun in ancient China. This acupoint is 5 cun proximal to the tip of the elbow, hence the name 五里 WuLi.

【Location】3 cun superior to the cubital crease, on the line connecting QuChi (LI-11) with JianYu (LI-15).

【Indications】①Scrofula; ②spasm of the elbow and arm.

14 臂臑 BiNao LI-14

【Source】《黄帝明堂经》 *Huangdi Mingtang Jing*

【Annotation】臂 Bi means the arm. 臑 Nao refers to muscles of the upper arm that bulge near the armpit. This acupoint is located 7 cun proximal to QuChi (LI-11) on the muscle of the upper arm, hence the name 臂臑 BiNao.

【Location】On the lateral side of the upper arm, 7 cun proximal to QuChi (LI-11), anterior to the border of the deltoid muscle.

【Indications】①Scrofula; ②eye disease; ③pain of the shoulder and arm, inability to raise the arm.

15 肩髃 JianYu LI-15

【Source】《黄帝明堂经》 *Huangdi Mingtang Jing*

【Annotation】肩 Jian means the shoulder. 骨 Gu means the bone. 禺 Yu means a corner formed with two sides. The Chinese character 髃 Yu combining 骨 with 禺 refers to the interosseous space. This acupoint is located between the acromion and the greater tubercles of the humerus, where depressed in front of the acromion when raising the arm. Hence it is named 肩髃 JianYu.

【Location】At shoulder girdle area, in the depression between the anterior end of lateral border of the acromion and the greater tubercle of the humerus.

【Indications】①Rubella; ②paralysis of the upper limbs, pain of the shoulder and arm.

16 巨骨 JuGu LI-16 (Meeting point of the Large Intestine channel with the Yang Motility vessel)

【Source】《素问·气府论》*Suwen: Qifu Lun*

【Annotation】巨骨 JuGu is an ancient anatomical noun meaning the clavicle. This acupoint is near the junction of the clavicle and the scapular spine, hence the name 巨骨 JuGu.

【Location】In the depression between the acromial end of the clavicle and the scapular spine.

【Indications】Pain of the shoulder and inability to raise the arm.

17 天鼎 TianDing LI-17

【Source】《黄帝明堂经》*Huangdi Mingtang Jing*

【Annotation】天 Tian means the sky. This acupoint is on the neck, which is the position of the sky of the human body. 鼎 Ding refers to an ancient cooking stove. The name of this acupoint can be explained from two aspects. Firstly, Ding is characterized by the shape of three feet and two ears. This acupoint is on the neck and above the QuePen (ST-12). It is named TianDing because the medial ends of the clavicle and the laryngeal prominence resemble a three-legged tripod, with two ears of a person forming the shape of a Ding. Secondly, the point can reconcile fire and water as a cooking stove can, mainly being used to treat sudden loss of voice, sour throat, and other diseases caused by fire invading the throat, hence the name 天鼎 TianDing.

【Location】At the same level as the cricoid cartilage, posterior to the border of the sternocleidomastoid muscle.

【Indications】①Swelling and pain of the throat, sudden loss of voice, hiccup; ②scrofula, goiter.

18 扶突 FuTu LI-18

【Source】《灵枢·本输》*Lingshu: Benshu*

【Annotation】扶 Fu is considered to be the width of four fingers together. Put four fingers except for the thumb together. Their width is about 3 cun. 突 Tu refers to a protuberance. This acupoint is 3 cun (1 Fu) lateral to the laryngeal prominence, hence it is named 扶突 FuTu.

【Location】At the same level as the laryngeal prominence, between the anterior and posterior borders of the sternocleidomastoid muscle.

【Indications】①Swelling and pain of the throat, sudden loss of voice, hiccup; ②cough, panting; ③goiter.

19 口禾髎 KouHeLiao LI-19

【Source】《黄帝明堂经》 Huangdi Mingtang Jing

【Annotation】禾 He refers to standing grain. 髎 Liao means a hole. This acupoint is located between the nose and the mouth, lateral to the philtrum. The nostril is shaped like a hole, and the mustache nearby looks like standing grain. Hence it is named 口禾髎 KouHeLiao.

【Location】Level with the junction of the upper one-third and lower two-thirds of the philtrum, inferior to the lateral margin of the nostril.

【Indications】①Nasal congestion, allergic rhinitis, nosebleed; ②deviation of the mouth and eye, lockjaw.

20 迎香 YingXiang LI-20

【Source】《黄帝明堂经》 Huangdi Mingtang Jing

【Annotation】迎 Ying means to be face to face. 香 Xiang means aroma and can generally refer to smell. The nose is an olfactory organ. This acupoint is about 0.5 cun lateral to the nasal ala and can treat loss of smell. It is named 迎 香 YingXiang because of the human nature of preferring aroma to foul odor.

【Location】On the face, at the same level as the midpoint of the lateral border of the nasal ala, in the nasolabial sulcus.

【Indications】Sinusitis, nosebleed, deviation of the mouth and eye, itching and swelling of the face.

Chapter 4

The Stomach Channel Points of Foot Yangming

1 承泣 **ChengQi ST-1** (Meeting point of the Stomach channel with the Yang Heel and Conception vessels)

【Source】《黄帝明堂经》 *Huangdi Mingtang Jing*

【Annotation】承 Cheng means carrying. 泣 Qi means weeping silently. Tears flow down the face while people cry. This acupoint is directly below the pupil on the infraorbital margin, a place that carries tears, hence it is named 承泣 ChengQi.

【Location】On the face, directly below the pupils between the eyeballs and the infraorbital margin.

【Indications】①Redness, swelling and pain of the eyes, lacrimation on exposure to wind, nyctalopia, myopia, twitching of the eyelids; ②deviation of the mouth and eye.

2 四白 **SiBai ST-2**

【Source】《黄帝明堂经》 *Huangdi Mingtang Jing*

【Annotation】四 Si means four and refers to all directions here. 白 Bai refers to bright. This acupoint is 1 cun inferior to the eyes and is mainly used to treat eye diseases. Needling at this point can make people have a bright sight in all directions, hence the name.

【Location】On the face, in the infraorbital foramen.

【Indications】①Redness, swelling and pain of the eyes, corneal nebula, lacrimation on exposure to wind, twitching of the eyelids, facial pain, facial convulsion, deviation of the mouth and eye; ②headache, dizziness.

3 巨髎 JuLiao ST-3 (Meeting point of the Stomach channel with the Yang Heel vessel)

【Source】《黄帝明堂经》 *Huangdi Mingtang Jing*

【Annotation】巨 Ju means enormous. 髎 Liao means a hole. This acupoint is in a huge depression on the inferior border of the zygomatic bone beside the nose, hence the name 巨髎 JuLiao.

【Location】Level with the inferior border of the nasal ala, directly below the pupil.

【Indications】Optic atrophy, blurred vision, corneal nebula, twitching of the eyelids, deviation of the mouth and eye, swelling of the lips and cheek.

4 地仓 DiCang ST-4 (Meeting point of the Stomach channel with the Yang Heel vessel)

【Source】《黄帝明堂经》 *Huangdi Mingtang Jing*

【Annotation】地 Di means ground and earth. Ancient Chinese divided one's face into three divisions, above the nose for the upper, the nose for the middle, and below the nose for the lower. These three divisions correspond to three levels of sky, human, and earth. This acupoint is lateral to the corner of the mouth under the nose, which belongs to the level of earth. 仓 Cang refers to a place for storing food. The mouth is to eat, where food is stored. That is the reason why this point is called 地仓 DiCang.

【Location】0.4 cun lateral to the corner of the mouth.

【Indications】Deviation of the mouth and eye, sluggish speech, drooling.

5 大迎 DaYing ST-5

【Source】《素问·气穴论》《素问·气府论》 *Suwen: Qixue Lun, Suwen: Qifu Lun*

【Annotation】迎 Ying means meeting. There are two meanings of the name. Firstly, the mandible was called 大迎骨 DaYing Bone by ancient Chinese, and this acupoint is near the bone, hence the name 大迎 DaYing. Secondly, the Large Intestine channel meets the Stomach channel at this point, hence the name.

【Location】Anterior to the angle of the mandible, in a depression anterior to the masseter attachment, over the facial artery.

【Indications】Deviation of the mouth and eye, facial convulsion, lockjaw, cheek swelling, toothache.

6 颊车 JiaChe ST-6

【Source】《黄帝明堂经》 *Huangdi Mingtang Jing*

【Annotation】颊 Jia means the cheek. 车 Che refers to wheels and is a metaphor for transportation and rotation. Ancient Chinese called the gum bone as 牙车 YaChe (牙 Ya means the teeth). This acupoint is located where the mandibular joint can rotate, a place in charge of the opening and closing of the mouth, hence it is named 颊车 JiaChe. It can treat lower toothache since it is close to the lower teeth.

【Location】Approximately 1 fingerbreadth (middle finger) anterior and superior to the angle of the mandible.

【Indications】Deviation of the mouth and eye, toothache, cheek swelling, lockjaw.

7 下关 XiaGuan ST-7 (Meeting point of the Stomach and Gall Bladder channels)

【Source】《素问·气穴论》《灵枢·本输》 *Suwen: Qixue Lun, Lingshu: Benshu*

【Annotation】下 Xia means being inferior to the zygomatic arch, opposite ShangGuan (GB-3). 关 Guan refers to a hub of opening and closing. This acupoint is close to the mandibular joint beneath the zygomatic arch that is in charge of the opening and closing of the joint, hence it is named 下关 XiaGuan.

【Location】In the depression between the midpoint of the lower border of the zygomatic arch and the mandibular notch.

【Indications】①Toothache, cheek swelling, deviation of the mouth and eye, dislocation of the jaw; ②deafness, tinnitus.

8 头维 TouWei ST-8 (Meeting point of the Stomach and Gall Bladder channels with the Yang Linking vessel)

【Source】《黄帝明堂经》 *Huangdi Mingtang Jing*

【Annotation】维 Wei refers to defending. This acupoint is within the anterior hairline at the corner of the forehead and mainly works like a horn defending the head from invasion by exogenous pathogens. Hence the name 头维 TouWei.

【Location】0.5 cun directly superior to the anterior hairline at the corner of the forehead, 4.5 cun lateral to the anterior midline.

【Indications】Headache, eye pain, lacrimation, blurred vision, twitching of the eyelids.

9 人迎 RenYing ST-9 (Meeting point of the Stomach and Gall Bladder channels)

【Source】《素问·气府论》《灵枢·本输》 *Suwen: Qifu Lun, Lingshu: Benshu*

【Annotation】This acupoint is over the carotid artery beside the thyroid cartilage, called RenYing Pulse in palpation. 人 Ren means human. 迎 Ying means to greet and welcome. The artery is called RenYing Pulse because ancient Chinese believed it was a place greeting the qi of five viscera and six bowels to nourish the human body.

【Location】Level with the thyroid cartilage, anterior to the sternocleidomastoid muscle, over the carotid artery.

【Indications】①Headache, dizziness; ②panting; ③swelling and pain of the throat, scrofula, goiter.

10 水突 ShuiTu ST-10

【Source】《黄帝明堂经》 *Huangdi Mingtang Jing*

【Annotation】水 Shui refers to the qi from water and food. 突 Tu means protruding and refers to the laryngeal prominence here. This acupoint is located on the anterior border of the sternocleidomastoid muscle beside the laryngeal prominence. When people eat and drink, qi at this acupoint will rush upward to meet with water and food. Furthermore, needling at this point can treat cough caused by water and qi ascending reversely. Hence it is named 水突 ShuiTu.

【Location】Anterior to the sternocleidomastoid muscle, midpoint between RenYing (ST-9) and QiShe (ST-11).

【Indications】①Cough, panting; ②swelling and pain of the throat, scrofula, goiter.

11 气舍 QiShe ST-11

【Source】《黄帝明堂经》*Huangdi Mingtang Jing*

【Annotation】气 Qi refers to stomach qi. 舍 She means a residence. This acupoint is the home for qi of the Stomach channel to stay, hence it is named 气舍 QiShe.

【Location】In the supraclavicular fossa, superior to the sternal end of the clavicle, in the depression between the sternal and clavicular heads of the sternocleidomastoid muscle.

【Indications】①Cough, panting; ②swelling and pain of the throat, scrofula, goiter, pain and stiffness of the neck and nape.

12 缺盆 QuePen ST-12

【Source】《素问·刺热》*Suwen: Cire*

【Annotation】缺盆 QuePen is the ancient name of the clavicle. This acupoint is in the center of the depression superior to the clavicle, directly above the nipple, hence the name 缺盆 QuePen.

【Location】In the supraclavicular fossa, in the depression superior to the clavicle, 4 cun lateral to the anterior midline.

【Indications】①Cough, panting; ②swelling and pain of the throat, scrofula, pain of the supraclavicular fossa.

13 气户 QiHu ST-13

【Source】《黄帝明堂经》*Huangdi Mingtang Jing*

【Annotation】户 Hu means a door. 气户 QiHu is located on the chest and corresponds to the lung. QiHu level with YunMen (LU-2), both refer to a door for qi absorption, treating diseases such as cough with dyspnea, chest pain, back pain, fullness of the chest and hypochondrium, and panting. Hence the name 气户 QiHu.

【Location】Inferior to the clavicle, 4 cun lateral to the anterior midline.

【Indications】①Cough, panting; ②pain of the chest, distending pain of the chest and lateral costal region.

14 库房 KuFang ST-14

【Source】《黄帝明堂经》 *Huangdi Mingtang Jing*

【Annotation】库房 KuFang refers to a storehouse. The chest stores the heart and lungs like a storehouse. This acupoint is located on the chest and can treat syndromes like fullness of the chest and hypochondrium and cough with dyspnea, hence it is named 库房 KuFang.

【Location】In the first intercostal space, 4 cun lateral to the anterior midline.

【Indications】①Cough, panting, coughing of pus and blood; ②distending pain of the chest and hypochondrium.

15 屋翳 WuYi ST-15

【Source】《黄帝明堂经》 *Huangdi Mingtang Jing*

【Annotation】翳 Yi refers to a canopy made of feathers, which has a denotative meaning of the shelter. This acupoint is between KuFang (ST-14), a storehouse, and YingChuang (ST-16), a window. As a point in the middle, it is like an eave providing shelter against external pathogens for the chest. That is why it mainly treats diseases such as cough and panting. Hence the name 屋翳 WuYi.

【Location】In the second intercostal space, 4 cun lateral to the anterior midline.

【Indications】Cough, panting; fullness of the chest, acute mastitis.

16 膺窗 YingChuang ST-16

【Source】《黄帝明堂经》 *Huangdi Mingtang Jing*

【Annotation】膺 Ying means the chest. 窗 Chuang means a window for ventilation. This acupoint is on the chest and is good at dredging. It can promote the movement of stagnated qi in the chest, like opening the window for ventilation, hence it is named 膺窗 YingChuang.

【Location】In the third intercostal space, 4 cun lateral to the anterior midline.

【Indications】Fullness of the chest, panting, acute mastitis.

17 乳中 RuZhong ST-17

【Source】《黄帝明堂经》*Huangdi Mingtang Jing*

【Annotation】乳 Ru means the breast. 中 Zhong means center. This acupoint is at the center of the nipple, hence it is named 乳中 RuZhong.

【Location】At the center of the nipple.

【Indications】①Mania-depression, epilepsy; ②prolonged labor; ③acute mastitis.

18 乳根 RuGen ST-18

【Source】《黄帝明堂经》*Huangdi Mingtang Jing*

【Annotation】乳 Ru means the breast. 根 Gen means root and base. This acupoint is beneath the nipple and on the base of the breast, hence the name 乳根 RuGen.

【Location】In the fifth intercostal space, 4 cun lateral to the anterior midline.

【Indications】①Cough, panting, fullness of the chest, chest pain; ②acute mastitis, mammary hyperplasia, scanty lactation.

19 不容 BuRong ST-19

【Source】《黄帝明堂经》*Huangdi Mingtang Jing*

【Annotation】不 Bu means not. 容 Rong means to hold and to contain. This acupoint is 6 cun superior to the umbilicus, corresponding to the cardia. BuRong indicates that water and food would overflow here, and the stomach cannot hold anymore, hence the name 不容 BuRong.

【Location】6 cun superior to the center of the umbilicus, 2 cun lateral to the anterior midline.

【Indications】①Abdominal distention and vomiting, poor appetite; ②abdominal pain leading to the back.

20 承满 ChengMan ST-20

【Source】《黄帝明堂经》*Huangdi Mingtang Jing*

【Annotation】This acupoint is under BuRong (ST-19), corresponding to the upper part of the stomach. BuRong indicates that water and food would overflow, while ChengMan means that the amount of water and food is full at this point, hence the name 承满 ChengMan.

【Location】5 cun superior to the center of the umbilicus, 2 cun lateral to the anterior midline.

【Indications】Borborygmus, abdominal pain, abdominal distention, dysphagia-occlusion, hematemesis.

21 梁门 LiangMen ST-21

【Source】《黄帝明堂经》 *Huangdi Mingtang Jing*

【Annotation】梁 Liang means a bridge important for water and land transportation and is a metaphor of a key point. It is also an interchangeable word of 粮 Liang, which refers to water and food. The ancients believed that the stomach is the reservoir of water and grain. This acupoint and GuanMen (ST-22) correspond to the stomach and are essential gateways for the stomach qi to enter and exit. Hence it is named 梁门 LiangMen.

【Location】4 cun superior to the center of the umbilicus, 2 cun lateral to the anterior midline.

【Indications】Epigastric stuffiness and distention, abdominal pain, diarrhea, poor appetite.

22 关门 GuanMen ST-22

【Source】《黄帝明堂经》 *Huangdi Mingtang Jing*

【Annotation】关 Guan means to close. 门 Men refers to a gateway for entrance and exit. This acupoint is the gateway of the stomach, an essential place for water and food entering to intestines, hence it is named 关门 GuanMen.

【Location】3 cun superior to the center of the umbilicus, 2 cun lateral to the anterior midline.

【Indications】①Abdominal pain, tympanites, borborygmus, diarrhea; ②edema, enuresis.

23 太乙 TaiYi ST-23

【Source】《黄帝明堂经》 *Huangdi Mingtang Jing*

【Annotation】 太 Tai is an interchangeable word of 大 Da, which means huge. 乙 Yi is a hieroglyphic of fish intestines, according to *Er Ya*. This acupoint is 2 cun superior to the umbilicus, corresponding to the transverse colon that bends like the figure of 乙. It can treat intestinal diseases such as borborygmus and abdominal distention, hence it is named 太乙 TaiYi.

【Location】 2 cun superior to the center of the umbilicus, 2 cun lateral to the anterior midline.

【Indications】 ①Epilepsy, protruding tongue; ②abdominal pain, abdominal distention, vomiting.

24 滑肉门 HuaRouMen ST-24

【Source】《黄帝明堂经》 *Huangdi Mingtang Jing*

【Annotation】 滑 Hua means to dredge. 肉 Rou means flesh. This acupoint is located on soft and tender flesh, corresponding to peritoneal fat inside the belly. Besides, it belongs to the Stomach channel and is good at dealing with spleen and stomach diseases. Since it is vital for dredging the spleen and stomach to dry dampness and dispel phlegm, it is also commonly used to lose weight. Hence the name 滑肉门 HuaRouMen.

【Location】 1 cun superior to the center of the umbilicus, 2 cun lateral to the anterior midline.

【Indications】 ①Epilepsy, protruding tongue; ②abdominal pain, abdominal distention, vomiting.

25 天枢 TianShu ST-25 (Front-*Mu* point of the Large Intestine channel)

【Source】《黄帝明堂经》 *Huangdi Mingtang Jing*

【Annotation】 天 Tian means the sky. 枢 Shu means a hub. 天枢 TianShu is the Chinese name of the first star of the Big Dipper, presiding over the operation of stars in the sky as a hub. This acupoint is located at a vital place of the human body where it works as a hub of the upward, downward, inward, and outward movement of qi of the middle and lower energizers, hence it is named 天枢 TianShu.

【Location】Level with the center of the umbilicus, 2 cun lateral to the anterior midline.

【Indications】①Abdominal pain, abdominal distention, borborygmus, diarrhea, constipation; ②irregular menstruation, dysmenorrhea.

26 外陵 WaiLing ST-26

【Source】《黄帝明堂经》 *Huangdi Mingtang Jing*

【Annotation】 外 Wai means outside. 陵 Ling means mountains. When the abdomen exerts, the rectus abdominis bulges and forms the shape of a mountain. Hence the name 外陵 WaiLing.

【Location】1 cun inferior to the center of the umbilicus, 2 cun lateral to the anterior midline.

【Indications】Abdominal pain, abdominal distention.

27 大巨 DaJu ST-27

【Source】《黄帝明堂经》 *Huangdi Mingtang Jing*

【Annotation】巨 Ju has the same meaning as 大 Da, which is huge. This acupoint is surrounded by huge muscles on the abdominal wall, hence it is named 大巨 DaJu.

【Location】2 cun inferior to the center of the umbilicus, 2 cun lateral to the anterior midline.

【Indications】①Abdominal distention, abdominal pain; ②inhibited urination, hernia, seminal emission.

28 水道 ShuiDao ST-28

【Source】《黄帝明堂经》 *Huangdi Mingtang Jing*

【Annotation】水 Shui means water and fluid. 道 Dao means a passage. This acupoint corresponds to the bladder and mainly treats diseases of the kidney, bladder, and triple energizers such as dysuria. It can regulate the waterways, making water seep into the bladder, hence the name 水道 ShuiDao.

【Location】3 cun inferior to the center of the umbilicus, 2 cun lateral to the anterior midline.

【Indications】①Inhibited urination, distention and fullness of the lower abdomen, hypogastric pain in women extending to the genitals, hernia; ②dysmenorrhea, infertility.

29 归来 GuiLai ST-29

【Source】《黄帝明堂经》 *Huangdi Mingtang Jing*

【Annotation】归来 GuiLai means to return and come back. These two Chinese characters have the extended meaning of 'come back (to life)'. Needling at this acupoint can recover various prolapse diseases, hence the name 归来 GuiLai.

【Location】4 cun inferior to the center of the umbilicus, 2 cun lateral to the anterior midline.

【Indications】①Pain of the lower abdomen, hernia; ②swelling, pain and cold of the vagina, irregular menstruation.

30 气冲 QiChong ST-30

【Source】《黄帝明堂经》 *Huangdi Mingtang Jing*

【Annotation】There are two explanations for this name. Firstly, 冲 Chong refers to the thoroughfare vessel. The ancients believed that the thoroughfare vessel comes from the qi thoroughfare and then goes up with the Kidney channel beside the umbilicus. The qi thoroughfare is over the femoral artery, where QiChong locates. This acupoint is not only the qi thoroughfare of the Stomach channel but also where the qi of the thoroughfare vessel rushes through, hence the name 气冲 QiChong. It is also called 气街 QiJie, the Chinese name of qi thoroughfare. Secondly, 冲 Chong means to move and rush. Secondly, this acupoint is named after its function. It can mainly treat syndromes caused by qi ascending counterflow, such as hernia, running piglet, and pregnancy suspension.

【Location】In the groin, superior to the pubic symphysis, 2 cun lateral to the anterior midline, over the femoral artery.

【Indications】Hernia, irregular menstruation, infertility.

31 髀关 BiGuan ST-31

【Source】《黄帝明堂经》 *Huangdi Mingtang Jing*

【Annotation】 髀 Bi means the thigh. 关 Guan refers to a joint and especially means the hip joint here. This acupoint is at the anterior and superior part of the thigh, close to the hip joint, hence it is named 髀关 BiGuan.

【Location】 On the line connecting the anterior superior iliac spine with the lateral end of the base of the patella, level with the perineum and in the depression lateral to the sartorius muscle when bending the thigh.

【Indications】 Flaccidity and impediment of the lower limbs, inability to extend and bend the knee.

32 伏兔 FuTu ST-32

【Source】《黄帝明堂经》 *Huangdi Mingtang Jing*

【Annotation】 伏 Fu means lying down. 兔 Tu refers to a rabbit. This acupoint is 6 cun above the knee, on the rectus femoris. While squatting, the muscle bulges like a lying rabbit, hence the name 伏兔 FuTu.

【Location】 On the line connecting the anterior superior iliac spine with the lateral end of the base of the patella, 6 cun proximal to the base of the patella.

【Indications】 Flaccidity and impediment of the lower limbs, coldness of the knee, beriberi.

33 阴市 YinShi ST-33

【Source】《黄帝明堂经》 *Huangdi Mingtang Jing*

【Annotation】 市 Shi means a market. Although this acupoint belongs to a yang channel, it is mainly used to treat yin and cold syndromes, such as heaviness of the low back and legs, cold abdominal colic, flaccidity and impediment of the lower limbs, yin-dampness, and menstrual irregularities. It serves as a market where yin qi gathers, hence it is named 阴 市 YinShi.

【Location】 On the line connecting the anterior superior iliac spine with the lateral end of the base of the patella, 3 cun proximal to the base of the patella.

【Indications】Cold abdominal colic leading to knee pain, flaccidity and impediment of the lower limbs, inability to extend and bend the knee.

34 梁丘 LiangQiu ST-34 (*Xi*-Cleft point)

【Source】《黄帝明堂经》*Huangdi Mingtang Jing*

【Annotation】梁 Liang means the protruding part of an object. 丘 Qiu refers to a small mound, which also means protrusion. This acupoint is 2 cun above the knee, in the cleft between the vastus lateralis and the rectus femoris muscles, where the muscles bulge like a highland, hence it is named 梁丘 LiangQiu.

【Location】On the line connecting the anterior superior iliac spine with the lateral end of the base of the patella, 2 cun proximal to the base of the patella.

【Indications】①Stomachache; ②acute mastitis, breast pain; ③swelling and pain of the knee, motor impairment of the lower limbs.

35 犊鼻 DuBi ST-35

【Source】《素问·气府论》《灵枢·本输》*Suwen: Qifu Lun, Lingshu: Benshu*

【Annotation】犊 Du refers to a calf. 鼻 Bi means the nose. This acupoint is in the depression lateral to the patellar ligament, hence it is also known as 外膝眼 WaiXiYan. (外 Wai means outer. 膝 Xi means the knee. 眼 Yan means the eye and can refer to depression in the Chinese context.) The kneecap is oval, and the inner and outer XiYan are at the lower border of the knee, similar to the nostrils of calves, hence the name 犊鼻 DuBi. The Stomach channel belongs to the earth (one of the five phases), and so does 坤 Kun in Bagua (the Eight Diagrams). It is named after a calf's nose instead of a pig's or a sheep's because *YiJing* says Kun corresponds to a cow.

【Location】In the depression lateral to the patellar ligament.

【Indications】Swelling and pain of the knee, inability to extend and bend the knee, beriberi.

36 足三里 ZuSanLi ST-36 (*He*-Sea point, Lower *He*-Sea point of the Stomach)

【Source】Presented as 三里 SanLi in《黄帝内经》*Huangdi Neijing*, and as 足三里 ZuSanLi in《太平圣惠方》*Taiping Shenghui Fang*.

【Annotation】三 San refers to three, there are two explanations for this name. First, 三里 SanLi means 3 cun. This acupoint is 3 cun inferior to the knee, on the lateral side of the tibia, hence the name. Second, 里 Li is an interchangeable word of 理 Li, which means to manage and to deal with. 三里 SanLi indicates that this acupoint can deal with symptoms of the upper, middle, and lower abdomen, such as stomachache, vomiting, abdominal distention, and diarrhea, thus enhance the function of spleen and stomach. So it is always used as a vital point for health care. This point is located on the lower limbs, so named 足三里 ZuSanLi to be distinguished from ShouSanLi (LI10).

【Location】3 cun inferior to ST-35, one fingerbreadth lateral to the anterior tibial crest.

【Indications】①Stomachache, vomiting, hiccup, abdominal distention, abdominal pain, borborygmus, diarrhea, constipation; ② febrile disease, mania-depression; ③ acute mastitis; ④weakness and thinness caused by consumptive diseases; ⑤swelling and pain of the knee and feet.

37 上巨虚 ShangJuXu ST-37 (Lower *He*-Sea point of the Large Intestine)

【Source】Presented as 巨虚上廉 JuXuShangLian in《黄帝内经》*Huangdi Neijing*, and as 上巨虚 ShangJuXu in《铜人腧穴针灸图经》*Tongren Shuxue Zhenjiu Tujing*.

【Annotation】上 Shang means the upper. 巨虚 JuXu refers to a big gap. In the big gap between the tibia and fibula on the lateral side of the shank, there are two acupoints on the upper and the lower end respectively. This acupoint is the former one, hence the name 上巨虚 ShangJuXu. As the lower *He*-Sea point of the Large Intestine, it is good at treating intestinal diseases such as borborygmus, diarrhea, constipation, and intestinal abscess.

【Location】6 cun inferior to ST-35, one fingerbreadth lateral to the anterior tibial crest.

【Indications】①Abdominal pain, diarrhea, constipation, borborygmus, acute mastitis; ②hemiplegia, flaccidity and impediment of the lower limbs, beriberi.

38 条口 TiaoKou ST-38

【Source】《黄帝明堂经》 *Huangdi Mingtang Jing*

【Annotation】条 Tiao describes long and narrow. 口 Kou means a gap. This acupoint is in the same narrow gap with ShangJuXu (ST-37) and XiaJuXu (ST-39), with the former on the upper end and the latter on the lower end. It is between them, hence the name 条　口 TiaoKou.

【Location】8 cun inferior to ST-35, one fingerbreadth lateral to the anterior tibial crest.

【Indications】Flaccidity and impediment of the lower limbs.

39 下巨虚 XiaJuXu ST-39 (Lower *He*-Sea point of the Small Intestine)

【Source】Presented as 巨虚下廉 JuXuXiaLian in《黄帝内经》 *Huangdi Neijing*, and as 上巨虚 XiaJuXu in《铜人腧穴针灸图经》 *Tongren Shuxue Zhenjiu Tujing*.

【Annotation】下 Xia means the lower. 巨虚 JuXu refers to a big gap. In the big gap between the tibia and fibula on the lateral side of the shank, there are two acupoints on the upper and the lower end respectively. This acupoint is the latter one, hence the name 下　巨虚 XiaJuXu. As the lower *He*-Sea point of the Small Intestine, it is good at treating small intestinal diseases such as abdominal pain and diarrhea, as well as flaccidity and impediment of lower limbs.

【Location】9 cun inferior to ST-35, one fingerbreadth lateral to the anterior tibial crest.

【Indications】①Lower abdominal pain, diarrhea, lumbar pain radiating to the testicles; ②acute mastitis; ③hemiplegia, flaccidity and impediment of the lower limbs.

40 丰隆 FengLong ST-40 (*Luo*-Connecting point of the Stomach channel)

【Source】《灵枢·经脉》 *LingShu: Jingmai*

【Annotation】There are two explanations for this name. Firstly, 丰 Feng means plump. 隆 Long refers to a bulge. This acupoint is between the tibialis anterior and extensor digitorum longus, where the muscles are plump and bulged. 丰 Feng also means plenty. This acupoint belongs to the Stomach channel, which contains plenty of qi and blood, hence the name 丰隆 FengLong. Secondly, the god of thunder in China used to be called 丰隆 FengLong, and the word was borrowed to represent thunder sounds. This acupoint is on the lower limbs of the human body. It can treat symptoms caused by diffused yin–qi, such as phlegm stagnation in the chest and diaphragm, dizziness, and headache, with a noticeable effect of dispelling phlegm and draining dampness like thunder. A thunder rises from the earth and becomes dark clouds that bring storms. After the storms, the dark clouds dissipate. Therefore, this acupoint is named 丰隆 FengLong, which implies clouds and thunder.

【Location】8 cun superior to the prominence of the lateral malleolus, lateral to ST–38, two fingerbreadths lateral to the anterior tibial crest.

【Indications】①Abdominal pain, abdominal distention, constipation; ②cough, asthma, copious phlegm, swelling and pain of the throat, chest pain; ③headache with dizziness, mania–depression; ④motor impairment, flaccidity and impediment of the lower limbs.

41 解溪 JieXi ST–41 (*Jing*–River point)

【Source】《灵枢·本输》 *Lingshu: Benshu*

【Annotation】解 Jie means to untie. 溪 Xi means a stream and refers to the small gap or depression between tendons here. This acupoint is on the ankle, where the shoelaces are untied, so it is named 解 Jie. It is in the depression at the center of the horizontal crease on the dorsum of the foot, between the tendons of the extensor hallucis longus and the extensor digitorum longus, like a stream, hence the name 溪 Xi.

【Location】On the ankle, in the depression at the center of the front surface of the ankle, between the tendons of extensor hallucis longus and extensor digitorum longus.

【Indications】①Headache, dizziness, mania–depression; ②abdominal distention, constipation; ③flaccidity and impediment of the lower limbs, weakness of the ankle joint.

42 冲阳 ChongYang ST–42 (*Yuan*–Source point)

【Source】《灵枢·本输》《灵枢·根结》 *Lingshu: Benshu, Lingshu: Genjie*

【Annotation】冲 Chong means impulse. 阳 Yang, here refers to the dorsum of the foot. This acupoint is over the dorsalis pedis artery (also known as 趺阳脉 anterior tibial pulse), where the impulse can be sensed by hand, hence the name 冲阳 ChongYang.

【Location】On the highest part of the dorsum of the foot, over the dorsalis pedis artery, between the tendons of extensor hallucis longus and extensor digitorum longus.

【Indications】①Stomachache, abdominal distention; ②deviation of the mouth and eye, toothache, swelling of the face; ③mania-depression; ④atrophy, weakness, swelling, and pain of the feet.

43 陷谷 XianGu ST-43 (*Shu*-Stream point)

【Source】《灵枢·本输》*Lingshu: Benshu*

【Annotation】陷 Xian means to sink. 谷 Gu refers to a valley between mountains. This acupoint is in front of the joint of the second and third metatarsal bones, sunken like a valley, hence it is named 陷谷 XianGu.

【Location】Between the second and third metatarsal bones, in the depression proximal to the second metatarsophalangeal joint.

【Indications】 ①Abdominal pain, borborygmus; ②swelling of the face, oedema; ③swelling and pain of the dorsum of the foot.

44 内庭 NeiTing ST-44 (*Ying*-Spring point)

【Source】《灵枢·本输》*Lingshu: Benshu*

【Annotation】内 Nei means internal. 庭 Ting means a hall. 内庭 NeiTing is a hall inside a door. The channel qi of the stomach passes to LiDui (ST-45) through this point, and then reaches YinBai (SP-1). LiDui is the next acupoint of this channel and according to *YiJing*, Dui corresponds to the door in the Eight Diagrams Theory. Hence the name 内庭 NeiTing. As the *Ying*-Spring point, a kind of point in charge of heat in the body, of the Stomach channel, this acupoint is good at clearing stomach fire, mainly treating toothache, swelling of the throat, nosebleed, constipation, and other diseases caused by stomach fire.

【Location】Between the second and third toes, at the border between the red and white flesh posterior to the web margin.

【Indications】①Toothache, swelling and pain of the throat, nosebleed, deviation of the mouth and eye; ②abdominal distention, diarrhea, poor appetite; ③febrile disease; ④swelling and pain of the dorsum of the foot.

45 厉兑 LiDui ST-45 (*Jing*-Well point)

【Source】《灵枢·本输》《灵枢·根结》*Lingshu: Benshu, Lingshu: Genjie*

【Annotation】There are two explanations for its name. First, 厉 Li refers to the dangous brink of shore. This acupoint is about 0.1 cun proximal-lateral to the corner of the second toenail, like being on the shore, hence the word 厉 Li. 兑 Dui refers to the door, according to *YiJing*. As the last point of the Stomach channel, this acupoint is a door for the entrance and exit of the channel qi. Hence it is named 厉兑 LiDui. Secondly, 厉 Li is the original word of 砺 Li, meaning a hard grindstone. 兑 Dui is an interchangeable word of 锐 Rui, which means sharp. As a *Jing*-Well point, this acupoint is located at the sharp point of the toe. Meanwhile, it corresponds to metal in the five phases theory, hence named 厉兑 LiDui.

【Location】On the lateral side to the distal phalanx of the second toe, 0.1 cun proximal-lateral to the lateral corner of the second toenail.

【Indications】 ①Nosebleed, toothache, swelling of the face, deviation of the mouth and eye, swelling and pain of the throat; ②febrile disease, mania-depression, dreaminess, easily frightened, loss of consciousness.

Chapter 5
The Spleen Channel Points of Foot Taiyin

1 隐白 YinBai SP-1 (*Jing*–Well point)

【Source】《灵枢·本输》*Lingshu: Benshu*

【Annotation】隐 Yin means to be hidden and bred. 白 Bai refers to white, a color corresponding to metal according to the five phases theory, thus indicating the Lung channel of Hand Taiyin. This acupoint is the *Jing*–Well point of the Spleen channel, from which the channel qi departs and then flows up to the chest to connect with the Lung channel through ZhongFu (LU-1). YinBai implies that metal is hidden in the earth, indicating that the spleen breeds the lung as a mother. Therefore, this acupoint can not only treat spleen and stomach diseases as well as symptoms of the spleen failing to control the blood, such as abdominal distention, hematochezia, and metrorrhagia, but also treat symptoms caused by lung qi ascending counterflow, such as panting and fullness of the chest leading to insomnia. Hence it is named 隐白 YinBai.

【Location】On the medial aspect of the great toe, 0.1 cun posterior to the corner of the nail.

【Indications】①Abdominal distention, diarrhea, vomiting; menorrhagia; ②hematochezia, hematuria, nosebleed; ③loss of consciousness.

2 大都 DaDu SP-2 (*Ying*–Spring point)

【Source】《灵枢·本输》*Lingshu: Benshu*

【Annotation】大 Da refers to great. 都 Du refers to a city which has an extended meaning of gathering. This acupoint is like a great city for the channel qi of the Spleen channel to gather and get abundant. Hence the name 大都 DaDu.

【Location】On the medial side of the foot, in the depression at the border between the red and white flesh distal and inferior to the first metatarsophalangeal joint.

【Indications】①Abdominal distention, stomachache, diarrhea, constipation; ②fever.

3 太白 TaiBai SP-3 (*Shu*-Stream and *Yuan*-Source point)

【Source】《灵枢·九针十二原》《灵枢·本输》*Lingshu: Jiuzhen Shieryuan, Lingshu: Benshu*

【Annotation】太 Tai refers to big and great. This acupoint is at the border between the red and white flesh proximal to the medial side of the big toe. 白 Bai is a color corresponding to metal according to the five phases theory. This acupoint is the *Shu*-Stream and Earth point of the Spleen channel, thus strengthening the earth (spleen) to generate metal (lung). Hence it is named 太白 TaiBai.

【Location】In the depression at the border between the red and white flesh proximal and inferior to the first metatarsophalangeal joint.

【Indications】①Stomachache, abdominal distention, borborygmus, diarrhea, constipation; ②heavy body with painful joints.

4 公孙 GongSun SP-4 (*Luo*-Connecting point, Confluent point of the thoroughfare vessel)

【Source】《灵枢·经脉》*Lingshu: JingMai*

【Annotation】公 Gong means the concourse, a collection of branches. 孙 Sun means branches and collaterals. This acupoint is the *Luo*-Connecting point of the Spleen channel, connecting the main channel of the Spleen (as the concourse) with the collateral vessels of the Stomach channel (as branches). Hence the name 公孙 GongSun.

【Location】At the border between the red and white flesh distal and inferior to the base of the first metatarsal bone.

【Indications】①Stomachache, vomiting, abdominal pain, abdominal distention, diarrhea; ②dysphoria.

5 商丘 ShangQiu SP-5 (*Jing*-River point)

【Source】《灵枢·本输》*Lingshu: Benshu*

【Annotation】商 Shang is one of the five notes of the ancient Chinese pentatonic scale, subsumed to metal according to the five phases theory. 丘 Qiu refers to a hill. This acupoint is the *Jing*-River point of the Spleen channel, which also corresponds to metal. It is in the depression anterior to the medial malleolus, which bulges like a hill. Hence it is named 商丘 ShangQiu.

【Location】In the depression distal and inferior to the medial malleolus, at the midpoint of the line connecting the tubercle of scaphoid bone with the tip of the medial malleolus. At the junction of the straight line drawn along the anterior border of the medial malleolus and the transverse line drawn along its inferior border.

【Indications】①Abdominal distention, diarrhea, constipation, hemorrhoids; ②ankle pain, hernia leading to pain of the knee and thigh.

6 三阴交 SanYinJiao SP-6 (Meeting point of the Spleen, Liver and Kidney channels)

【Source】《千金翼方·针灸》*QianJinYiFang: ZhenJiu*

【Annotation】三阴 SanYin refers to three yin channels of the foot, to be specific, the spleen, liver and kidney channels. 交 Jiao means to meet. This acupoint is the meeting point of the three yin channels mentioned above, treating diseases they govern. Meanwhile, it is the first choice for genitourinary system diseases relating to menstruation, labor[①], uterus, and spermary. Hence the name 三阴交 SanYinJiao.

【Location】3 cun superior to the prominence of the medial malleolus, posterior to the medial border of the tibia.

【Indications】①Irregular menstruation, flooding and spotting, leucorrhoea disease, uterine prolapse, infertility, prolonged labor; ②seminal emission, impotence, enuresis, difficult urination, hernia; ③abdominal distention, borborygmus, diarrhea; ④flaccidity and

---

① Do not needle at this acupoint for pregnant women. Since this acupoint and HeGu (LI-4) can promote uterine contraction, electro-acupuncture at these two points to promote labor has been reported in the literature.

impediment of the lower limbs.

7 漏谷 LouGu SP-7

【Source】《黄帝明堂经》 *Huangdi Mingtang Jing*

【Annotation】 There are two explanations for this name. Firstly, 漏 Lou means to leak. 谷 refers to depression. This acupoint is considered the *Luo*-Connecting point of the Spleen channel[①], whose collateral vessels leak from this point to another channel, hence named 漏 Lou. Since this acupoint is in the depression posterior to the medial border of the tibia, it is named 谷 Gu. Secondly, 谷 Gu also refers to corn. 漏谷 LouGu means leaking corns, indicating that this acupoint can treat indigestion, abdominal distension, and borborygmus caused by dyspepsia. Therefore, the ancients believed in using DiJi (SP-8), LouGu, and GongSun (SP-4) to treat malnutrition caused by dyspepsia.

【Location】 On the medial side of the shank, on the line connecting the prominence of the medial malleolus and YinLingQuan (SP-9), 6 cun superior to the prominence of the medial malleolus, posterior to the medial border of the tibia.

【Indications】 ①Abdominal distention, borborygmus; ②difficult urination, seminal emission, hernia; ③flaccidity and impediment of the lower limbs.

8 地机 DiJi SP-8 (*Xi*-Cleft point)

【Source】《黄帝明堂经》 *Huangdi Mingtang Jing*

【Annotation】 地 Di means land, the carrier of the earth, and the spleen is subsumed to earth according to the five phases theory. Therefore, 地 Di refers to the Spleen channel here. 机 Ji means the key point. As the *Xi*-Cleft point of the Spleen channel, this acupoint is the key point where qi and blood of this channel accumulate deeply. Hence it is named 地机 DiJi.

【Location】 3 cun below YinLingQuan (SP-9), posterior to the medial border of the tibia.

【Indications】 ①Abdominal distention, diarrhea; ②irregular menstruation, hernia.

---

① 《针灸穴名解》 *Zhenjiu Xuemingjie* says this acupoint is also called the *Luo*-Connecting point of Taiyin. Since it is located on the opposite side of FengLong (ST-40), the *Luo*-Connecting point of the Foot Yangming, it is suspected of connecting with the Stomach channel. Hence the name.

9 阴陵泉 YinLingQuan SP-9 (*He*-Sea point)

【Source】Presented as 阴之陵泉 LingQuan of Yin in《灵枢》*Lingshu*, and as 阴陵泉 YinLingQuan in《黄帝明堂经》*Huangdi Mingtang Jing*.

【Annotation】阴 Yin means yin side. 陵 Ling means a peak. 泉 Quan means a spring. This acupoint is in the depression posterior and inferior to the medial condyle of the tibia, like a deep spring on the yin side of a peak. Hence the name 阴陵泉 YinLingQuan.

【Location】In the depression formed by the inferior border of the medial condyle of the tibia and the posterior border of the tibia.

【Indications】①Abdominal pain, abdominal distention, diarrhea; ②pain of the genitals of women, dysmenorrhea, difficult urination, enuresis, seminal emission; oedema; ③aching pain of the lumbar and knee.

10 血海 XueHai SP-10

【Source】《黄帝明堂经》*Huangdi Mingtang Jing*

【Annotation】血 Xue means blood. 海 Hai means a sea where hundreds of streams converge. This acupoint mainly treats blood disorders and syndromes of blood failing to stay in the channels, such as flooding and spotting, irregular menstruation and amenorrhea, with the function of guiding blood back to its channel, like guiding the torrent into the sea. Hence the name 血海 XueHai.

【Location】2 cun proximal to the medial and superior border of the patella, on the bulge of the vastus medialis muscle.

【Indications】①Irregular menstruation, amenorrhea, flooding and spotting; ②eczema, rubella.

11 箕门 JiMen SP-11

【Source】《黄帝明堂经》*Huangdi Mingtang Jing*

【Annotation】箕 Ji refers to a dustpan. 门 Men means a gateway. This acupoint is on the inner side of the thigh. Since it needs to be selected with two legs spread apart, with the front large and the rear small, resembling a dustpan, it is named 箕门 JiMen.

【Location】On the line connecting XueHai (SP–10) and ChongMen (SP–12), 6 cun superior to XueHai.

【Indications】①Obstructed urination, enuresis; ②pain and swelling of the inguinal region.

12 冲门 ChongMen SP-12 (Meeting point of the Spleen and Liver channels with the Yin Linking vessel)

【Source】《黄帝明堂经》*Huangdi Mingtang Jing*

【Annotation】冲 Chong means to rush. 门 Men means a gateway. This acupoint is lateral to the pulsating external iliac artery in the groin, parallel to QiChong (ST–30), and is the gateway for the qi of the Spleen channel to rush into the abdomen. Hence the name 冲 门 ChongMen.

【Location】Lateral to the groin, 3.5 cun lateral to the midpoint on the superior margin of the public symphysis, lateral to the external iliac artery.

【Indications】①Abdominal distention, pain caused by abdominal masses; ②hernia, dribbling and retention of urine; ③prolonged labor.

13 府舍 FuShe SP-13 (Meeting point of the Spleen and Liver channels with the Yin Linking vessel)

【Source】《黄帝明堂经》*Huangdi Mingtang Jing*

【Annotation】府舍 FuShe refers to a house. This acupoint is located on the lower abdomen, serving as a house that stores the source qi of viscera and bowels. Hence it is named 府舍 FuShe.

【Location】4 cun inferior to the center of the umbilicus, 0.7 cun superior to ChongMen (SP–12), 4 cun lateral to the anterior midline.

【Indications】①Hernia of women; ②abdominal pain, abdominal distention, abdominal masses, vomiting, diarrhea.

14 腹结 FuJie SP-14

【Source】《黄帝明堂经》*Huangdi Mingtang Jing*

【Annotation】腹 Fu means the abdomen. 结 Jie means a hard knot. When the lower abdomen is exerted, the muscles at this acupoint become hard as a knot. Meanwhile, it is good at treating syndromes of aggregation–accumulation in the abdomen, such as abdominal pain, constipation, and hernia. Hence the name 腹结 FuJie.

【Location】1.3 cun inferior to DaHeng (SP–15), 4 cun lateral to the anterior midline.

【Indications】Periumbilical pain, diarrhea.

15 大横 DaHeng SP–15 (Meeting point of the Spleen channel with the Yin Linking vessel)

【Source】《黄帝明堂经》 Huangdi Mingtang Jing

【Annotation】横 Heng means to be flush with something. This acupoint is 4 cun lateral to the umbilicus and is flush with it. Hence it is named 大横 DaHeng.

【Location】4 cun lateral to the center of the umbilicus.

【Indications】Abdominal pain, diarrhea, constipation.

16 腹哀 FuAi SP–16 (Meeting point of the Spleen channel with the Yin Linking vessel)

【Source】《黄帝明堂经》 Huangdi Mingtang Jing

【Annotation】哀 Ai refers to moan, which indicates bowel sounds here. Located at the upper abdomen, this acupoint is mainly used to treat dyspepsia, abdominal pain, and borborygmus, like the moan of the abdomen. Hence the name 腹哀 FuAi.

【Location】3 cun superior to the center of the umbilicus, 4 cun lateral to the anterior midline.

【Indications】Dysentery with pus and blood, abdominal pain, constipation, undigested food in the stool.

17 食窦 ShiDou SP–17

【Source】《黄帝明堂经》 Huangdi Mingtang Jing

【Annotation】食 Shi means food. 窦 Dou means a hole where something goes through. The Spleen channel goes through this point onto the chest and lungs, with the essential qi from food penetrating the diaphragm to enhance the lung qi. Hence the name 食 窦 ShiDou. This acupoint has the function of soothing the chest and diaphragm and unclogging the esophagus, so its name can also be understood as the esophagus.

【Location】In the fifth intercostal space, 6 cun lateral to the anterior midline.

【Indications】Fullness of the chest, hypochondriac pain.

18 天溪 TianXi SP-18

【Source】《黄帝明堂经》 *Huangdi Mingtang Jing*

【Annotation】天 Tian refers to the upper part of human body above the diaphragm. 溪 Xi means a stream. This acupoint is located on the chest, in the depression of the intercostal space lateral to the breast. It is named 天溪 TianXi because the depression is long and narrow, like a stream.

【Location】In the fourth intercostal space, 6 cun lateral to the anterior midline.

【Indications】①Pain of the chest, cough, panting; ②acute mastitis.

19 胸乡 XiongXiang SP-19

【Source】《黄帝明堂经》 *Huangdi Mingtang Jing*

【Annotation】胸 Xiong refers to the chest. 乡 Xiang means a location. This acupoint is located on the flat part of the lateral thorax and is named 胸乡 XiongXiang because of its location.

【Location】In the third intercostal space, 6 cun lateral to the anterior midline.

【Indications】Pain and swelling of the chest and lateral costal region extending to the back.

20 周荣 ZhouRong SP-20

【Source】《黄帝明堂经》 *Huangdi Mingtang Jing*

【Annotation】周 Zhou refers to the whole body. 荣 Rong, an interchangeable word for 营 Ying, means nutrition. This acupoint belongs to the Spleen channel. Since the spleen governs muscles and controls the blood, acupuncturing at this point can control the blood and spread the essence to nourish our whole body. Hence the name 周荣 ZhouRong.

【Location】In the second intercostal space, 6 cun lateral to the anterior midline.

【Indications】Distention and fullness of the chest and lateral costal region, panting, coughing with pus and blood.

21 大包 DaBao SP-21 (Great *Luo*-Connecting point of the Spleen)

【Source】《灵枢·经脉》*Lingshu: Jingmai*

【Annotation】大 Da means great and vast. 包 Bao means to hold and contain. This acupoint is called the Great *Luo*-Connecting point of the Spleen because it can hold everything by governing yin and yang collaterals and then dispersing essence to irrigate five viscera and six bowels with spleen qi. Stimulating this point can invigorate the spleen qi, promoting the function of transportation and transformation, governing the intake and metabolism of nutrition, and regulating the reasonable distribution of water and fluid. Therefore, it can treat unexplained heaviness, pain, and weakness of the whole body, as well as obesity and edema caused by spleen dysfunction.

【Location】In the sixth intercostal space, on the mid-axillary line.

【Indications】Hypochondriac pain, pain in the whole body, weariness of the limbs.

Chapter 6
The Heart Channel Points of Hand Shaoyin

1 极泉 JiQuan HE-1

【Source】《黄帝明堂经》 *Huangdi Mingtang Jing*

【Annotation】极 Ji means extremely high. 泉 Quan means spring, the source of water. The acupoint is located at the summit of the Heart channel of Hand Shaoyin, which is a metaphor for the meridian qi flowing down like water from a very high spring, hence it is named 极泉 JiQuan.

【Location】In the depression at the center of the axilla, where the axillary artery pulsates.

【Indications】①Heart pain; ②retching, dry throat; ③scrofula; ④hypochondriac pain, pain of the shoulder and arm.

2 青灵 QingLing HE-2

【Source】《太平圣惠方·明堂》 *Taiping Shenghui Fang: Mingtang*

【Annotation】青 Qing means the color of the first birth of all things. 灵 Ling means spirit, which is stored in the heart. This acupoint belongs to the Heart channel of Hand Shaoyin. *Su Wen: Liujie Zangxiang Lun* mentioned that the heart is the root of life and the place where the spirit resides, hence the name 青灵 QingLing.

【Location】3 cun proximal to the medial end of the transverse cubital crease, in the groove medial to the biceps brachii muscle.

【Indications】①Goiter; ②axillary pain, pain of the shoulder and arm.

3 少海 ShaoHai HE-3 (*He*-Sea point)

【Source】《黄帝明堂经》 *Huangdi Mingtang Jing*

【Annotation】少 Shao means the Heart channel of Hand Shaoyin. 海 Hai, the place where rivers confluence. 少海 ShaoHai, is the He-Sea and Water point of the Heart channel of Hand Shaoyin, where the channel qi of this channel converges, hence it is named 少海 ShaoHai, a metaphor for the sea of Shaoyin.

【Location】At the same level as the transverse cubital crease, anterior to the medial epicondyle of humerus.

【Indications】①Heart pain; ②vomiting; ③scrofula; ④hypochondriac pain, axillary pain, spasm pain of the elbow and arm.

4 灵道 LingDao HE-4 (*Jing*-River point)

【Source】《黄帝明堂经》 *Huangdi Mingtang Jing*

【Annotation】灵 Ling means spirit, which is stored in the heart, hence it is named 灵 Ling. 道 Dao means passage. This acupoint is the river point of the Heart channel of Hand Shaoyin, where the channel qi travels like water flowing in an unobstructed river, and refers to the passage through which the channel qi of the Heart channel passes, hence it is named 灵道 LingDao. It is an important acupoint for the treatment of coronary atherosclerotic heart disease and angina pectoris.

【Location】On the radial side of the tendon of flexor carpi ulnaris, 1.5 cun proximal to the palmar wrist crease.

【Indications】①Heart pain, moody and restless; ②sudden loss of voice; ③spasm of the elbow and arm.

5 通里 TongLi HE-5 (*Luo*-Connecting point)

【Source】《灵枢·经脉》 *Lingshu: Jingmai*

【Annotation】通 Tong means to pass through or penetrate. 里 Li means inside. This acupoint is the connecting point of the Heart channel of Hand Shaoyin. Its collateral vessel branches out from this acupoint, turns upwards and follows the meridian into the heart, where it is associated with the tongue and attributed to the eye. It also leads to the corresponding superficial and internal meridian, bridging the two meridians and supplementing the circulation of the meridians, hence it is named 通里 TongLi.

【Location】On the radial side of the tendon of flexor carpi ulnaris, 1 cun proximal to the palmar wrist crease.

【Indications】①Palpitation, heart pain; ②swelling and pain in throat, sudden loss of voice; ③contraction of the elbow and arm.

6 阴郄 **YinXi HE-6** (*Xi*-Cleft point)

【Source】《黄帝明堂经》 *Huangdi Mingtang Jing*

【Annotation】阴 Yin means the Heart channel of Hand Shaoyin. 郄 Xi, same as 隙 Xi in Chinese, means cleft aperture and void, also means the cleft point. This acupoint is the cleft point of the Heart channel of Hand Shaoyin. It is the cleft where the qi and blood of the Heart channel gather deeply, hence it is named 阴郄 YinXi. It has the capability of enriching yin and nourishing the blood, so it is mostly used for symptoms of heart yin deficiency such as steaming bone and night sweating, insomnia due to vexation.

【Location】On the radial side of the tendon of flexor carpi ulnaris, 0.5 cun proximal to the palmar wrist crease.

【Indications】①Heart pain, palpitation; ②hemoptysis, steaming bone and night sweating; epistaxis.

7 神门 **ShenMen HE-7** (*Shu*-Stream point and *Yuan*-Source point)

【Source】《黄帝明堂经》 *Huangdi Mingtang Jing*

【Annotation】神 Shen means spirit and consciousness, which is stored in the heart. 门 Men means a gate for entry and exit. This acupoint is the source point of the Heart channel of Hand Shaoyin, where the heart qi enters and exits. It also treats fear, palpitation, dullness, dementia, forgetfulness, madness, epilepsy, and other disorders of the mind, hence it is named 神门 ShenMen.

【Location】At the wrist joint, ulnar to the palmar wrist crease, on the radial side of flexor carpi ulnaris.

【Indications】Heart pain, vexation, palpitation, dementia, forgetfulness, insomnia, manic psychosis, epilepsy.

8 少府 ShaoFu HE-8 (*Ying*–Spring point)

【Source】《黄帝明堂经》*Huangdi Mingtang Jing*

【Annotation】少 Shao means Shaoyin, also means small. 府 Fu means to gather. This acupoint is where the channel qi of the Heart channel of Hand Shaoyin gathers, hence it is named 少府 ShaoFu.

【Location】At the same level as the fifth metacarpophalangeal joint, in the depression between the forth and fifth metacarpal bones, where the tip of the little finger rests when a fist is made. At the same level as 劳宫 LaoGong.

【Indications】①Palpitation, agitation and fullness, chest pain; ②pain of the arm and elbow, heat of the palms, spasm of fingers.

9 少冲 ShaoChong HE-9 (*Jing*–Well point)

【Source】《黄帝明堂经》*Huangdi Mingtang Jing*

【Annotation】少 Shao means the Heart channel of Hand Shaoyin, also means small, a metaphor for the meridian qi being young. 冲 Chong means important place, and here refers to the place where meridian qi of Yin and Yang pass through. This acupoint is the well point of the Heart channel of Hand Shaoyin. The acupoint where the channel qi emerges is like the source of water, indicating that the channel qi is young and not yet in abundance. This acupoint is where the Heart channel of Hand Shaoyin and the Small Intestine channel of Hand Taiyang meet, hence it is named 少冲 ShaoChong. Besides, a well is a place where water pumps out, so 冲 Chong also means to pump and to rush through. The acupoint treats diseases including agitation and fullness, qi going upward, heart deficiency, heat stagnation, halitosis, and throat impediment with its functions of flushing and harmonizing.

【Location】On the little finger, radial to the distal phalanx, approximately 0.1 cun from the corner of the nail.

【Indications】①Heart pain, palpitation, vexation, loss of consciousness; ②pain of the lateral costal region.

Chapter 7
The Small Intestine Channel Points of Hand Taiyang

1 少泽 **ShaoZe SI-1** (*Jing*–Well point)

【Source】《灵枢·本输》*Lingshu: Benshu*

【Annotation】少 Shao means small. 泽 Ze means glossy and moist. This acupoint is the *Jing*-Well point of the Small Intestine channel of Hand Taiyang, located at the end of the little finger of the hand, from which the channel qi emanates with weak strength. Hence it is named 少 泽 ShaoZe. By virtue of its capability to moisten, 少 泽 ShaoZe has the capability of treating symptoms such as heat in the mouth, vexation, throat impediment, corneal opacity, stiff tongue, etc.

【Location】On the little finger, ulnar to the distal phalanx, approximately 0.1 cun from the corner of the nail.

【Indications】①Acute mastitis, oligogalactia; ②corneal opacity, sore throat; ③heat disease, coma; ④headache, stiffness and pain of the neck.

2 前谷 **QianGu SI-2** (*Ying*–Spring point)

【Source】《灵枢·本输》*Lingshu: Benshu*

【Annotation】前 Qian means before, as opposed to after. 谷 Gu means valley refers to a place between two mountains. This acupoint is located in front of the metacarpophalangeal joint of the little finger of the hand, where the depression is like a valley, hence it is named 前 谷 QianGu.

【Location】On the ulnar border of the little finger, in a depression just distal to the metacarpophalangeal joint, at the border between the red and white flesh.

【Indications】①Eye pain, tinnitus, sore throat; ②acute mastitis, oligogalactia; ③heat disease, mania–depression; ④headache, stiffness and pain of the neck; ⑤swelling and pain of finger.

3 后溪 HouXi SI–3 (*Shu*–Stream point, Confluent point of the Governor vessel)

【Source】《灵枢·本输》*Lingshu: Benshu*

【Annotation】后 Hou, an orientation word which means behind the phalanx of the little finger of the hand. 溪 Xi means stream. This acupoint is located at the top of the transverse crease behind the metacarpophalangeal joint of the little finger of the hand. The flesh on the outside of the metacarpophalangeal joint of the little finger rises like a peak when clenched in a fist and looks like a small stream when pressed, hence it is named 后溪 HouXi.

【Location】On the ulnar border of the hand, in the depression proximal to the fifth metacarpophalangeal joint, at the border between the red and white flesh.

【Indications】①Deafness, redness and pain of the eyes, epistaxis; ②mania–depression; ③malaria; ④headache, stiffness and pain of the neck, pain of the elbow and arm.

4 腕骨 WanGu SI–4 (*Yuan*–Source point)

【Source】《灵枢·本输》*Lingshu: Benshu*

【Annotation】腕骨 WanGu means wrist bone. This acupoint is in the depression in front of the wrist, near the wrist bone (known as the pisiform bone in anatomy). The acupoint and the bone are of the same name. Hence the name 腕骨 WanGu.

【Location】In the depression between the base of the fifth metacarpal bone and the triquetral bone, at the border between the red and white flesh.

【Indications】①Tinnitus, corneal opacity; ②jaundice; ③heat disease, convulsion, hy perspasmia; ④malaria; ⑤headache, stiffness and pain of the neck, pain of the shoulder, arm, wrist and finger.

5 阳谷 YangGu SI–5 (*Jing*–River point)

【Source】《灵枢·本输》*Lingshu: Benshu*

【Annotation】阳 Yang means yang side, here means lateral of the arm. 谷 Gu means a valley between two mountains. This acupoint is in the depression between the styloid process of the ulna and the triquetral bone in the lateral wrist of the hand. And the depression is not as wide and deep as 阳溪 YangXi and 阳池 YangChi, shaped like a small valley. Hence the name 阳谷 YangGu.

【Location】At the ulnar border of the wrist, in the depression between the styloid process of the ulna and the triquetral bone.

【Indication】①Headache, vertigo, tinnitus, deafness; ②heat disease, mania–depression, epilepsy; ③swelling of the neck and submandibular region, pain of the wrist and arm.

6 养老 YangLao SI–6 (*Xi*–Cleft point)

【Source】《黄帝明堂经》*Huangdi Mingtang Jing*

【Annotation】养老 YangLao means support for the aged. This acupoint is often used for the treatment of senile diseases such as blurred vision, deafness, pain of the shoulder and arm. Acupuncture at this acupoint is beneficial to the health and longevity of the elderly, and is the key point for the treatment of senile diseases, hence it is named 养老 YangLao.

【Location】In the depression radial to the head of ulna, 1 cun proximal to the dorsal wrist crease.

【Indication】①Blurred vision; ②inability to raise due to pain of the shoulder and arm.

7 支正 ZhiZheng SI–7 (*Luo*–Connecting point)

【Source】《灵枢·经脉》*Lingshu: Jingmai*

【Annotation】支 Zhi means branch and detachment. 正 Zheng means main channel. This acupoint is the *Luo*–Connecting point, the collateral of the Small Intestine channel of Hand Taiyang branches from here towards the Heart channel of Hand Shaoyin, hence it is named 支正 ZhiZheng. Therefore, it can treat neck pain caused by the Small Intestine channel of Hand Taiyang disorders as well as calm the mind and treat the Heart channel of Hand

Shaoyin disorders such as epilepsy and forgetfulness.

【Location】5 cun proximal to the dorsal wrist crease, in the groove between the anterior border of the ulna and the muscle belly of flexor carpi ulnaris.

【Indication】①Heat disease, mania–depression; ②wart; ③headache, stiffness and pain of the neck, soreness and pain of the elbow and arm.

8 小海 XiaoHai SI-8 (*He*–Sea point)

【Source】《灵枢·本输》*Lingshu: Benshu*

【Annotation】小 Xiao refers to the Small Intestine channel. 海 Hai means sea, the place where rivers confluence. This acupoint is the *He*–Sea of the Small Intestine channel of Hand Taiyang, a metaphor for channel qi of the Small Intestine channel reaching here as if it is a river merging into the sea, hence it is named 小海 XiaoHai.

【Location】In the depression between the tip of the olecranon process of the ulna and the tip of the medial epicondyle of the humerus. With the elbow slightly flexed, the acupoint is taken in the sulcus for the ulnar nerve between the tip of the olecranon process of the ulna and the tip of the medial epicondyle of the humerus. When tapping this acupoint with the finger, there is an electric shock numbness straight to the little finger.

【Indication】①Epilepsy; ②headache, stiffness and pain of the neck, pain of the elbow and arm.

9 肩贞 JianZhen SI-9

【Source】《素问·气穴论》*Suwen: Qixue Lun*

【Annotation】肩 Jian means shoulder. 贞 Zhen means middle firstly. This acupoint is located directly below the middle of the shoulder joint. Secondly, 贞 Zhen refers to healthy qi. Acupuncture on this point can reinforce the healthy qi and eliminate the pathogenic qi. It is used to treat all shoulder discomforts such as inability to raise the arm due to wind obstruction, heat sensation and pain of the supraclavicular fossa, hence it is named 肩贞 JianZhen.

【Location】On the posterior aspect of the shoulder, 1 cun superior to the posterior axillary crease.

【Indication】①Scrofula; ②pain of the shoulder, numbness with inability to raise the arm.

10 臑俞 NaoShu SI-10

【Source】《黄帝明堂经》*Huangdi Mingtang Jing*

【Annotation】臑 Nao means upper arm. 俞 Shu, an interchangeable word for 腧 Shu, refers to acupoint. This acupoint is located near the axilla, directly superior to the posterior axillary crease, inferior to the scapular spine. It is used to treat local symptoms such as weakness and pain of the arm, pain of scapula. Hence it is named 臑俞 NaoShu.

【Location】In the depression inferior to the scapular spine, directly superior to the posterior axillary crease.

【Indication】Pain of the shoulder and arm.

11 天宗 TianZong SI-11

【Source】《黄帝明堂经》*Huangdi Mingtang Jing*

【Annotation】天 Tian means sky, here it refers to the upper part of the body. 宗 Zong means to respect and esteem, here it refers to the sun, moon and stars. This acupoint together with several other acupoints such as 臑俞 NaoShu, 曲垣 QuYuan, 秉风 BingFeng are arranged like a constellation, hence it is named 天宗 TianZong.

【Location】In the depression between the upper 1/3 and lower 2/3 of the line connecting the midpoint of the spine of the scapula with the inferior angle of the scapula.

【Indication】Pain and inability to raise the shoulder and arm.

12 秉风 BingFeng SI-12

【Source】《黄帝明堂经》*Huangdi Mingtang Jing*

【Annotation】秉 Bing means to govern. 风 Feng means wind refers to the pathogenic wind here. This acupoint is used to treat diseases such as pain of the shoulder with inability to raise the arm, pain and numbness of the upper arm and cough, which are caused by the invasion of pathogenic wind, as if in charge of pathogenic wind. Hence it is named 秉风 BingFeng.

【Location】In the scapular region, in the supraspinous fossa, superior to the midpoint of the spine of the scapula.

【Indication】Pain of the shoulder with inability to raise the arm.

13 曲垣 QuYuan SI-13

【Source】《黄帝明堂经》 *Huangdi Mingtang Jing*

【Annotation】曲 Qu means curve. 垣 Yuan means parapet. This acupoint is located in the central curved depression of the scapula, surrounded by bones that protrude like a parapet, hence it is named 曲垣 QuYuan.

【Location】In the tender depression superior to the medial end of the scapular spine.

【Indication】Inability to raise arm due to pain of shoulder.

14 肩外俞 JianWaiShu SI-14

【Source】《黄帝明堂经》 *Huangdi Mingtang Jing*

【Annotation】外 Wai means lateral side. This acupoint is located in the medial end of the scapula, and is called " 肩外俞 JianWaiShu" because it is located lateral to the 肩中俞 JianZhongShu.

【Location】3 cun lateral to the lower border of the spinous process of T1.

【Indication】Pain of the shoulder and back extending to the neck and arm.

15 肩中俞 JianZhongShu SI-15

【Source】《黄帝明堂经》 *Huangdi Mingtang Jing*

【Annotation】中 Zhong means middle. This acupoint is medial to the scapula, between 大椎 DaZhui and 肩井 JianJing, hence it is named 肩中俞 JianZhongShu.

【Location】2 cun lateral to the lower border of the spinous process of C7.

【Indication】①Chills and fever, cough, dyspnea; ②dimness of vision; ③pain of the shoulder and back.

16 天窗 TianChuang SI-16

【Source】《灵枢·本输》 *Lingshu: Benshu*

【Annotation】天 Tian means the sky. This acupoint is at the top of the head, corresponding to the sky. 窗 Chuang, the place for ventilation of the house. This acupoint can treat deafness, loss of voice, sore throat, trismus and other diseases of the five sense organs of head, just like opening windows for ventilation, hence it is named 天窗 TianChuang.

【Location】On the posterior border of the sternocleidomastoid muscle, level with the laryngeal prominence.

【Indication】①Tinnitus, deafness, sore throat; ②sudden loss of voice; ③stiffness and pain of the neck.

17 天容 TianRong SI–17

【Source】《灵枢·本输》 *Lingshu: Benshu*

【Annotation】天 Tian means the sky. The area above the shoulder corresponds to the sky. 容 Rong means face and appearance. This acupoint is located behind the angle of mandible, where the Small Intestine channel of Hand Taiyang goes upwards into the face. It is almost at the place where the earring, which is to enhance appearance, always hangs.

【Location】In the depression between the angle of mandible and the anterior border of the sternocleidomastoid muscle.

【Indication】①Chest pain, dyspnea; ②deafness; ③sore throat, goiter, stiffness and pain of the neck.

18 颧髎 QuanLiao SI–18 (Meeting point of the Small Intestine and Sanjiao channels)

【Source】《黄帝明堂经》 *Huangdi Mingtang Jing*

【Annotation】颧 Quan means cheekbone. 髎 Liao means the crevice on or beside the bone. This acupoint is named after its location. It is in the depression at the lower border of the zygomatic bone, hence it is named 颧髎 QuanLiao.

【Location】Directly below the outer canthus, in the depression at the lower border of the zygomatic bone.

【Indication】Deviation of the mouth and eye, ceaseless twitching of the eyelids, red eyes, yellow eyes, toothache, swelling of the cheek.

19 听宫 TingGong SI-19 (Meeting point of the Small Intestine, Sanjiao and Gall Bladder channels)

【Source】《灵枢·刺节真邪》 *Lingshu: Cijie Zhenxie*

【Annotation】听 Ting means to hear. 宫 Gong, the first note of the five tones of traditional Chinese music. This acupoint is located in front of the ear, and can help the ear hear sounds and restore hearing while acupunctured, which is an important acupoint for treating ear diseases, hence it is named 听宫 TingGong.

【Location】In the depression between the middle of the tragus and the condyloid process of the mandible.

【Indication】①Tinnitus, deafness, suppurative otitis media; ②mania-depression.

Chapter 8
The Bladder Channel Points of Foot Taiyang

1 睛明 **JingMing BL-1** (Meeting point of the Small Intestine, Bladder, Stomach with the Yin Heel and Yang Heel vessels)

【Source】《黄帝明堂经》 *Huangdi Mingtang Jing*

【Annotation】睛 Jing means eyes. 明 Ming means brightness. This acupoint is located at the inner canthus and is used to treat eye diseases and has the capability of brightening the eyes, hence it is named 睛明 JingMing.

【Location】Medial and superior to the inner canthus, in the depression of the medial wall of the orbit. (When the eye is closed, it is located in the depression 0.1 cun superomedial to the inner canthus.)

【Indications】①Redness and swelling of the eyes, lacrimation on exposure to wind, blurred vision, night blindness, dimness of vision; ②visual dizziness.

2 攒竹 **CuanZhu BL-2**

【Source】《黄帝明堂经》 *Huangdi Mingtang Jing*

【Annotation】攒 Cuan means to gather. 竹 Zhu means bamboo. 攒竹 CuanZhu means clusters of bamboo. This acupoint is located in the depression of the eyebrow, where the eyebrows resemble clustered newborn bamboo leaves, hence it is named 攒竹 CuanZhu.

【Location】In the depression on the eyebrow, close to its medial end, at the frontal notch.

【Indications】①Headache, pain of the eyebrow; ②redness and swelling of the eyes, blurred vision, lacrimation, twitch of the eyelids, eyelid ptosis, deviated eye and mouth.

3 眉冲 MeiChong BL-3

【Source】《脉经·平三关病候并治宜第三》*Maijing: Ping Sanguan Binghou Bing Zhiyi the third*

【Annotation】眉 Mei means eyebrow. 冲 Chong means to go upward straightly. This acupoint is located on the hairline directly above the medial end of eyebrow , hence it is named 眉冲 MeiChong.

【Location】Directly superior to the frontal notch, 0.5 cun within the anterior hairline.

【Indications】①Headache, dizziness; ②nasal congestion; ③epilepsy.

4 曲差 QuCha BL-4

【Source】《黄帝明堂经》*Huangdi Mingtang Jing*

【Annotation】曲 Qu means inflecting. 差 Cha means jagged. This acupoint is located at the lateral side of 眉冲 MeiChong, as the channel here is convoluted and jagged, hence it is named 曲差 QuCha.

【Location】0.5 cun within the anterior hairline, 1.5 cun lateral to the midline.

【Indications】①Headache, dizziness; ②blurred vision; ③nasal congestion.

5 五处 WuChu BL-5

【Source】《黄帝明堂经》*Huangdi Mingtang Jing*

【Annotation】五 Wu means five. 处 Chu means location. This acupoint is the 5th point of the Bladder channel of Foot Taiyang, hence it is named 五处 WuChu.

【Location】1 cun within the anterior hairline, 1.5 cun lateral to the midline.

【Indications】①Headache, heaviness of the head, dizziness; ②epilepsy, tetany, heat disease.

6 承光 ChengGuang BL-6

【Source】《黄帝明堂经》 *Huangdi Mingtang Jing*

【Annotation】承 Cheng means to carry. 光 Guang means sunlight. 承光 ChengGuang means to carry sunlight. This acupoint is located close to the top of the head and is used to treat eye diseases such as optic atrophy and dimness of vision. It can restore light to the eyes, meaning to carry the grace of light.

【Location】2.5 cun within the anterior hairline, 1.5 cun lateral to the midline.

【Indications】①Headache, dizziness; ②nasal congestion.

7 通天 TongTian BL-7

【Source】《黄帝明堂经》 *Huangdi Mingtang Jing*

【Annotation】通 Tong means access. 天 Tian means sky. This acupoint is 4 cun within the anterior hairline, almost the highest point on the body, and is a metaphor for the channel qi being connected to the sky, hence it is named 通 天 TongTian. The main function of this acupoint is to open the upper orifices and treat headache, heaviness of the head, nasal congestion and discharge, deviation of the mouth, blindness and other symptoms of upper orifice failure.

【Location】4 cun within the anterior hairline, 1.5 cun lateral to the midline.

【Indications】①Headache, dizziness; ②nasal congestion, sinusitis, nosebleed.

8 络却 LuoQue BL-8

【Source】《黄帝明堂经》 *Huangdi Mingtang Jing*

【Annotation】络 Luo means connection. 却 Que means to retreat, here refers to run towards the back of the head. The Bladder channel of Foot Taiyang enters at the top of the head, connects with the brain, and then turns to the back of the head as it returns downstream, where the acupoint is located. Hence the name 络却 LuoQue.

【Location】5.5 cun within the anterior hairline, 1.5 cun lateral to the midline.

【Indications】①Headache, dizziness; ②tinnitus, mania-depression.

9 玉枕 YuZhen BL-9

【Source】《黄帝明堂经》*Huangdi Mingtang Jing*

【Annotation】玉 Yu means jade, which is the essence of stone, a metaphor for preciousness. The brain is where the body's central nervous system is located and the skull protects it as if it is holding a jade. The occipital bone is the part that holds the head when lying on the back, hence the name 玉枕骨 YuZhen Bone for the part of the occipital bone that protrudes on either side. This acupoint is located in that area, hence it is named 玉枕 YuZhen.

【Location】At the same level as the external occipital protuberance, 1.3 cun lateral to the posterior midline.

【Indications】①Headache, stiffness and pain of the neck; ②eye pain, nasal congestion.

10 天柱 TianZhu BL-10

【Source】《灵枢·本输》*Lingshu: Benshu*

【Annotation】天 Tian means sky, refers to upper part and head. 柱 Zhu means pillars. The head is on the upper part of human body, considered as the sky. The cervical spine is like a pillar up to the sky, hence the name 天柱骨 TianZhu Bone. This acupoint is located at the beginning of the trapezius of the neck, on either side of the TianZhu Bone, hence it is named 天柱 TianZhu.

【Location】At the same level as the superior border of the spinous process of C2, in the depression lateral to the trapezius (0.5 cun within the posterior hairline, in the depression lateral to the trapezius).

【Indications】①Headache, dizziness; ②eye pain; ③mania–depression, epilepsy, heat disease; ④stiffness and pain of the neck, pain of the shoulder and back.

11 大杼 DaZhu BL-11 (*Hui*–Meeting point of bones, Meeting point of the Small Intestine channel and the Bladder channel)

【Source】《素问·水热穴论》《灵枢·刺节真邪》*Suwen: Shuirexue Lun, Lingshu: Cijie Zhenxie*

【Annotation】杼 Zhu means the shuttle of a loom. The transverse processes of the vertebrae are shaped like shuttles on a loom, and the first thoracic transverse process is particularly large. This acupoint is located on both side of the first thoracic vertebra below the spinous process, hence it is named 大杼 DaZhu.

【Location】At the lower border of the spinous process of the T1, 1.5 cun lateral to the posterior midline.

【Indications】①Cough, asthma; ②fever; ③stiffness and pain of the neck, pain of the shoulder and back.

12 风门 FengMen BL–12 (Meeting point of the Bladder channel with the Governor vessel)

【Source】《黄帝明堂经》*Huangdi Mingtang Jing*

【Annotation】风 Feng means pathogenic wind, which is one of the six external pathogenic factors. This acupoint is the gateway to the invasion of wind into body and can treat all diseases caused by wind, hence it is named 风门 FengMen.

【Location】Below the spinous process of the T2, 1.5 cun lateral to the posterior midline.

【Indications】①Cough, fever, headache, nasal congestion, runny nose; ②stiffness and pain of the back, pain of the chest and back.

13 肺俞 FeiShu BL–13 (Back–*Shu* point of the Lung)

【Source】《灵枢·背腧》*Lingshu: Beishu*

【Annotation】肺 Fei refers to the lung. 俞 Shu, same as 输 Shu in Chinese, means to transport and infuse. This acupoint is located close to the lung and is where the lung qi infuses to the back. It has the capabilities of diffusing the lung to calm panting, resolving phlegm to suppress cough, clearing heat and regulating qi. It is an important acupoint in the treatment of lung diseases, hence it is named 肺俞 FeiShu.

【Location】Below the spinous process of T3, 1.5 cun lateral to the posterior midline.

【Indications】①Cough, asthma, consumption, spitting blood, tidal fever, night sweating; ②turtle back in children.

14 厥阴俞 JueYinShu BL-14 (Back-*Shu* point of the Pericardium)

【Source】《千金要方·肺脏方·积气第五》 *Qianjin Yaofang: Feizang Fang: Jiqi the fifth*

【Annotation】厥阴 JueYin means to the Pericardium channel of Hand Jueyin. This acupoint is where the Pericardium qi is infused into the back and has the capability of regulating qi and relieving depression in the chest. It is an important acupoint in the treatment of pericardium diseases, hence it is named 厥阴俞 JueYinShu.

【Location】Below the spinous process of the T4, 1.5 cun lateral to the posterior midline.

【Indications】①Heartache, oppression of the chest; ②cough; ③vomiting.

15 心俞 XinShu BL-15 (Back-*Shu* point of the Heart)

【Source】《灵枢·背腧》 *Lingshu: Beishu*

【Annotation】心 Xin means heart. This acupoint is located close to the heart and is where the heart qi is infused into the back. It has the capability of freeing the collaterals of heart, regulating qi and blood, calming heart and tranquilizing, and is an important acupoint in the treatment of heart diseases, hence it is named 心俞 XinShu.

【Location】Below the spinous process of the T5, 1.5 cun lateral to the posterior midline.

【Indications】①Heartache, fright palpitation, insomnia, forgetful, nocturnal emission; ②cough, hemoptysis, night sweating; ③epilepsy.

16 督俞 DuShu BL-16

【Source】《太平圣惠方》 *Taiping Shenghui Fang*

【Annotation】督 Du refers to the Governor vessel. This acupoint is where the qi of the Governor vessel is infused into the back and can treat diseases in areas where the GV passes through, such as the waist, spine, head and brain, hence it is named 督俞 DuShu.

【Location】Below the spinous process of the T6, 1.5 cun lateral to the posterior midline.

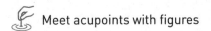

【Indications】①Heartache; ②abdominal pain, abdominal distention, borborygmus, qi counterflow.

17 膈俞 GeShu BL-17 (*Hui*–Meeting point of Blood)

【Source】《灵枢·背腧》*Lingshu: Beishu*

【Annotation】膈 Ge means the diaphragm. This acupoint is located below the spinous process of the T7 on either side, corresponding to the diaphragm internally. This acupoint has the capabilities of regulating qi to soothe the chest, harmonizing the stomach to direct qi downward, and is an important acupoint for treating diaphragmatic diseases such as hiccup, choke and eruption, hence it is named 膈俞 GeShu. Moreover, this acupoint is located between BL-15and BL-18, which are the back–Shu points of the heart and liver respectively. The heart governs blood and the liver stores blood, which has the capabilities of activating blood and dispelling wind. It can be used to treat blood syndrome such as hemoptysis, epistaxis and urticaria, hence it is the *Hui*–Meeting point of Blood.

【Location】Below the spinous process of the T7, 1.5 cun lateral to the posterior midline.

【Indications】①Vomiting, hiccup, spitting blood; ②asthma.

18 肝俞 GanShu BL-18 (Back–*Shu* point of the Liver)

【Source】《灵枢·背腧》*Lingshu: Beishu*

【Annotation】肝 Gan means liver. This acupoint is located close to the liver and is where the liver qi is infused into the back. It is an important acupoint in the treatment of liver diseases as it has the capabilities of relieving liver and regulating qi, cooling blood and brightening eyes, hence it is named 肝俞 GanShu.

【Location】Below the spinous process of the T9, 1.5 cun lateral to the posterior midline.

【Indications】①Hypochondriac pain, jaundice; ②redness of eyes, blurred vision, night blindness, lacrimation; ③spitting blood; ④mania–depression.

19 胆俞 DanShu BL-19 (Back–*Shu* point of the Gallbladder)

【Source】《黄帝明堂经》 *Huangdi Mingtang Jing*

【Annotation】胆 Dan means gall bladder. This acupoint is located close to the gallbladder and is where the gallbladder qi is infused into the back. It has the capability of soothing and draining liver and gallbladder, clearing and purging liver–gallbladder dampness–heat, and is an important acupoint in the treatment of gallbladder diseases, hence it is named 胆俞 DanShu.

【Location】Below the spinous process of the T10, 1.5 cun lateral to the posterior midline.

【Indications】Vomiting, bitter taste in the mouth, jaundice, hypochondriac pain.

20 脾俞 PiShu BL-20 (Back–*Shu* point of the Spleen)

【Source】《灵枢·背腧》 *Lingshu: Beishu*

【Annotation】脾 Pi means spleen. This acupoint is located close to the spleen and is where the spleen qi is infused into the back. It has the capability of fortifying the spleen and draining dampness, and is an important acupoint in the treatment of spleen diseases, hence it is named 脾俞 PiShu.

【Location】Below the spinous process of the T11, 1.5 cun lateral to the posterior midline.

【Indications】①Abdominal distention, vomiting, diarrhea; ②oedema, jaundice; ③swift digestion with rapid hungering, emaciation.

21 胃俞 WeiShu BL-21 (Back–*Shu* point of the Stomach)

【Source】《黄帝明堂经》 *Huangdi Mingtang Jing*

【Annotation】胃 Wei means stomach. This acupoint is located close to the stomach and is where the stomach qi is infused into the back. It has the capability of fortifying the spleen and harmonizing the stomach, promoting digestion and removing food stagnation, and is an important acupoint in the treatment of stomach diseases, hence it is named 胃俞 WeiShu.

【Location】Below the spinous process of the T12, 1.5 cun lateral to the posterior midline.

【Indications】①Pain of abdomen, vomiting, abdominal distention, borborygmus; ②swift digestion with rapid hungering, emaciation.

22 三焦俞 SanJiaoShu BL-22 (Back-*Shu* point of the Sanjiao)

【Source】《黄帝明堂经》*Huangdi Mingtang Jing*

【Annotation】三焦 SanJiao means triple energizers. This acupoint is where the qi of sanjiao is infused into the waist. It has the capability of regulating the waterways, and is an important acupoint in the treatment of sanjiao diseases, such as oedema, difficult urination and other water metabolism disorders, hence it is named 三焦俞 SanJiaoShu.

【Location】Below the spinous process of the L1, 1.5 cun lateral to the posterior midline.

【Indications】①Abdominal distention, vomiting, borborygmus, diarrhea; ②difficult urination, oedema; ③low back pain.

23 肾俞 ShenShu BL-23 (Back-*Shu* point of the Kidney)

【Source】《灵枢·背腧》*Lingshu: Beishu*

【Annotation】肾 Shen means kidney. This acupoint is located close to the kidney and is where the kidney qi is infused into the back. It has the capability of tonifying the kidney and assisting yang, strengthening the waist and promoting urination, improving the hearing and brightening the eyes. It is an important acupoint in the treatment of kidney diseases, hence it is named 肾俞 ShenShu.

【Location】Below the spinous process of the L2, 1.5 cun lateral to the posterior midline.

【Indications】①Tinnitus, deafness; ②enuresis, spermatorrhea, impotence, prospermia; ③irregular menstruation, leukorrhagia, infertility; ④swift digestion with rapid hungering, emaciation; ⑤lumbago.

24 气海俞 QiHaiShu BL-24

【Source】《太平圣惠方》*Taiping Shenghui Fang*

【Annotation】This acupoint corresponds to 气海 QiHai (CV-5) on abdomen, which is where the body's original qi is infused into the waist and back. It has the capability of assisting the kidney to promote qi absorption, hence it is named 气海俞 QiHaiShu, which treats a variety of symptoms slightly similar to those of 气海 QiHai (CV-5).

【Location】Below the spinous process of the L3, 1.5 cun lateral to the posterior midline.

【Indications】①Lumbago, dysmenorrhea; ②hemorrhoid.

25 大肠俞 DaChangShu BL-25 (Back-*Shu* point of the Large Intestine)

【Source】《黄帝明堂经》*Huangdi Mingtang Jing*

【Annotation】大肠 DaChang means large intestine. This acupoint is where the large intestine qi is infused into the waist and back. It has the capabilities of soothing and harmonizing the intestine, regulating qi and removing stagnation, and is an important acupoint in the treatment of large intestine diseases, hence it is named 大肠俞 DaChangShu.

【Location】Below the spinous process of the L4, 1.5 cun lateral to the posterior midline.

【Indications】①Abdominal distention, abdominal pain, borborygmus, diarrhea, constipation; ②lumbago.

26 关元俞 GuanYuanShu BL-26

【Source】《太平圣惠方》*Taiping Shenghui Fang*

【Annotation】This acupoint corresponds to 关元 GuanYuan (CV-4), which is where the body's original qi is infused into the waist and back. It has the capability of cultivating and tonifying the original qi, and treats impotence, spermatorrhea, leukorrhagia, diarrhea, similar to 关元 GuanYuan (CV-4), hence it is named 关元俞 GuanYuanShu.

【Location】Below the spinous process of the L5, 1.5 cun lateral to the posterior midline.

【Indications】①Abdominal distention, diarrhea; ②frequent urination, enuresis, difficult urination; ③lumbar pain.

27 小肠俞 XiaoChangShu BL-27 (Back-*Shu* point of the Small Intestine)

【Source】《黄帝明堂经》 *Huangdi Mingtang Jing*

【Annotation】小肠 XiaoChang means small intestine. This acupoint is where the small intestine qi is infused into the waist and back. It has the capability of regulating the intestine, and is an important acupoint in the treatment of small intestine diseases, hence it is named 小肠俞 XiaoChangShu.

【Location】At the level of the 1st posterior sacral foramen, 1.5 cun lateral to the posterior midline.

【Indications】①Spermatorrhea, enuresis, blood in the urine, stranguria, hernia, leukorrhagia; ②diarrhea; ③lumbar pain.

28 膀胱俞 PangGuangShu BL-28 (Back-*Shu* point of the Bladder)

【Source】《黄帝明堂经》 *Huangdi Mingtang Jing*

【Annotation】膀胱 PangGuang means bladder. This acupoint is located close to the bladder and is where the bladder qi is infused into the waist and back. It is an important acupoint in the treatment of bladder diseases, hence it is named 膀胱俞 PangGuangShu.

【Location】At the level of the 2nd posterior sacral foramen, 1.5 cun lateral to the posterior midline.

【Indications】①Difficult urination, enuresis; ②diarrhea, constipation; ③lumbar pain.

29 中膂俞 ZhongLvShu BL-29

【Source】《黄帝明堂经》 *Huangdi Mingtang Jing*

【Annotation】中 Zhong means the midpoint. 膂 Lv means the muscle of the back, lumbar region and buttock next to the spine. This acupoint is located at the middle of the full length of the body and on the gluteus maximus next to the spine, hence it is named 中膂俞 ZhongLvShu.

【Location】At the level of the 3rd posterior sacral foramen, 1.5 cun lateral to the posterior midline.

【Indications】①Abdominal distention, diarrhea, dysentery; ②lumbar pain.

30 白环俞 BaiHuanShu BL-30

【Source】《黄帝明堂经》 *Huangdi Mingtang Jing*

【Annotation】白环 BaiHuan means the jade ring, is believed by Taoists to be the place where the body stores essence. This acupoint is where the essence qi of jade ring is infused into the lumbar region, and treats symptoms of essence deficiency, such as gonorrhea, leukorrhagia, spermatorrhea, irregular menstruation, consumptive disease and steaming bone, hence it is named 白环俞 BaiHuanShu.

【Location】At the level of the 4th posterior sacral foramen, 1.5 cun lateral to the posterior midline (1.5 cun lateral to the sacralhiatus).

【Indications】①Enuresis, spermatorrhea, gonorrhea, sanguineous leukorrhea, irregular menstruation; ②lumbar pain.

31 上髎 ShangLiao BL-31

【Source】《黄帝明堂经》 *Huangdi Mingtang Jing*

【Annotation】髎 Liao means cleft aperture, here refers to the posterior sacral foramen. This acupoint is located at the 1st sacral foramen, in a superior position, hence it is named 上 髎 ShangLiao. This acupoint is on the same level as BL-26(GuanYuanShu) and has the capabilities of regulating menstruation, boosting qi and treating prolapse. It is used to treat diseases of the reproductive system and lumbosacral region such as irregular menstruation, leukorrhagia, spermatorrhea, soreness and weakness of the waist and knees.

【Location】Over the 1st posterior sacral foramen.

【Indications】①Irregular menstruation, leukorrhagia, uterine prolapse, scrotocele; ②lumbar pain.

32 次髎 CiLiao BL-32

【Source】《黄帝明堂经》 *Huangdi Mingtang Jing*

【Annotation】次 Ci means the second. 髎 Liao means cleft aperture, here refers to the posterior sacral foramen. This acupoint is located at the 2nd sacral foramen, just below BL-31(ShangLiao), hence it is named 次髎 CiLiao. This acupoint treats diseases same as 上髎

ShangLiao (BL–31) and is the preferred point of treating dysmenorrhea.

【Location】Over the 2nd posterior sacral foramen.

【Indications】①Irregular menstruation, dysmenorrhea, leukorrhagia, spermatorrhea, difficult urination, hernia; ②lumbago, paralysis of the lower limb.

33 中髎 ZhongLiao BL–33

【Source】《黄帝明堂经》 *Huangdi Mingtang Jing*

【Annotation】中 Zhong means middle. 髎 Liao means cleft aperture, here refers to the posterior sacral foramen. The acupoint is located in the 3rd sacral foramen and is in a central position, hence it is named 中髎 ZhongLiao.

【Location】Over the 3rd posterior sacral foramen.

【Indications】①Irregular menstruation, leukorrhagia, difficult urination; ②constipation, diarrhea; ③lumbar pain.

34 下髎 XiaLiao BL–34

【Source】《黄帝明堂经》 *Huangdi Mingtang Jing*

【Annotation】髎 Liao means cleft aperture, here refers to the posterior sacral foramen. This acupoint is located at the 4th sacral foramen, in a lower position, hence it is named 下髎 XiaLiao.

【Location】Confront the 4th posterior sacral foramen.

【Indications】①Leucorrhea, constipation, blood in the stool, difficult urination; ②hernia pain radiating to the lower abdomen, pain of the waist.

35 会阳 HuiYang BL–35

【Source】《黄帝明堂经》 *Huangdi Mingtang Jing*

【Annotation】会 Hui means a rendezvous. 阳 Yang refers to yang channels. This acupoint is where the Bladder channel of Foot Taiyang and the Governor vessel meet, both of which are yang channels, hence it is named 会阳 HuiYang.

【Location】0.5 cun lateral to the tip of the coccyx.

【Indications】①Hemorrhoid, dysentery; ②impotence, leucorrhea.

36 承扶 ChengFu BL-36

【Source】《黄帝明堂经》*Huangdi Mingtang Jing*

【Annotation】承 Cheng means to undertake. 扶 Fu means to support. This acupoint is below the buttock and above the thigh, just in the center of the transverse gluteal crease. It has the capability of undertaking the upper body and supporting the lower limbs, hence it is named 承扶 ChengFu.

【Location】Midpoint of the gluteal sulcus.

【Indications】①Hemorrhoid, prolapse, constipation, difficult urination; ②lumbago, pain of sacrum, buttock and thigh.

37 殷门 YinMen BL-37

【Source】《黄帝明堂经》*Huangdi Mingtang Jing*

【Annotation】殷 Yin means grand, refers to the richness of the muscles where the acupoint is located. 门 Men means a gateway for entrance and exit, refers to the capability of this acupoint to drain stagnation. This acupoint treats pain of the waist and legs that makes it difficult to stretch and lift, and has a capability of relieving and draining, like an entrance for pathogen. Hence it is named 殷门 YinMen.

【Location】6 cun below the gluteal sulcus, in the depression between the biceps femoris muscle and semitendinosus.

【Indications】Lumbago, painful obstruction and atrophy disorder of the lower limb.

38 浮郄 FuXi BL-38

【Source】《黄帝明堂经》*Huangdi Mingtang Jing*

【Annotation】浮 Fu means superficial. 郄 Xi means cleft aperture. This acupoint is located 1 cun above BL-39(WeiYang), at the aperture of the biceps femoris tendon. Compared with BL-37(YinMen), the muscles at this acupoint are shallow and thin. Hence the name 浮郄 FuXi.

【Location】1 cun superior to the popliteal crease, medial to the biceps femoris tendon.

【Indications】①Constipation; ②pain of the buttock and thigh, numbness.

39 委阳 WeiYang BL-39 (Lower *He*–Sea point of the Sanjiao)

【Source】《灵枢·本输》*Lingshu: Benshu*

【Annotation】委 Wei means flexion. The popliteal fossa is formed by flexion of the thigh and calf. This acupoint is at the lateral end of the popliteal crease, and the attribute of outside is yang, hence it is named 委阳 WeiYang.

【Location】On the popliteal crease, medial to the biceps femoris tendon.

【Indications】①Fullness of the abdomen, difficult urination; ②low back pain, pain of the leg and foot.

40 委中 WeiZhong BL-40 (*He*–Sea point, Lower *He*–Sea point of the Bladder)

【Source】《灵枢·背腧》*Lingshu: Beishu*

【Annotation】委 Wei means flexion. The popliteal fossa is formed by flexion of the thigh and calf. 中 Zhong means middle. This acupoint is in the center of the popliteal fossa, hence the name.

【Location】At the midpoint of the popliteal crease.

【Indications】①Pain of the lower abdomen, difficult urination, enuresis; ②low back pain, painful obstruction and atrophy disorder of the lower limb.

41 附分 FuFen BL-41 (Meeting point of the Small Intestine channel and the Bladder channel)

【Source】《黄帝明堂经》*Huangdi Mingtang Jing*

【Annotation】附 Fu means attach to. 分 Fen means branch. This acupoint is the first acupoint on the second lateral line of the Bladder channel of Foot Taiyang. The second lateral line is a branch of the Bladder channel of Foot Taiyang and is attached to the first lateral line, with two lateral lines running in parallel down the back. Hence the name 附分 FuFen.

【Location】Below the spinous process of the T2, 3 cun lateral to the posterior midline.

【Indications】Contraction of the shoulder and back, stiffness and pain of the neck, numbness of the elbow and upper arm.

42 魄户 PoHu BL-42

【Source】《黄帝明堂经》*Huangdi Mingtang Jing*

【Annotation】魄 Po means corporeal soul. 户 Hu means gateway. This acupoint is located on either side below the spinous process of the T3, flush with BL-13(FeiShu), and is the gateway to the entry and exit of lung qi. It treats deficiency–consumption, lung atrophy, cough, asthma and other lung diseases. The lung stores corporeal soul. Hence the name 魄户 PoHu.

【Location】Below the spinous process of the T3, 3 cun lateral to the posterior midline.

【Indications】Cough, asthma, lung consumption; pain of the shoulder and back, stiffness and pain of the neck.

43 膏肓 GaoHuang BL-43

【Source】《千金要方·针灸下·杂病第七》*Qianjin Yaofang: Zhenjiu Xia: Zabing the seventh*

【Annotation】In ancient Chinese medicine, the fat at the heart's tip refers to 膏 Gao, and the area between the heart and the diaphragm is called 肓 Huang. 膏肓 GaoHuang refers to the area above the diaphragm and below the heart, where the effect of medicine cannot reach. This acupoint is flush with the Back–shu point of the pericardium, BL-14(JueYinShu), and is used for treating various chronic deficiency–consumption diseases, hence it is named 膏肓 GaoHuang.

【Location】Below the spinous process of the T4, 3 cun lateral to the posterior midline.

【Indications】①Cough, asthma, night sweating, lung consumption; ②spermatorrhea; ③deficiency–consumption, emaciation.

44 神堂 ShenTang BL-44

【Source】《黄帝明堂经》*Huangdi Mingtang Jing*

【Annotation】神 Shen means spirit. 堂 Tang means hall. This acupoint is located on either side below the spinous process of the T5, flush with BL-15(XinShu), where the heart qi stays and gathers. It treats all kinds of heart diseases. The heart stores spirit. Hence the name

神堂 ShenTang.

【Location】Below the spinous process of the T5, 3 cun lateral to the posterior midline.

【Indications】①Cough, asthma, chest tightness; ②low back pain.

45 谚谑 YiXi BL-45

【Source】《素问·骨空论》*Suwen: Gukong Lun*

【Annotation】谚 Yi and 谑 Xi are both intonational exclamations, expressing sighs or grief. This acupoint is located on either side of the spinous process of the T6. The patient often sighs in fear of pain when the wind invades the Bladder channel of Foot Taiyang by pressing on the acupoint, hence it is named 谚谑 YiXi.

【Location】Below the spinous process of the T6, 3 cun lateral to the posterior midline.

【Indications】①Cough, asthma; ②malaria, heat disease; ③contracture of the shoulder and back radiating to the lateral costal region.

46 膈关 GeGuan BL-46

【Source】《黄帝明堂经》*Huangdi Mingtang Jing*

【Annotation】膈 Ge means the diaphragm. 关 Guan means the boundary. This acupoint is located on either side of the spinous process of the T7, flush with BL-17(GeShu), and corresponds to the diaphragm internally, which is the boundary of the thorax and abdomen. Besides, it treats belch, hiccup, the same as BL-17(GeShu). Hence it is named 膈关 GeGuan.

【Location】Below the spinous process of the T7, 3 cun lateral to the posterior midline.

【Indications】①Vomiting, hiccup, belch; ②chest tightness, low back pain.

47 魂门 HunMen BL-47

【Source】《黄帝明堂经》*Huangdi Mingtang Jing*

【Annotation】魂 Hun means the ethereal soul. 门 Men means gateway. This acupoint is located on either side of the spinous process of the T9, flush with BL-18(GanShu). The liver stores the ethereal soul, and this acupoint is the gateway for the soul of liver to enter and exit the body. It is used to treat liver diseases such as fullness and distention of the chest and lateral costal region, hence it is named 魂门 HunMen.

【Location】Below the spinous process of the T9, 3 cun lateral to the posterior midline.

【Indications】①Vomiting, diarrhea; ②pain of the lateral costal region, back pain.

48 阳纲 YangGang BL-48

【Source】《黄帝明堂经》*Huangdi Mingtang Jing*

【Annotation】纲 Gang means order and law. This acupoint is located on either side of the spinous process of the T10, flush with BL-19(DanShu). The gallbladder is the organ similar to an official of justice and is responsible for decision and is the outline of healthy qi. The healthy qi represents yang as opposed to pathogen, hence it is named 阳纲 YangGang. It is used to treat syndromes such as heat in the body, wasting-thirst, difficult ingestion, yellow eyes and other inability to soothe and drain liver and gallbladder of Shaoyang, and has the same effect as BL-19(DanShu).

【Location】Below the spinous process of the T10, 3 cun lateral to the posterior midline.

【Indications】①Borborygmus, diarrhea, indigestion; ②reddish-yellow urination.

49 意舍 YiShe BL-49

【Source】《黄帝明堂经》*Huangdi Mingtang Jing*

【Annotation】意 Yi means the thought. 舍 She means shelter. This acupoint is located on either side below the spinous process of the T11, flush with BL-20(PiShu), where the spleen qi stays. It is used for treating abdominal distention, diarrhea and other spleen diseases. The spleen stores thought. Hence the name 意舍 YiShe.

【Location】Below the spinous process of the T11, 3 cun lateral to the posterior midline.

【Indications】①Abdominal distention, diarrhea, wasting-thirst; ②fever; ③yellow eyes.

50 胃仓 WeiCang BL-50

【Source】《黄帝明堂经》*Huangdi Mingtang Jing*

【Annotation】胃 Wei means stomach. 仓 Cang means granary. This acupoint is located on either side below the spinous process of the T12, flush with BL-21(WeiShu). It is used to treat abdominal fullness, difficult ingestion and other stomach diseases. The stomach is the organ similar to the granary. Hence the name 胃仓 WeiCang.

【Location】Below the spinous process of the T12, 3 cun lateral to the posterior midline.

【Indications】①Stomachache, abdominal distention, oedema, infantile indigestion; ②low back pain.

51 肓门 HuangMen BL–51

【Source】《黄帝明堂经》*Huangdi Mingtang Jing*

【Annotation】肓 Huang means the membrane tissue among the five viscera, such as pleura and peritoneum. Space among the membrane tissue of the body is the passage for the flow of qi of sanjiao. This acupoint is located on both sides below the spinous process of the L1, flush with BL–22(SanJiaoShu). It is the gateway for qi of sanjiao to enter and exit the body, hence it is named 肓门 HuangMen.

【Location】In the lumbar region, below the spinous process of the L1, 3 cun lateral to the posterior midline.

【Indications】①Abdominal pain, abdominal mass; ②postpartum diseases.

52 志室 ZhiShi BL–52

【Source】《黄帝明堂经》*Huangdi Mingtang Jing*

【Annotation】志 Zhi means will and memory. 室 Shi means room. This acupoint is flush with BL–23(ShenShu). It is where the kidney qi stays and gathers so that can be used to treat kidney diseases such as lumbago, spermatorrhea. Kidney stores will. Hence the name 志室 ZhiShi.

【Location】Below the spinous process of the L2, 3 cun lateral to the posterior midline.

【Indications】①Spermatorrhea, impotence, difficult urination; ②low back pain.

53 胞肓 BaoHuang BL–53

【Source】《黄帝明堂经》*Huangdi Mingtang Jing*

【Annotation】胞肓 BaoHuang means the lipid membrane that surrounds the bladder.

This acupoint is located on both sides of the 2nd sacral foramen, flush with BL-28(PangGuangShu), and is used to treat bladder diseases, hence it is named 胞肓 BaoHuang.

【Location】At the level of the 2nd sacral foramen, 3 cun lateral to the posterior midline.

【Indications】①Dribbling and retention of urine; ②borborygmus, abdominal distention, constipation; ③pain of the lumbar region and spine.

54 秩边 ZhiBian BL-54

【Source】《黄帝明堂经》 *Huangdi Mingtang Jing*

【Annotation】秩 Zhi means orderly and organized. 边 Bian means edge. The various acupoints on the back of the Bladder channel of Foot Taiyang are arranged in sequence and order. This acupoint is located on either side of the 21st vertebrae and is the last acupoint on the second lateral line of the back, at the edge, hence it is named 秩边 ZhiBian.

【Location】At the level of the 4th sacral foramen, 3 cun lateral to the posterior midline (3 cun lateral to the sacral hiatus).

【Indications】①Hemorrhoid, constipation, difficult urination, pain of the genital; ②lumbar pain, painful obstruction and atrophy disorder of the lower limb.

55 合阳 HeYang BL-55

【Source】《黄帝明堂经》 *Huangdi Mingtang Jing*

【Annotation】A branch of the Bladder channel of Foot Taiyang runs from the waist down through the buttocks and into the popliteal fossa. Another branch passes straight down through the inner edge of the scapula, passes down through the buttocks, runs along the posterior-lateral side of the thigh, and meets the branch coming down from the waist in the popliteal fossa. This acupoint is below the popliteal crease, where the two branches of the Bladder channel of Foot Taiyang meet, hence it is named 合阳 HeYang.

【Location】2 cun inferior to the popliteal crease, between the two heads of the gastrocnemius muscle.

【Indications】①Hernia, menorrhagia; ②low back pain, painful obstruction and atrophy disorder of the lower limb.

56 承筋 ChengJin BL-56

【Source】《黄帝明堂经》*Huangdi Mingtang Jing*

【Annotation】承 Cheng means to undertake. 筋 Jin means meridian sinew. This acupoint is located in the bellies of the gastrocnemius muscle, where the meridian sinews of the Bladder channel of Foot Taiyang coalesce. It is used to treat sinew diseases such as clonic spasm and cramp of calf, hence it is named 承筋 ChengJin.

【Location】5 cun inferior to the popliteal crease, between the two bellies of the gastrocnemius muscle.

【Indications】① Hemorrhoid; ② lumbago, clonic spasm of calf.

57 承山 ChengShan BL-57

【Source】《黄帝明堂经》*Huangdi Mingtang Jing*

【Annotation】承 Cheng means to undertake and carry. 山 Shan means body weight here. This acupoint is in the depression at the lower end of the two bellies of the gastrocnemius muscle, as if it was in the canyon of a mountain, and could undertake a body as heavy as a mountain. Hence it is named 承山 ChengShan.

【Location】The angle of intersection of the two bellies of the gastrocnemius muscle with the tendon. When the calf is straightened or the heel is lifted, it appears in an angled depression that appears under the bellies of the gastrocnemius muscle.

【Indications】① Hemorrhoid, constipation; ② low back pain, clonic spasm of calf.

58 飞扬 FeiYang BL-58 (*Luo*–Connecting point)

【Source】Presented as 飞阳 FeiYang in《灵枢·经脉》*Lingshu: Jingmai* and as 飞扬 FeiYang in《黄帝明堂经》*Huangdi Mingtang Jing*.

【Annotation】飞扬 FeiYang means to lift up, to branch off diagonally, to get off the right track. This acupoint is the *Luo*–Connecting point of the Bladder channel, from which the channel qi travels separately to the Kidney channel of Foot Taiyin, linking the two channels. This acupoint can therefore treat diseases of both channels, such as urinary tract infection, nephritis and weakness of the knee and tibia, hence it is named 飞扬 FeiYang. In addition, this acupoint is a common acupoint for treating weakness in the legs, thus why it is also described as an acupoint that enables one to walk as if on wings.

【Location】 7 cun directly superior to BL-60(KunLun), where the lateral lower side of the gastrocnemius muscle migrates with the Achilles tendon.

【Indications】 ①Headache, dizziness; ②nosebleed; ③hemorrhoid; ④pain of the waist and legs.

59 跗阳 FuYang BL-59 (*Xi*-Cleft point of the Yang Heel vessel)

【Source】《黄帝明堂经》*Huangdi Mingtang Jing*

【Annotation】 跗 Fu, same as 附 Fu in Chinese, means to attach. This acupoint is located 3 cun superior to the lateral malleolus of the foot and lateral to the tarsal bones. It is also the *Xi*-Cleft point of the Yang Heel vessel, which passes through this acupoint and then moves upwards, meaning that the Yang Heel is dependent on the Bladder channel of Foot Taiyang's acupoint.

【Location】 3 cun superior to BL-60(KunLun), between the perone and Achilles tendon.

【Indications】 ①Headache; ②lumbar pain, painful obstruction and atrophy disorder of the lower limb, swelling and pain of foot and malleolus.

60 昆仑 KunLun BL-60 (*Jing*-River point)

【Source】《灵枢·本输》*Lingshu: Benshu*

【Annotation】 昆仑 KunLun, name of a mountain. The ancients considered KunLun Mountain to be the highest mountain, and here the metaphor is that the lateral malleolus is high and protruding like KunLun Mountain. This acupoint is behind the tip of the lateral malleolus, hence it is named 昆仑 KunLun.

【Location】 In the depression between the prominence of the lateral malleolus and the Achilles tendon.

【Indications】 ①Headache, eye pain, nosebleed; ②difficult labor; ③epilepsy; ④stiffness and pain of the neck, lumbago, swelling and pain of foot and malleolus.

61 仆参 PuCan BL-61

【Source】《黄帝明堂经》*Huangdi Mingtang Jing*

【Annotation】仆 Pu, an ancient term for a person of low rank. 参 Can means to worship. In ancient times, servants paid homage to their masters by curtsying. The point where the finger hangs down is this acupoint, hence it is named 仆参 PuCan.

【Location】Directly inferior to BL-60(KunLun), on the lateral side of the calcaneus, at the border between the red and white flesh.

【Indications】①Epilepsy; ②lumbago, atrophy disorder of the leg, cramp and pain of the foot, swelling and pain of the heel.

62 申脉 ShenMai BL-62 (Confluent point of the Yang Heel vessel)

【Source】《黄帝明堂经》*Huangdi Mingtang Jing*

【Annotation】The name of this acupoint has two meanings. Firstly, 申 Shen refers to the Shen hour(one of the 12 two-hour periods in ancient), which is between 3 and 5 pm. This time period is when the qi and blood flow into the Bladder channel of Foot Taiyang, hence it is named 申脉 ShenMai. Secondly, 申 Shen is an interchangeable word for 伸 Shen, meaning flexion and extension. 脉 Mai refers to the Yang Heel vessel. This acupoint is the Confluent point of the Yang Heel vessel, where it originates. The Yang Heel vessel controls the movement of the lower limbs and is the vessel that maintains normal function and activities such as flexion and extension. It treats limb dysfunctions such as stiffness and difficulty in extending the back, difficulty in extending and flexing the joint and cramps, hence it is named 申脉 ShenMai.

【Location】Directly inferior to the lateral malleolus, in the depression between the lower border of the lateral malleolus and calcaneus.

【Indications】①Insomnia, headache, dizziness, mania-depression, epilepsy; ②pain of the lumbar region and leg.

63 金门 JinMen BL-63 (*Xi*-Cleft point)

【Source】《黄帝明堂经》*Huangdi Mingtang Jing*

【Annotation】金 Jin means metal, which is one of the five phases. 门 Men means portal and gateway. The previous acupoint of this acupoint is BL-62(ShenMai). The attribute of 申 Shen is metal. The qi and blood of the Bladder channel of Foot Taiyang infuse this portal at the Shen hour, hence it is named 金门 JinMen. Also, because 金 Jin represents change, it has a subdued, harsh and convergency nature. The Bladder channel of Foot Taiyang passes through this acupoint, approaching the end, and will meet the qi of Shaoyin just as yang qi changes into yin qi during windy late fall. Hence it is named 金门 JinMen.

【Location】Directly inferior to the lateral malleolus, in the depression of the lower border of the cuboid.

【Indications】①Headache; ②infantile convulsion; ③lumbago, painful obstruction and atrophy disorder of the lower limb, swelling and pain of the foot and malleolus.

64 京骨 JingGu BL-64 (*Yuan*-Source point)

【Source】《灵枢·本输》*Lingshu: Benshu*

【Annotation】京 Jing means big. 骨 Gu means bone. This acupoint is located near a significant prominence at the base of lateral side of the 5th metatarsal bone, known to the ancients as the 京骨 Jing Bone, hence it is named 京骨 JingGu.

【Location】Anterior and inferior to the tuberosity of the 5th metatarsal bone, at the border between the red and white flesh.

【Indications】①Headache; ②epilepsy; ③stiffness and pain of the neck, pain of the lumbar region and leg.

65 束骨 ShuGu BL-65 (*Shu*-Stream point)

【Source】《灵枢·本输》*Lingshu: Benshu*

【Annotation】束 Shu means to bring together. 骨 Gu means bone. This acupoint is located just posterior and inferior to the metatarsalis of the 5th metatarsal bone, which tapers to a constricted shape from BL-64(JingGu) to this acupoint, hence it is named 束骨 ShuGu.

【Location】Proximal to the 5th metatarsophalangeal joint, at the border between the red and white flesh.

【Indications】①Headache, dizziness; ②mania-depression; ③stiffness and pain of the neck, pain of the lumbar region and leg.

66 足通谷 ZuTongGu BL-66 (*Ying*–Spring point)

【Source】《灵枢·本输》 *Lingshu: Benshu*

【Annotation】通 Tong means to pass through. 谷 Gu means valley. This acupoint is in the depression anterior and inferior to the 5th metatarsophalangeal joint on the lateral side of the foot, shaped like a valley. This acupoint is the *Ying*–Spring point, meaning the channel qi emanates from *Jing*–Well point and flows through this acupoint. The name 足通谷 ZuTongGu is given in order to distinguish it from KD-20(TongGu, the Kidney channel of Foot Shaoyin) on the abdomen with the same name.

【Location】Distal to the 5th metatarsophalangeal joint, at the border between the red and white flesh.

【Indications】①Headache, stiffness and pain of the neck; ②nosebleed; ③epilepsy.

67 至阴 ZhiYin BL-67 (*Jing*–Well point)

【Source】《灵枢·本输》 *Lingshu: Benshu*

【Annotation】至 Zhi means to arrive. 阴 Yin refers to the Kidney channel of Foot Shaoyin. This acupoint is located at the end of the little toe of the foot, where the qi of the Bladder channel of Foot Taiyang meets the Kidney channel of Foot Shaoyin, indicating that yang qi is disappearing and yin qi is about to arise, hence it is named 至阴 ZhiYin.

【Location】Lateral to the distal phalanx, 0.1 cun proximal to the lateral corner of the toenail.

【Indications】①Malposition of fetus, bradytocia; ②headache, eye pain, nasal congestion, nosebleed; ③swelling and pain of the foot and knee.

Chapter 9
The Kidney Channel Points of Foot Shaoyin

1 涌泉 YongQuan KI–1 (*Jing*–Well point)

【Source】《灵枢·本输》*Lingshu: Benshu*

【Annotation】涌 Yong means upwelling and gushing. 泉 Quan means water ejected from the ground. This acupoint is located at the central depression of the bottom of the foot and is the *Jing*–Well point of the Kidney channel of Foot Shaoyin, where the channel qi emerges as if from a spring, hence it is named 涌泉 YongQuan.

【Location】In a depression formed when the foot is plantar flexed.

【Indications】①Fever, agitation, infantile convulsion; ②sore throat, cough, dyspnea; ③constipation, difficult urination; ④heat in the soles of the feet, pain of lumbar and spine.

2 然谷 RanGu KI–2 (*Ying*–Spring point)

【Source】《灵枢·本输》*Lingshu: Benshu*

【Annotation】The name of this acupoint has two meanings. Firstly, this acupoint is named after the ancient anatomical nomenclature which called the navicular tuberosity 然骨 Ran Bone, and which is located in the depression of the lower edge of the navicular bone, hence it is named 然谷 RanGu. Secondly, 然 Ran is an interchangeable word for 燃 Ran. This point is the *Ying*–spring and Fire point of the Kidney channel, which is found in the depression medial to the lower edge of the navicular bone, like dragon fire[①] burning in the valley. This

---

① Dragon fire refers to kidney fire.

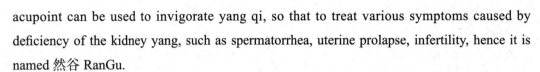

acupoint can be used to invigorate yang qi, so that to treat various symptoms caused by deficiency of the kidney yang, such as spermatorrhea, uterine prolapse, infertility, hence it is named 然谷 RanGu.

【Location】On the medial side of the foot, inferior to the navicular tuberosity, at the border between the red and white flesh.

【Indications】Coughing blood, sore throat; wasting-thirst, jaundice, diarrhea; irregular menstruation, uterine prolapse, itching of the genitals, spermatorrhea, impotence; neonatal tetanus; pain and swelling of the instep.

3 太溪 TaiXi KI-3 (*Shu*-Stream and *Yuan*-Source point)

【Source】《灵枢·九针十二原》《灵枢·本输》*Lingshu: Jiuzhen Shieryuan, Lingshu: Benshu*

【Annotation】太 Tai means big. 溪 Xi means running water in the mountains. This acupoint is the *Shu*-Stream point of the Kidney channel. The channel qi originates from 涌泉 YongQuan and comes out of 然谷 RanGu, and gradually flourishes at this acupoint as if it is a stream in the mountains. Moreover, this acupoint is located at a deep and large depression between the medial malleolus and the Achilles tendon, hence it is named 太溪 TaiXi.

【Location】In the depression between the medial malleolus and the Achilles tendon.

【Indications】①Spermatorrhea, impotence; ②irregular menstruation; ③cough, dyspnea, coughing blood, chest pain; ④sore throat, toothache; ⑤wasting-thirst, constipation; ⑥pain of the waist and back, coldness of the lower limbs.

4 大钟 DaZhong KI-4 (*Luo*-Connecting point)

【Source】《灵枢·经脉》*Lingshu: Jingmai*

【Annotation】There are two explanations for this name. Firstly, 钟 Zhong is an interchangeable word for 踵 Zhong, refers to the heel. This acupoint is located at the heel, hence the name. Secondly, 钟 Zhong means injection and convergence. This acupoint is the *Luo*-Connecting point of the Kidney channel of Foot Shaoyin, means that it is the place where the collateral of the Kidney channel converges and separates. Channels gather here and then separate, hence it is named 大钟 DaZhong.

【Location】Posteroinferior to the medial malleolus, superior to the calcaneus, in the depression anterior to the attachment of the calcaneal tendon.

【Indications】①Dribbling and retention of urine, constipation; ②coughing blood, dyspnea; ③dementia, somnolence; ④pain of the waist and back, pain of the heel.

5 水泉 ShuiQuan KI–5 (*Xi*–Cleft point)

【Source】《黄帝明堂经》*Huangdi Mingtang Jing*

【Annotation】This acupoint is the *Xi*–Cleft point of the Kidney channel of Foot Shaoyin, the place where the qi and blood of Kidney channel gather deeply, like a deep water source, hence it is named 水泉 ShuiQuan.

【Location】1 cun inferior to 太溪 Taixi KI–3, in a depression medial to the calcaneal tuberosity.

【Indications】①Irregular menstruation, dysmenorrhea, uterine prolapse, difficult urination; ②cloudy vision.

6 照海 ZhaoHai KI–6 (Confluent point of the Yin Motility vessel)

【Source】《黄帝明堂经》*Huangdi Mingtang Jing*

【Annotation】照 Zhao means light. 海 Hai is the sea. The property of the Kidney is water, and 然谷 RanGu is the *Ying*–spring and Fire point of the Kidney channel, like the dragon fire in water. This acupoint is close to 然谷 RanGu, like the light of dragon fire shining on the surface of the sea, hence it is named 照海 ZhaoHai.

【Location】1 cun below the prominence of the medial malleolus, in the depression inferior to the medial malleolus.

【Indications】①Insomnia, redness and pain of the eyes, dry throat, sore throat; ②irregular menstruation, sanguinous leukorrhea, uterine prolapse, dribbling and retention of urine, hernia; ③epilepsy.

7 复溜 FuLiu KI–7 (*Jing*–River point)

【Source】《灵枢·本输》*Lingshu: Benshu*

【Annotation】复 Fu means to resume. 溜 Liu means flow. There are two explanations for this name. Firstly, it is named after the running course of the channel. This channel travels diagonally from the center of the foot towards the medial malleolus, circling around and passing through 大钟 DaZhong and 水泉 ShuiQuan before converging on 照海 ZhaoHai, and then resuming its positive direction after travelling diagonally to this acupoint (water flowing downstream is the positive direction), hence it is named 复溜 FuLiu. Secondly, the acupoint is named according to its function. This acupoint is used to treat sweating, oedema, diarrhea and other disorders of water distribution and has the capability of regulating the waterways, maintaining and restoring the normal flow of water, hence the name.

【Location】2 cun superior to the prominence of the medial malleolus, anterior to the calcaneal tendon.

【Indications】①Abdominal distension, diarrhea; ②hyperhidrosis, absence of sweating, oedema; ③pain of the lumbar and back, atrophy disorder of the leg.

8 交信 JiaoXin KI-8 (*Xi*-Cleft point of the Yin Motility vessel)

【Source】《黄帝明堂经》 *Huangdi Mingtang Jing*

【Annotation】交 Jiao means meeting and intersecting. 信 Xin means faith, which is one of the five virtues. The ancients believed that the five virtues of benevolence, righteousness, manner, wisdom and faith were compatible with the five phases, and the attribute of faith is earth, which is also the attribute of the spleen, referring to the Spleen channel of Foot Taiyin here. Although this acupoint belongs to the Kidney channel of Foot Shaoyin, it is on the route of the Spleen channel of Foot Taiyin, and they meet via this acupoint at 三阴交 SanYinJiao. Therefore, This acupoint has the capability of storing and controlling the blood, and can be used to treat menstrual disorders such as irregular menstruation and menorrhagia. Hence it is named 交信 JiaoXin.

【Location】2 cun superior to the prominence of the medial malleolus, in the depression posterior to the medial border of the tibia.

【Indications】①Dribbling and retention of urine, hernia pain involving thighs and knees, irregular menstruation; ②diarrhea, constipation.

9 筑宾 ZhuBin KI-9 (*Xi*-Cleft point of the Yin Link vessel)

【Source】《黄帝明堂经》 *Huangdi Mingtang Jing*

【Annotation】筑 Zhu means construction. 宾 Bin means guests, here refers to the house where the guests live. This acupoint belongs to the Kidney channel of Foot Shaoyin and is also the *Xi*–Cleft point of the Yin Link vessel. This acupoint takes the Kidney channel of Foot Shaoyin as the host and takes the Yin Link vessel as guest, like building an inn on the Kidney channel of Foot Shaoyin to welcome the arrival of the Yin Link vessel, hence it is named 筑宾 ZhuBin.

【Location】5 cun superior to 太溪 TaiXi KI–3, between the soleus muscle and the calcaneal tendon.

【Indications】①Epilepsy, protruding tongue; ②vomiting; ③hernia; ④pain of calf.

10 阴谷 YinGu KI–10 (*He*–Sea point)

【Source】《灵枢·本输》*Lingshu: Benshu*

【Annotation】阴 Yin refers to medial side here. 谷 Gu means valley. This acupoint is on the medial side of the knee joint, between the tendons of semitendinosus and semimembranosus, in a depression shaped like a valley, hence it is named 阴谷 YinGu.

【Location】At the medial end of the popliteal fossa, between the tendons of semitendinosus and semimembranosus when slightly flexing the knee.

【Indications】①Impotence, difficult urination, irregular menstruation, menorrhagia; ②mania–depression; ③pain of the waist and spine, pain radiating to the lower abdomen and genitals and knee and thigh.

11 横骨 HengGu KI–11 (Meeting point of the Kidney channel with the thoroughfare vessel)

【Source】《黄帝明堂经》*Huangdi Mingtang Jing*

【Annotation】横骨 HengGu, the bone that runs horizontally between the legs, namely the pubis. This acupoint is located just above the pubis, and on the same level as 曲骨 QuGu, hence it is named 横骨 HengGu.

【Location】5 cun below the umbilicus, 0.5cun lateral to the midline.

【Indications】Hypogastric pain, retention of urine, enuresis, spermatorrhea, impotence, hernia.

12 大赫 DaHe KI-12 (Meeting point of the Kidney channel with the thoroughfare vessel)

【Source】《黄帝明堂经》 *Huangdi Mingtang Jing*

【Annotation】There are two explanations for this name. Firstly, 赫 He means exuberance. This acupoint is located where the thoroughfare vessel and Kidney channel meet, and the channel qi is exuberant, hence it is named 大赫 DaHe. Secondly, 赫 He refers to extreme heat. This acupoint is on the same level as 中极 ZhongJi (CV-3), and corresponds to the genital system. It can treat deficiency of the uterus and some other genitalia, such as uterine prolapse and impotence, and is effective in helping to generate heat and yang, hence it is named 大赫 DaHe.

【Location】4 cun below the umbilicus, 0.5cun lateral to the midline.

【Indications】Spermatorrhea, impotence, uterine prolapse, leucorrhea, retraction of scrotum.

13 气穴 QiXue KI-13 (Meeting point of the Kidney channel with the thoroughfare vessel)

【Source】《黄帝明堂经》 *Huangdi Mingtang Jing*

【Annotation】气 Qi means source qi. This acupoint is located next to 关元 GuanYuan (CV-4), where kidney yin and kidney yang meet. This acupoint is the place where the source qi generated and is also a key acupoint for absorbing qi, hence it is named 气穴 QiXue.

【Location】3 cun below the umbilicus, 0.5 cun lateral to the midline.

【Indications】①Irregular menstruation, leucorrhea; ②infertility; ③hypogastric pain radiating to the lumbar spine.

14 四满 SiMan KI-14 (Meeting point of the Kidney channel with the thoroughfare vessel)

【Source】《黄帝明堂经》 *Huangdi Mingtang Jing*

【Annotation】满 Man means satiation and turgor. This acupoint is the 4th acupoint on the Kidney channel of Foot Shaoyin after it enters the abdomen, where the lower abdomen is full. It treats swelling of the lower abdomen, hernia and other symptoms of turgor, hence it is named 四满 SiMan.

【Location】2 cun below the umbilicus, 0.5 cun lateral to the midline.

【Indications】①Irregular menstruation, leucorrhea, spermatorrhea, enuresis; ②diarrhea, abdominal pain, abdominal masses, oedema.

15 中注 ZhongZhu KI-15 (Meeting point of the Kidney channel with the thoroughfare vessel)

【Source】《黄帝明堂经》 *Huangdi Mingtang Jing*

【Annotation】中 Zhong means internality. 注 Zhu means to inject. There are two explanations for this name. Firstly, this acupoint is located around the umbilicus and corresponds to the intestinal tract. The essence of the kidney is injected inwards from this acupoint, thus using the kidney water to fluence and lubricate the dry intestinal tract. It is used for treating heat in the abdomen, dry stools and other heat syndromes, hence it is named 中注 ZhongZhu. Secondly, this acupoint corresponds to uterus and testicle, where the essence of the kidney is injected, hence the name.

【Location】1 cun below the umbilicus, 0.5 cun lateral to the midline.

【Indications】Abdominal pain, constipation.

16 肓俞 HuangShu KI-16 (Meeting point of the Kidney channel with the thoroughfare vessel)

【Source】《黄帝明堂经》 *Huangdi Mingtang Jing*

【Annotation】肓 Huang means the membrane tissue between the five viscera. This acupoint is located next to the umbilicus, within the peritoneum, and corresponds to 肓门 HuangMen (BL-51) on the back, hence it is named 肓俞 HuangShu.

【Location】0.5 cun lateral to the center of the umbilicus.

【Indications】Abdominal pain, constipation.

17 商曲 ShangQu KI-17 (Meeting point of the Kidney channel with the thoroughfare vessel)

【Source】《黄帝明堂经》 *Huangdi Mingtang Jing*

【Annotation】 This acupoint is located at the upper abdomen and corresponds to the intestines. The attribute of the large intestine is metal in five phases, which corresponds to 商 Shang in the five tones of traditional Chinese music. 曲 Qu means curved, which is the shape of intestine. Hence it is named 商曲 ShangQu.

【Location】 2 cun above the umbilicus, 0.5 cun lateral to the midline.

【Indications】 Abdominal pain, diarrhea, constipation, abdominal masses.

18 石关 ShiGuan KI-18 (Meeting point of the Kidney channel with the thoroughfare vessel)

【Source】《黄帝明堂经》 *Huangdi Mingtang Jing*

【Annotation】 There are two explanations for this name. Firstly, 石 Shi is a description of hardness. 关 Guan refers to an important area in the body. This acupoint is good for treating symptoms of firmness and fullness, such as constipation, epigastric fullness, and qi strangury, hence it is named 石关 ShiGuan. Besides, 石 Shi is an interchangeable word for 食 Shi, means food. This acupoint is at the stomach, which is an important organ to receiving food and water, hence the name.

【Location】 3 cun above the umbilicus, 0.5 cun lateral to the midline.

【Indications】 Abdominal pain, constipation, much spittle, hiccup.

19 阴都 YinDu KI-19 (Meeting point of the Kidney channel with the thoroughfare vessel)

【Source】《黄帝明堂经》 *Huangdi Mingtang Jing*

【Annotation】 都 Du means convergence. This acupoint belongs to the Kidney channel of Foot Shaoyin, the attribute of kidney is yin within yin. The location of this acupoint corresponds to the stomach, which is known as "the sea of food and water". Hence it is named 阴都 YinDu.

【Location】4 cun above the umbilicus, 0.5 cun lateral to the midline.

【Indications】Abdominal pain, abdominal distention, borborygmus.

20 腹通谷 FuTongGu KI-20 (Meeting point of the Kidney channel with the thoroughfare vessel)

【Source】《黄帝明堂经》 *Huangdi Mingtang Jing*

【Annotation】通 Tong means to pass through and to run through. 谷 Gu, a channel for the flow of water between mountains. This acupoint is on the abdomen, level with 上脘 ShangWan (CV-13) of the Conception vessel, at the upper part of the stomach, and is a pathway for food and drink. It is used for treating abdominal pain, abdominal distention, vomiting, as well as heartache, palpitation. Its therapeutic effect runs thorough chest and abdomen, that is, runs thorough up and down, hence it is named 腹通谷 FuTongGu.

【Location】5 cun above the umbilicus, 0.5 cun lateral to the midline.

【Indications】Abdominal pain, abdominal distention, abdominal masses, vomiting.

21 幽门 YouMen KI-21 (Meeting point of the Kidney channel with the thoroughfare vessel)

【Source】《黄帝明堂经》 *Huangdi Mingtang Jing*

【Annotation】门 Men means door. 幽 You means dark and quiet, both of which are yin images. Here it refers to the intersection of two Yin channels, the Kidney channel of Foot Shaoyin and the thoroughfare vessel. Specifically, the Kidney channel enters the abdomen and goes up with the thoroughfare vessel together. The thoroughfare vessel will deviate from the Kidney channel and then disperses in the thorax after this acupoint, where the Kidney channel also goes from the abdomen to the thorax, that is, from yin-position to yang-position, like a door where Yin and Yang meet. Hence the name 幽门 YouMen.

【Location】6 cun above the umbilicus, 0.5 cun lateral to the midline.

【Indications】Abdominal pain, abdominal distention, vomiting, hiccup, diarrhea.

22 步廊 BuLang KI-22

【Source】《黄帝明堂经》 *Huangdi Mingtang Jing*

【Annotation】步 Bu means walking. 廊 Lang means corridor. This acupoint is level with 中庭 ZhongTing (CV–16) of the Conception vessel. From this acupoint, the Kidney channel of Foot Shaoyin moves from the abdomen towards the chest and follows the sides of the ribs, just like stepping into the gallery on either side of the front courtyard, hence it is named 步廊 BuLang.

【Location】In the fifth intercostal space, 2 cun lateral to the midline.

【Indications】①Cough, asthma, fullness and pain of the chest and hypochondrium; ②vomiting.

23 神封 ShenFeng KI–23

【Source】《黄帝明堂经》 Huangdi Mingtang Jing

【Annotation】神 Shen means spirit, which stored in the heart, here it refers to the heart. 封 Feng means storing. This acupoint corresponds to the heart internally and is flush with 膻中 DanZhong (CV–17). CV–17 is the palace of the pericardium, which is a metaphor for this acupoint as a place where the spirit are stored, hence it is named 神封 ShenFeng.

【Location】In the fourth intercostal space, 2 cun lateral to the midline.

【Indications】①Cough, asthma, fullness and pain of the chest and hypochondrium; ②vomiting, no pleasure in eating; ③breast abscess.

24 灵墟 LingXu KI–24

【Source】《黄帝明堂经》 Huangdi Mingtang Jing

【Annotation】灵 Ling means spirit, which is the same as 神 Shen in Chinese. 墟 Xu means dwelling. This acupoint is in the third intercostal space, corresponding to the heart, as if the residence of the heart, hence it is named 灵墟 LingXu. The implication of the name and main treatment is the same as 神封 ShengFeng.

【Location】In the third intercostal space, 2 cun lateral to the midline.

【Indications】①Cough, asthma, fullness and pain of the chest and hypochondrium; ②vomiting; ③breast abscess.

25 神藏 ShenCang KI–25

【Source】《黄帝明堂经》 Huangdi Mingtang Jing

【Annotation】神 Shen means spirit, which stored in the heart, here it refers to the heart. 藏 Cang means storing. This acupoint is in the second intercostal space, corresponding to the heart, as if it is a place where the spirit is stored, hence it is named 神藏 ShenCang. The implication of the name and main treatment is the same as 神封 ShengFeng and 灵墟 LingXu.

【Location】In the second intercostal space, 2 cun lateral to the midline.

【Indications】①Cough, asthma, fullness and pain of the chest and hypochondrium; ②vomiting, loss of appetite.

26 彧中 YuZhong KI-26

【Source】《黄帝明堂经》 *Huangdi Mingtang Jing*

【Annotation】彧 Yu, describes a literary talent. The lung is compared to canopy, which is the organ similar to the official position of 相傅 XiangFu. 相傅 XiangFu is the prime minister, a man of great knowledge and literary talent, hence the use of 彧 Yu as a metaphor for lung. This acupoint corresponds to the lung internally and is flush with 华盖 HuaGai (CV-20). This acupoint is used to treat lung diseases such as cough, asthma, fullness and pain of the chest and ribs, hence it is named 彧中 YuZhong.

【Location】In the first intercostal space, 2 cun lateral to the midline.

【Indications】Cough, asthma, accumulation of phlegm, fullness and pain of the chest and hypochondrium.

27 俞府 ShuFu KI-27

【Source】《黄帝明堂经》 *Huangdi Mingtang Jing*

【Annotation】俞 Shu, an interchangeable word for 输 Shu, means transfer. 府 Fu, an interchangeable word for 腑 Fu, means inside of body. The channel qi travels from the foot to the chest, where it is transmitted into the lung. This acupoint is used to treat coughing, dyspnea and other symptoms of fullness in the chest, hence it is named 俞府 ShuFu.

【Location】Inferior to the clavicle, 2 cun lateral to the midline.

【Indications】①Cough, asthma, chest pain; ②vomiting.

Chapter 10
The Pericardium Channel Points of Hand Jueyin

1 天池 TianChi PC-1

【Source】《灵枢·本输》*Lingshu:* Benshu

【Annotation】天 Tian generally means the sky and specifically refers to areas above the waist. 池 Chi means a pond. This acupoint is located above the waist (position of the sky of the human body) where sags like a pond, hence it is named 天池 TianChi.

【Location】In the fourth intercostal space, 5 cun lateral to the anterior midline.

【Indications】①Cough, panting, copious phlegm, chest distress, chest pain; ②axillary swelling, scrofula.

2 天泉 TianQuan PC-2

【Source】《黄帝明堂经》*Huangdi Mingtang Jing*

【Annotation】天 Tian refers to areas above the waist. 泉 Quan means a spring where water comes to the surface. This acupoint is located at the medial side of the upper arm, above the waist (position of the sky of the human body). The Pericardium channel circulates down along this acupoint, like a spring flows down, hence it is named 天泉 TianQuan.

【Location】2 cun distal to the anterior axillary fold, between the long head and short head of the biceps brachii muscle.

【Indications】①Heartache, cough, distending pain in the chest and hypochondrium; ②brachial pain.

3 曲泽 QuZe PC-3 (*He*-Sea point)

【Source】《灵枢·本输》*Lingshu:* Benshu

【Annotation】曲 Qu means to bend. This acupoint is located in the depression medial to the elbow and can be selected when the elbow bend. 泽 Ze refers to the place where water converges. Being the *He*-Sea point of the Pericardium channel, this acupoint is like the sea where the channel qi converges, hence it is named 曲泽 QuZe.

【Location】On the cubital crease, in the depression medial to the biceps brachii tendon.

【Indications】①Heartache, palpitations, propensity to fright; ②stomach duct pain, hematemesis, vomiting; ③fever, dry mouth; ④pain of the elbow and arm.

4 郄门 XiMen PC-4(*Xi*-Cleft point)

【Source】《黄帝明堂经》*Huangdi Mingtang Jing*

【Annotation】郄 Xi, an interchangeable word of 隙 Xi, refers to a cleft. 门 Men refers to a door. This acupoint is the *Xi*-Cleft point of the Pericardium channel, and is located in the cleft between the radius and the ulna which are like doors on both sides, hence it is named 郄门 XiMen.

【Location】5 cun proximal to the palmar wrist crease, between the tendons of the palmaris longus and the flexor carpi radialis.

【Indications】①Heartache, palpitations, vexation, chest pain; ②hemoptysis, hematemesis, epistaxis.

5 间使 JianShi PC-5(*Jing*-River point)

【Source】《灵枢·本输》*Lingshu:* Benshu

【Annotation】间 Jian means middle. This acupoint is located in the depression between two tendons, 3 cun proximal to the palmar wrist crease. 使 Shi refers to an envoy. The heart is an organ similar to the monarch. The pericardium is an organ similar to the envoy because it is the periphery of the heart, preventing the heart from being attacked by exterior pathogenic factors and performing the functions of the heart. This acupoint is the *Jing*-River point of the Pericardium channel, and is mainly used for treating heart and mind disorders, hysteria and epilepsy. Since its location is consistent with the meaning of 间 , and its indications are consistent with the meaning of 使 , this acupoint is named 间使 JianShi.

【 Location 】 3 cun proximal to the palmar wrist crease, between the tendons of the palmaris longus and the flexor carpi radialis.

【 Indications 】 Heartache, palpitations, vexation; stomach duct pain, vomiting; depression, mania, epilepsy; loss of voice; febrile disease, malaria.

6 内关 NeiGuan PC-6 (*Luo*–Connecting point, Confluent point of the Yin Linking vessel)

【 Source 】《灵枢·经脉》 *Lingshu:* Jingmai

【 Annotation 】 内 Nei means medial. 关 Guan refers to an important place for contacting. As the *Luo*-Connecting point of the Pericardium channel, this acupoint contacts with the Sanjiao channel and is located at the medial side of the forearm which corresponds to WaiGuan (SJ–5), hence it is named 内关 NeiGuan.

【 Location 】 2 cun proximal to the palmar wrist crease, between the tendons of the palmaris longus and the flexor carpi radialis.

【 Indications 】 ①Heartache, palpitations, chest distress; ②stomach duct pain, vomiting, hiccup; ③depression, mania, epilepsy; ④pain and contraction of the upper limb.

7 大陵 DaLing PC-7 (*Shu*–Stream and *Yuan*–Source point)

【 Source 】《灵枢·九针十二原》《灵枢·本输》 *Lingshu: Jiuzhen Shieryuan, Lingshu: Benshu*

【 Annotation 】 大 Da means big. 陵 Ling refers to a hill. This acupoint is in the depression between two tendons on the palmar wrist crease. Since the place is relatively uneven and the metacarpal bone is like a big hill, it is named 大陵 DaLing.

【 Location 】 On the palmar wrist crease, between the tendons of the palmaris longus and the flexor carpi radialis.

【 Indications 】 ①Pain in the chest and lateral costal region, heartache, palpitations; ②stomach duct pain, vomiting, hematemesis; ③depression, mania, epilepsy; ④pain and contraction of the upper limb; ⑤swollen sore.

8 劳宫 LaoGong PC-8 (*Ying*-Spring point)

【Source】《灵枢·本输》 *Lingshu:* Benshu

【Annotation】劳 Lao means to labor. There are two explanations for this name. Firstly, this acupoint is located in the center of the palm and our hands are the main organs for laboring. 宫 Gong symbolizes the residence of monarchs. Considering the heart is an organ similar to the monarch, LaoGong means that this acupoint is located in the palm, the palace where the heart spirit resides. Secondly, according to TCM theory, the Pericardium channel belongs to fire. This point is the *Ying*-Spring and Fire point of the channel, therefore it is the Fire point of the Fire channel, mainly used for treating febrile diseases of the Heart channel such as aphtha and fetid mouth odor as well as mental disorders such as epilepsy and coma.

【Location】Proximal to the third metacarpophalangeal joint, in the depression between the second and third metacarpal bones and close to the latter. When clenching the fist and flexing the fingers, the point is under the tip of the middle finger.

【Indications】①Aphtha, fetid mouth odor; ②hand tinea; ③depression, mania, epilepsy; ④heartache, vexation; ⑤vomiting, hematemesis; ④febrile diseases, thirst.

9 中冲 ZhongChong PC-9 (*Jing*-Well point)

【Source】《灵枢·本输》 *Lingshu:* Benshu

【Annotation】中 Zhong means middle and specifically refers to the middle finger here. 冲 Chong means to rush out. This acupoint is at the center of the tip of the middle finger where channel qi of the Pericardium channel rushes out, hence it is named 中冲 ZhongChong.

【Location】At the center of the tip of the middle finger.

【Indications】①Stroke, stiff tongue with aphasia; ②loss of consciousness; ③heartache, vexation; ④heat stroke, febrile diseases; ⑤infantile convulsion.

Chapter 11
The Sanjiao Channel Points of Hand Shaoyang

1 关冲 GuanChong SJ–1 (*Jing*–Well point)

【Source】《灵枢·本输》 *Lingshu: Benshu*

【Annotation】 关 Guan refers to a key passage. 冲 Chong refers to important traffic channels or important places. This acupoint locates at the important channel of the exterior Sanjiao channel and the interior Pericardium channel, hence it is named 关冲 GuanChong.

【Location】 On the ring finger, ulnar to the distal phalanx, 0.1 cun proximal to the ulnar corner of the fingernail.

【Indications】 ①Headache, tinnitus, deafness, swelling and pain of throat; ②Corneal nebula; ③febrile disease, thirst, dry lips.

2 液门 YeMen SJ–2 (*Ying*–Spring point)

【Source】《灵枢·本输》 *Lingshu: Benshu*

【Annotation】液 Ye means fluid and humor. In TCM theory, the triple energizer (Sanjiao) is the organ similar to the official in charge of dredging and is responsible for regulating water passage. This acupoint is the *Ying*–Spring point of the Sanjiao channel. It can be used to treat symptoms of fluid damage such as throat pain and dry eyes, hence its name includes the word 液 . 门 Men, originating from the shape of traditional Chinese characters 門 , refers to a gate. Since this point locates in the depression between the ring and little fingers, a position shaping like 門 , it is named 液门 YeMen.

【Location】On the dorsum of the hand, in the depression superior to the web margin between the ring and little fingers, at the border between the red and white flesh.

【Indications】①Headache, red eyes, tinnitus, deafness, swelling and pain of throat; ②febrile disease, malaria; ③swelling and pain of the arm.

3 中渚 ZhongZhu SJ-3 (*Shu*-Stream point)

【Source】《灵枢·本输》*Lingshu: Benshu*

【Annotation】中 Zhong means in the middle. 渚 Zhu refers to an islet in the water. In TCM theory, the triple energizer (Sanjiao) is the organ similar to the official in charge of dredging and is responsible for regulating water passage. Therefore the Sanjiao channel is like a river. In addition, the acupoint locates between the fourth and fifth metacarpal bones, which seem like an islet in the river, hence it is named 中渚 ZhongZhu.

【Location】On the dorsum of the hand, between the fourth and fifth metacarpal bones, in the depression proximal to the fourth metacarpophalangeal joint.

【Indications】①Headache, pain of the eyes, tinnitus, deafness, swelling and pain of throat; ②pain of the elbow, upper arm, shoulder and upper back, inability to flex and extend the fingers; ③febrile disease.

4 阳池 YangChi SJ-4 (*Yuan*-Source point)

【Source】《灵枢·本输》*Lingshu: Benshu*

【Annotation】池 Chi refers to a pool. This acupoint locates at the dorsal wrist crease, where the depression is like a pool. In addition, according to the yin–yang theory, the dorsal wrist belongs to yang, hence the acupoint is named 阳池 YangChi.

【Location】On the dorsal wrist crease, in the depression ulnar to the extensor digitorum tendon.

【Indications】①Pain of the wrist, pain of the shoulder and arm; ②malaria; ③dry mouth.

5 外关 WaiGuan SJ-5 (*Luo*-Connecting point, confluent point of the Yang Linking vessel)

【Source】《灵枢·经脉》《灵枢·根结》*Lingshu: Jingmai, Lingshu: GenJie*

【Annotation】外 Wai means lateral. 关 Guan refers to an important place for contacting. As the *Luo*-Connecting point of the Sanjiao channel, this acupoint contacts with the Pericardium channel and is located at the lateral side of the forearm, which corresponds to NeiGuan (PC-6), hence it is named 外关 WaiGuan.

【Location】On the lateral side of the forearm, 2 cun proximal to the dorsal wrist crease, at the midpoint of the interosseous space between the ulna and the radius.

【Indications】①Tinnitus, deafness; ②pain of the chest and lateral costal region; ③obstructive pain of the upper limb.

6 支沟 ZhiGou SJ-6 (*Jing*-River point)

【Source】《灵枢·本输》*Lingshu: Benshu*

【Annotation】支 Zhi, an interchangeable word of 肢 Zhi, means the upper limbs. 沟 Gou refers to a ditch. As the *Jing*-River point of the Sanjiao channel, this acupoint locates in the depression between the ulna and the radius, 3 cun proximal to the wrist. The channel qi flows through this place as if water flows into the ditch, hence it is named 支沟 ZhiGou.

【Location】On the lateral side of the forearm, 3 cun proximal to the dorsal wrist crease, at the midpoint of the interosseous space between the ulna and the radius.

【Indications】①Tinnitus, deafness, loss of voice; ②scrofula; ③pain of the chest and lateral costal region; ④vomiting, constipation; ⑤febrile disease.

7 会宗 HuiZong SJ-7 (*Xi*-Cleft point)

【Source】《黄帝明堂经》*Huangdi Mingtang Jing*

【Annotation】会 Hui means gathering. 宗 Zong represents basis. This acupoint is located 3 cun proximal to the wrist, 0.5 cun next to ZhiGou (SJ-6), and distal to SanYangLuo (SJ-8). The qi of the Sanjiao channel gathers at this acupoint through ZhiGou (SJ-6) and then travels into SanYangLuo (SJ-8), thereby making the qi of three yang channels of the hand contact, hence it is named 会宗 HuiZong.

【Location】On the lateral side of the forearm, 3 cun proximal to the dorsal wrist crease, just radial to the ulna.

【Indications】①Deafness; ②epilepsy; ③dermatic pain of the upper limb.

8 三阳络 SanYangLuo SJ-8

【Source】《黄帝明堂经》*Huangdi Mingtang Jing*

【Annotation】三 San refers to three. 络 Luo means to contact. This acupoint is located where the yang qi of the Sanjiao channel, Small Intestine channel and Large Intestine channel contact, hence it is named 三阳络 SanYangLuo.

【Location】On the lateral side of the forearm, 4 cun proximal to the dorsal wrist crease, at the midpoint of the interosseous space between the ulna and the radius.

【Indications】①Deafness, sudden aphonia, toothache; ②pain of lumbago and lateral costal region, obstructive pain of the upper limb.

9 四渎 SiDu SJ-9

【Source】《黄帝明堂经》*Huangdi Mingtang Jing*

【Annotation】四 Si means four. 渎 Du refers to great rivers. In ancient times, the Yangtze River, the Yellow River, the Huai River and the Ji River are called SiDu. These four rivers all flow into the sea. The qi of the Sanjiao channel circulates from SanYangLuo (SJ-8), where the yang qi of three hand yang channels contact, to this acupoint and then flows into TianJing (SJ-9), the *He*-Sea point of the Sanjiao channel. In this case, this acupoint is like where streams converge into a large river and then flow into the sea, hence it is named 四渎 SiDu.

【Location】On the lateral side of the forearm, 5 cun distal to the prominence of the olecranon, at the midpoint of the interosseous space between the ulna and the radius.

【Indications】①Deafness, toothache; ②pain of the forearm.

10 天井 TianJing SJ-10(*He*-Sea point)

【Source】《灵枢·本输》*Lingshu: Benshu*

【Annotation】天 Tian refers to the heaven. 井 Jing means a well. This acupoint is the *He*-Sea point of the Sanjiao channel, and according to the five-element theory, it belongs to earth. In TCM theory, the triple energizer (Sanjiao) is responsible for regulating water passage, and where the water comes out from the earth is called 井 Jing. Furthermore, this acupoint is proximal to the olecranon, in the depression between two tendons which looks like a well.

Meanwhile, it locates on the upper limb, which belongs to the heaven location, hence it is named 天井 TianJing. With the capability of moving qi to relieve depression, the acupoint is often used to treat scrofula and goiter. Therefore it is considered a qi–elimination acupoint on the arm.

【Location】In the depression 1 cun proximal to the prominence of the olecranon.

【Indications】①Chest pain, heartache; ②deafness, migraine; ③epilepsy; ④scrofula, goiter; ⑤pain of the chest and lateral costal region, pain of the shoulder and arm.

11 清泠渊 QingLingYuan SJ–11

【Source】《黄帝明堂经》 Huangdi Mingtang Jing

【Annotation】清泠渊 QingLingYuan is the name of an ancient pool. 清 Qing means to clear and specific means to clear heat here. 渊 Yuan refers to a deep pool. The qi and blood of the Sanjiao channel flow into this acupoint like the water flows into a deep pool. The three words of its name give the impression of seeing a cold pond. Furthermore, the acupoint is used to treat syndrome of toxic heat in the clinic, hence it is named 清泠渊 QingLingYuan. In ancient China, people were vaccinated on QingLingYuan and XiaoLuo (SJ–12) due to their ability to outthrust and clear the toxin of obstructive–heat.

【Location】On the line connecting the prominence of the olecranon with the acromial angle, 2 cun proximal to the prominence of the olecranon.

【Indications】①Headache, pain of the eyes, hypochondriac pain; ②obstructive pain of the upper limb.

12 消泺 XiaoLuo SJ–12

【Source】《黄帝明堂经》 Huangdi Mingtang Jing

【Annotation】消 Xiao means to dissipate. 泺 Luo is the name of a river. This acupoint is good at clearing the heat of sanjiao, as if cool water dissipates heat, hence it is named 消泺 XiaoLuo. Besides, 泺 Luo and 止 泺 ZhiLuo are also aliases of the Chinese medicine Guanzhong (Rhizoma Cyrtomii), which is bitter and astringent. Its function is similar to this acupoint, namely heat–clearing and detoxication.

【Location】On the line connecting the prominence of the olecranon with the acromial angle, 5 cun proximal to the prominence of the olecranon.

【Indications】①Toothache; ②headache, pain of the neck.

13 臑会 NaoHui SJ–13

【Source】《黄帝明堂经》*Huangdi Mingtang Jing*

【Annotation】 臑 Nao means the upper arm. 会 Hui means to meet. The acupoint is posteroinferior to the border of the deltoid muscle. The Sanjiao channel and the Yang Linking vessel meet here, hence it is named 臑会 NaoHui.

【Location】On the line connecting the prominence of the olecranon with JianLiao (SJ–14), 3 cun inferior to JianLiao (SJ–14), and posteroinferior to the border of the deltoid muscle.

【Indications】①Goiter, scrofula; ②flaccid obstruction of the upper limbs.

14 肩髎 JianLiao SJ–14

【Source】《黄帝明堂经》*Huangdi Mingtang Jing*

【Annotation】 肩 Jian refers to the shoulder. 髎 Liao means the space of scleromere. When the upper arms abduct, two depressions can be found anterior and posterior to the acromion. The former is JianYu (LI–15), and the latter is JianLiao. These two acupoints are often combined to treat the pain and heaviness of the shoulder and arms with inability to raise up, hence it is named 肩髎 JianLiao.

【Location】Posterior to JianYu (LI–15), in the depression posteroinferior to the acromion when the arms abduct.

【Indications】Pain and restricted movement of the shoulder.

15 天髎 TianLiao SJ–15

【Source】《黄帝明堂经》*Huangdi Mingtang Jing*

【Annotation】髎 Liao means the space of scleromere. This acupoint locates at the uppermost part of the thoracic cavity, a position like the heaven. Meanwhile, it locates in the depression of the bone margin superior to the superior angle of scapula, hence it is named 天髎 TianLiao.

【Location】In the depression of the bone margin superior to the superior angle of scapula.

【Indications】Pain of the shoulder and arms, stiffness and pain of the neck.

16 天牖 TianYou SJ-16

【Source】《灵枢·本输》 *Lingshu: Benshu*

【Annotation】天 Tian refers to the heaven-part, namely the upper areas of the body. 牖 You means windows. This acupoint can relieve stagnant qi of the ears and eyes, being used to treat blurred vision and deafness, like a window of the heaven-part, hence it is named 天牖 TianYou.

【Location】At the same level as the angle of mandible, in the depression posterior to the sternocleidomastoid muscle.

【Indications】①Blurred vision, deafness, swelling and pain of throat; ②headache, dizziness; ③scrofula; ④stiffness and pain of the neck.

17 翳风 YiFeng SJ-17

【Source】《黄帝明堂经》 *Huangdi Mingtang Jing*

【Annotation】翳 Yi means to shield. 风 Feng refers to the pathogenic wind. This acupoint locates in the depression behind the ear, and the ear is like a barrier to shield it from the wind. Meanwhile, with the capacity to dispel pathogenic wind, the acupoint is good at treating wind patterns and is commonly used in the treatment of facial paralysis and facial spasm, hence it is named 翳风 YiFeng.

【Location】In the depression anterior to the inferior end of the mastoid process.

【Indications】①Tinnitus, deafness; ②deviated eye and mouth, lockjaw; ③swelling of the cheek, scrofula; ④swelling and pain of throat, hoarseness.

18 瘈脉 ChiMai SJ-18

【Source】《黄帝明堂经》 *Huangdi Mingtang Jing*

【Annotation】瘈 Chi means convulsion. 脉 Mai refers to cyan collateral vessels. This acupoint locates where the cyan collateral vessel is shaped like a chicken claw behind the ear root and is mainly used to treat symptoms of frightened epilepsy and convulsions such as infantile convulsion, thus it is named 瘈脉 ChiMai.

【Location】At the junction of the upper two-thirds and lower one-third of the curved line from YiFeng (SJ-17) to JiaoSun (SJ-20).

【Indications】Infantile frightened epilepsy, convulsion, headache, tinnitus, deafness.

19 颅息 LuXi SJ-19

【Source】《黄帝明堂经》 *Huangdi Mingtang Jing*

【Annotation】颅 Lu refers to the head. 息 Xi means to breathe. This acupoint locates at the cyan collateral vessel behind the ear, which corresponds to breathing, like the place the head breathes, hence it is named 颅息 LuXi.

【Location】At the junction of the upper one-third and lower two-thirds of the curved line from YiFeng (SJ-17) to JiaoSun (SJ-20).

【Indications】①Tinnitus, headache; ②infantile convulsion.

20 角孙 JiaoSun SJ-20 (Meeting point of the Sanjiao, Gall Bladder and Large Intestine channels)

【Source】《黄帝明堂经》 *Huangdi Mingtang Jing*

【Annotation】角 Jiao refers to the superior cornu of the ear. 孙 Sun means branches and refers explicitly to the sub-collateral vessels here. The acupoint is above the cornu of the ear. When the helix is folded towards the tragus, it locates just superior to the auricular apex where the sub-collateral vessels of the Sanjiao, Small Intestine and Gall Bladder channels meet, hence it is named 角孙 JiaoSun.

【Location】Just superior to the auricular apex.

【Indications】Toothache, swelling of the cheek, corneal nebula.

21 耳门 ErMen SJ-21

【Source】《黄帝明堂经》 *Huangdi Mingtang Jing*

【Annotation】耳 Er means the ear. 门 Men refers to a door or a key entrance. This acupoint locates in the depression anterior to the supratragic notch. The branch of the Sanjiao channel separates from the main track behind the ear, enters the ear and then comes out from this acupoint to the front of the ear, hence it is named 耳门 ErMen.

【Location】In the depression between the supratragic notch and the condylar process of the mandible.

【Indications】①Tinnitus, deafness, toothache; ②swelling of the cheek, swelling of the neck.

22 耳和髎 ErHeLiao SJ–22 (Meeting point of the Sanjiao, Gall Bladder and Small Intestine channels)

【Source】《黄帝明堂经》*Huangdi Mingtang Jing*

【Annotation】和 He means to harmonize the sound and music. 髎 Liao refers to the space of scleromere. This acupoint is mainly used to treat ear disorders such as deafness so that the ear can hear the sound of five tones harmoniously. Furthermore, it locates in the depression anterior to the auricular root, hence it is named 耳和髎 ErHeLiao.

【Location】Posterior to the earlock, anterior to the auricular root, posterior to the superficial temporal artery.

【Indications】Headache, tinnitus, lockjaw.

23 丝竹空 SiZhuKong SJ–23

【Source】《黄帝明堂经》*Huangdi Mingtang Jing*

【Annotation】There are two explanations for this name. Firstly, 丝 Si means tiny. 竹 Zhu refers to bamboo leaves. 空 Kong means depressions and cavities. This acupoint locates in the depression at the lateral end of the eyebrow, and the shape of the eyebrows is like bamboo leaves, hence it is named 丝竹空 SiZhuKong. Secondly, understanding from the perspective of musical instruments, stringed instruments are called 丝 Si and wind instruments are called 竹 Zhu. Therefore, Si and Zhu together are called 丝 竹 SiZhu, representing the music. The eyebrows are slender and curved, like the xiao (a Chinese vertical bamboo flute) or bowstring, and the acupoint is like a hole in the xiao or the bowstring, hence the name.

【Location】In the depression at the lateral end of the eyebrow.

【Indications】①Headache, dizziness, redness and pain of the eyes, twitching of the eyelids; ②epilepsy, upward staring eyes.

Chapter 12
The Gall Bladder Channel Points of Foot Shaoyang

1 瞳子髎 TongZiLiao GB–1 (Meeting point of the Small Intestine, Sanjiao and Gall Bladder channels)

【Source】《黄帝明堂经》*Huangdi Mingtang Jing*

【Annotation】瞳子 Tong Zi refers to an eyeball where the essence of an eye is. 髎 means a cleft. This acupoint locates at the interosseous space lateral to the outer canthus and has the capability of brightening eyes, hence it is named 瞳子髎 Tong Zi Liao.

【Location】In the depression 0.5 cun lateral to the outer canthus of the eye.

【Indications】①Headache; ②redness and pain of the eyes, internal visual obstruction (cataracts), bluish blindness (optic atrophy), corneal nebula, lacrimation.

2 听会 TingHui GB–2

【Source】《黄帝明堂经》*Huangdi Mingtang Jing*

【Annotation】听 Ting means hearing. 会 Hui means gathering. This acupoint locates in front of the ear, and is mainly used to treat ear diseases such as tinnitus and deafness, acting like the governor of hearing, hence it is named 听会 TingHui.

【Location】In the depression between the intertragic notch and the condylar process of the mandible.

【Indications】①Tinnitus, deafness; ②toothache; ③dislocation of the temporomandibular joint; ④deviated eye and mouth.

3 上关 ShangGuan GB-3 (Meeting point of the Sanjiao, Gall Bladder and Stomach channels)

【Source】《素问·气穴论》《灵枢·本输》 *Suwen: Qixue Lun, Lingshu: Benshu*

【Annotation】上 Shang means above. 关 Guan represents a pivot of opening and closing and specifically refers to the mandibular joint here. Opposite to XiaGuan (ST-7), which locates inferior to the zygomatic arch, this acupoint is above the arch, hence it is named 上关 ShangGuan. Furthermore, it is the meeting point of the Sanjiao, Gall bladder and Stomach channels, with the Sanjiao and Gall bladder channels as the master and the Stomach channel as the guest. Since this acupoint is where the guest and master meet, it is also called 客主人 Ke (guest) ZhuRen (master).

【Location】In the depression superior to the midpoint of the zygomatic arch.

【Indications】①Tinnitus, deafness, suppurative otitis media, toothache, deviated eye and mouth; ②dislocation or dysfunction of the temporomandibular joint; epilepsy.

4 颔厌 HanYan GB-4 (Meeting point of the Sanjiao, Gall Bladder and Stomach channels)

【Source】《黄帝明堂经》 *Huangdi Mingtang Jing*

【Annotation】颔 Han refers to the frontal eminence. 厌 Yan means to close. When chewing food, this acupoint locates where it moves under the influence of the opening and closing of the mandible joint near the frontal eminence, hence it is named 颔厌 HanYan.

【Location】At the junction of the upper one-fourth and lower three-fourths of the curved line from TouWei (ST-8) to QuBin (GB-7). To select the point, draw a curved line from TouWei (ST-8) to QuBin (GB-7) along the temple. The midpoint of the line is XuanLu (GB-5). HanYan is in the middle of TouWei (ST-8) and XuanLu (GB-5). Besides, the midpoint of XuanLu (GB-5) and QuBin (GB-7) is XuanLi (GB-6).

【Indications】Pain of the outer canthus, tinnitus; migraine, dizziness.

5 悬颅 XuanLu GB-5

【Source】《黄帝明堂经》 *Huangdi Mingtang Jing*

【Annotation】悬 Xuan means hanging. 颅 Lu refers to the head. There are two explanations for this name. Firstly, the acupoint is named after its location, which is suspended on the side of the head. Secondly, it is named after its indications. When dizzy, people feel that their feet are rootless and their head is hanging in the air. This acupoint is mainly used to treat dizziness, hence it is named 悬颅 Xuan Lu.

【Location】At the midpoint of the curved line from TouWei (ST-8) to QuBin (GB-7).

【Indications】①Migraine extending to the eyes, jaw and teeth; ②febrile disease.

6 悬厘 XuanLi GB-6 (Meeting point of the Sanjiao, Gall Bladder and Stomach channels)

【Source】《黄帝明堂经》 Huangdi Mingtang Jing

【Annotation】悬 Xuan means hanging. 厘 Li, describes a small distance. This acupoint locates at the head's lateral side, very close to XuanLu (GB-5). With a similar action to XuanLu (GB-5), it is mainly used to treat dizziness and headache, hence it is named 悬 厘 Xuan Li.

【Location】At the junction of the upper three-fourths and lower one-fourth of the curved line from TouWei (ST-8) to QuBin (GB-7).

【Indications】①Migraine, pain of the eyes; ②febrile disease.

7 曲鬓 QuBin GB-7 (Meeting point of the Gall Bladder and Bladder channels)

【Source】《黄帝明堂经》 Huangdi Mingtang Jing

【Annotation】曲 Qu means curved. 鬓 Bin refers to the earlock. This acupoint locates at the curved earlock, hence it is named 曲鬓 QuBin.

【Location】At the junction of the vertical line of the posterior border of the earlock and the horizontal line of the apex of the auricle.

【Indications】Headache, toothache, swelling of the cheek, lockjaw.

8 率谷 ShuaiGu GB-8 (Meeting point of the Gall Bladder and Bladder channels)

【Source】《黄帝明堂经》 Huangdi Mingtang Jing

【Annotation】There are two explanations for this name. Firstly, 率 Shuai means along. 谷 Gu refers to a valley. This acupoint can be found superior to QuBin (GB-7) along the ear, with a shape like a valley, hence it is named 率谷 ShuaiGu. Secondly, 率 Shuai also means to lead. Among all the acupoints named after 谷 Gu, ShuaiGu is the only one on the head, as if the leader of others, hence the name.

【Location】Directly superior to the auricular apex, 1.5 cun superior to the earlock.

【Indications】①Migraine, dizziness, vomiting; ②infantile convulsion.

9 天冲 TianChong GB-9 (Meeting point of the Gall Bladder and Bladder channels)

【Source】《黄帝明堂经》 *Huangdi Mingtang Jing*

【Annotation】 天 Tian, represents the heaven-part, specifically referring to the head here. 冲 Chong means contacting or making something unobstructed. This acupoint locates 2 cun superior to the hairline behind the ear. It is vertical to TongTian (BL-7) and contacts with the qi of the Bladder channel, hence it is named 天冲 Tian Chong, the name of a star, to describe the qi of this acupoint can contact with the sky. Furthermore, the acupoint is mainly used to treat head and facial disorders such as headache, epilepsy and swelling and pain of the gingiva, with an action of unblocking, hence the name.

【Location】Directly superior to the posterior border of the auricular root, 2 cun superior to the hairline. Almost 0.5 cun posterior to ShuaiGu (GB-8).

【Indications】①Headache, swelling and pain of the gingiva; ②epilepsy.

10 浮白 FuBai GB-10 (Meeting point of the Gall Bladder and Bladder channels)

【Source】《素问·气穴论》 *Suwen: Qixue Lun*

【Annotation】There are two explanations for this name. Firstly, 浮 Fu means to surface. 白 Bai refers to white hairs. Regular staying up late, insomnia and emotional depression may lead to the deficiency of yin-blood, resulting in insufficient blood to nourish the hair and the ascendant hyperactivity of liver yang. Therefore, white hair appears at the earlocks, with associated symptoms like headache, deafness and tinnitus. This acupoint can be used to treat such a syndrome, hence it is named 浮白 Fu Bai. Secondly, Fu Bai can also represent unrestrained drinking. This acupoint is mainly used to treat symptoms like a drunken state, such as inability to walk, headache, fullness of chest and expectoration of phlegm and foam, hence the name.

【Location】Posterior and superior to the mastoid process, at the junction of the upper one-third and lower two-thirds of the curved line from TianChong (BG-9) to WanGu (GB-12). Almost behind the auricular apex, 1 cun superior to the hairline.

【Indications】 ①Headache, pain of the eyes, toothache; ②flaccid obstruction of the lower limbs.

11 头窍阴 TouQiaoYin GB-11 (Meeting point of the Gall Bladder and Bladder channels)

【Source】《黄帝明堂经》*Huangdi Mingtang Jing*

【Annotation】头 Tou refers to the head. 窍 Qiao is understood as 空 Kong, meaning hollow. This acupoint is superior to WanGu (GB-12) and below the occipital bone. By pressing, an depression can be found at its location. According to the yin-yang theory, the front belongs to yang, and the back belongs to yin. Since the acupoint locates in the hollow at the yin side of the ear, it is named 头窍阴 TouQiaoYin.

【Location】Posterior and superior to the mastoid process, at the junction of the upper two-thirds and lower one-third of the curved line from TianChong (GB-9) to WanGu (GB-12).

【Indications】Headache, stiffness and pain of the neck.

12 完骨 Wan Gu GB-12 (Meeting point of the Gall Bladder and Bladder channels)

【Source】《素问·气穴论》*Suwen: Qixue Lun*

【Annotation】完 Wan means high and solid. 骨 Gu refers to the bone. WanGu refers to the mastoid process. It is named because the skull is tough, protecting the brain as the city wall. This acupoint locates in the depression posteroinferior to the mastoid process, which is the highest part of the skull, hence it is named 完骨 WanGu.

【Location】In the depression posteroinferior to the mastoid process.

【Indications】Headache, stiffness and pain of the neck; swelling and pain of the throat, swelling of the cheek, toothache; mania-depression; wind stroke, deviated eye and mouth.

13 本神 BenShen GB-13 (Meeting point of the Gall Bladder channel with the Yang Linking vessel)

【Source】《黄帝明堂经》 *Huangdi Mingtang Jing*

【Annotation】本 Ben means the origin and basis. 神 Shen refers to the original spirit. The head stores the original spirit. This acupoint locates at the head, level with ShenTing (GV-24), and corresponds to the brain. Meanwhile, it is mainly used to treat mental disorders with the spirit leaving its origin such as epilepsy, infantile convulsion and wind stroke, hence it is named 本神 BenShen.

【Location】On the head, 0.5 cun superior to the anterior hairline, 3 cun lateral to the anterior median line.

【Indications】①Headache, stiffness and pain of the neck, dizziness; ②infantile convulsion, epilepsy.

14 阳白 Yang Bai GB-14 (Meeting point of the Gall Bladder channel with the Yang Linking vessel)

【Source】《黄帝明堂经》 *Huangdi Mingtang Jing*

【Annotation】阳 Yang here refers to the head. 白 Bai means brightness. This acupoint locates at the forehead, directly superior to the pupil. Meanwhile, with an capability of brightening the eyes, it is mainly used to treat eye diseases, hence it is named 阳白 YangBai.

【Location】1 cun superior to the eyebrow, directly superior to the center of the pupil.

【Indications】Headache, pain of the eyes, itching of the eyes, corneal nebula.

15 头临泣 Tou Lin Qi GB-15 (Meeting point of the Gall Bladder and Bladder channels with the Yang Linking vessel)

【Source】Presented as 临泣 LinQi in《黄帝明堂经》 *Huangdi Mingtang Jing* and as 头临泣 TouLinQi in《针灸资生经》 *ZhenJiu ZiSheng Jing*.

【Annotation】头 Tou refers to the head. 临 Lin means looking down from a high place. 泣 Qi means to weep. Eyes are where the tears come out. This acupoint locates near the anterior hairline, directly superior to the center of the pupil, and is mainly used to treat head and eye diseases such as headache, dizziness, redness and pain of the eyes, and corneal nebula. Hence it is named 头临泣 TouLinQi.

【Location】0.5 cun within the anterior hairline, directly superior to the center of the pupil.

【Indications】①Headache, dizziness; ②pain of the eyes, dacryorrhea, corneal nebula; ③nasal congestion, sinusitis; ④infantile convulsion, upward staring eyes.

16 目窗 MuChuang GB-16 (Meeting point of the Gall Bladder channel with the Yang Linking vessel)

【Source】《黄帝明堂经》 Huangdi Mingtang Jing

【Annotation】目 Mu refers to the eyes. 窗 Chuang means the windows. This acupoint locates directly superior to the center of the pupil, 1.5 cun within the anterior hairline. It is mainly used to treat eye disorders such as redness and pain of the eyes, bluish blindness (optic atrophy) and blurred vision, like opening a window to brighten the house, hence it is named 目窗 MuChuang.

【Location】1.5 cun within the anterior hairline, directly superior to the center of the pupil.

【Indications】①Headache, dizziness; ②pain of the eyes, myopia.

17 正营 ZhengYing GB-17 (Meeting point of the Gall Bladder channel with the Yang Linking vessel)

【Source】《黄帝明堂经》 Huangdi Mingtang Jing

【Annotation】There are two explanations for this name. Firstly, 正 Zheng means central. 营 Ying means to contact. This acupoint locates on the top of the head, where the qi of the Gall Bladder channel and the Yang Linking vessel contact, hence it is named 正营 ZhengYing. Secondly, 营 Ying also refers to the horizontal line. ese, a north-south longitudinal line was called 经 Jing, and an east-west horizontal line was called 营 Ying. The acupoint is near the horizontal line of BaiHui (GV-20), which locates at the center of the head, hence the name.

【Location】2.5 cun within the anterior hairline, directly superior to the center of the pupil.

【Indications】Headache, dizziness; toothache.

18 承灵 ChengLing GB-18 (Meeting point of the Gall Bladder channel with the Yang Linking vessel)

【Source】《黄帝明堂经》 *Huangdi Mingtang Jing*

【Annotation】承 Cheng means holding. 灵 Ling refers to the god. The ancients believed that the god residents three feet above the head. This acupoint is 4 cun within the anterior hairline, a high position that holds the essence from the god, hence it is named 承灵 ChengLing.

【Location】4 cun within the anterior hairline, directly superior to the center of the pupil.

【Indications】Headache, aversion to cold, nasal congestion, epistaxis.

19 脑空 NaoKong GB-19 (Meeting point of the Gall Bladder channel with the Yang Linking vessel)

【Source】《黄帝明堂经》 *Huangdi Mingtang Jing*

【Annotation】脑 Nao refers to the brain. 空 Kong means the cleft. This acupoint locates at the level of the superior border of the external occipital protuberance, below which is the cleft in the occipital bone, hence it is named 脑空 Nao Kong.

【Location】At the level of the superior border of the external occipital protuberance, directly superior to FengChi (GB-20).

【Indications】①Pain of the eyes, deafness, epistaxis, nasal sore and ulcer; ②headache, dizziness, mania-depression and epilepsy; ③fever; ④stiffness and pain of the neck.

20 风池 FengChi GB-20 (Meeting point of the Gall Bladder channel with the Yang Linking vessel)

【Source】《灵枢·热病》 *Lingshu: Rebing*

【Annotation】风 Feng means the wind. 池 Chi refers to a pond. This acupoint locates inferior to the occipital bone, which is depressed like a pond and is easy for the pathogenic wind to invade. Meanwhile, it is a key acupoint for treating wind patterns, hence it is named 风池 FengChi.

【Location】In the depression between the origins of sternocleidomastoid and trapezius muscles.

【Indications】①Wind stroke, epilepsy, depression, mania; ②dizziness, tinnitus, deafness; ③redness and pain of the eyes, blurred vision; ④epistaxis; ⑤fever, headache, nasal congestion, stiffness and pain of the neck.

21 肩井 JianJing GB-21 (Meeting point of the Sanjiao, Gall Bladder and Stomach channels with the Yang Linking vessel)

【Source】《黄帝明堂经》*Huangdi Mingtang Jing*

【Annotation】There are two explanations for this name. Firstly, 肩 Jian refers to the shoulder. 井 Jing means a well. This acupoint locates in the depression at the center of the shoulder, under which is the thoracic cavity like a deep well, hence it is named 肩井 JianJing. Secondly, 井 Jing also refers to a city in ancient Chinese, implying that the roads extend in all directions. The Gall Bladder channel contacts with other yang channels through this acupoint, like an extensive traffic hub, hence the name.

【Location】At the midpoint of the line connecting the spinous process of the seventh cervical vertebra (C7) with the lateral end of the acromion.

【Indications】①Stiffness and pain of the neck, pain of the shoulder and upper back; ②wind stroke, upper limbs paralysis; ③scrofula; ④dystocia, mastitis, postpartum hypogalactia.

22 渊腋 YuanYe GB-22

【Source】《黄帝明堂经》*Huangdi Mingtang Jing*

【Annotation】渊 Yuan means deep. 腋 Ye refers to the axilla. This acupoint locates 3 cun inferior to the axilla, hiding deeply under the armpit, hence it is named 渊腋 YuanYe.

【Location】In the fourth intercostal space, on the midaxillary line.

【Indications】①Distending pain of the chest and lateral costal region, swelling of the axilla; ②pain and contraction of the upper limbs.

23 辄筋 ZheJin GB-23

【Source】《黄帝明堂经》*Huangdi Mingtang Jing*

【Annotation】辄 Zhe, an interchangeable word of 辙 Zhe, means the track of a wheel.

筋 Jin refers to the sinews. This acupoint locates at the lateral costal region, where the large sinews on either side are like the ruts, hence it is named 辄筋 ZheJin.

【 Location 】 In the fourth intercostal space, 1 cun anterior to the midaxillary line.

【 Indications 】 Insomnia caused by sudden fullness of the chest, panting.

24 日月 RiYue GB-24 (Front-*Mu* point of the Gall Bladder, Meeting point of the Gall Bladder and Spleen Channels)

【 Source 】《黄帝明堂经》 *Huangdi Mingtang Jing*

【 Annotation 】 日 Ri refers to the sun. 月 Yue represents the moon. This acupoint is the front-*Mu* point of the Gall Bladder. According to TCM theory, the gallbladder is an organ similar to an official of justice and is responsible for the decision. Decision-makers need to discover the minutest detail in everything. In Chinese, 日 Ri and 月 Yue form the character 明 Ming, which means perceived, hence it is named 日月 RiYue.

【 Location 】 In the seventh intercostal space, 4 cun lateral to the anterior median line.

【 Indications 】①Pain of the lateral costal region, profuse spittle, acid regurgitation, hiccup; ②jaundice.

25 京门 JingMen GB-25 (Front-*Mu* point of the Kidneys)

【 Source 】《黄帝明堂经》 *Huangdi Mingtang Jing*

【 Annotation 】 京 Jing, an interchangeable word of 原 Yuan in ancient Chinese, means the source. 门 Men refers to the door. Kidney qi is the source qi of the human body. Being the front-*Mu* point of the Kidneys, this acupoint is where the source qi of kidneys gathers and can boost the kidneys to promote urination, hence it is named 京门 JingMen.

【 Location 】 Inferior to the free extremity of the 12th rib.

【 Indications 】①Pain of the waist and lateral costal region; ②borborygmus, diarrhea, abdominal distention; ③difficult urination, edema.

26 带脉 DaiMai GB-26 (Meeting point of the Gall Bladder channel with the Belt vessel)

【 Source 】《黄帝明堂经》 *Huangdi Mingtang Jing*

【Annotation】带脉 Dai Mai refers to the Belt vessel. Being the meeting point of the Gall Bladder channel with the Belt vessel, this acupoint is mainly used to treat disorders of menstruation and vaginal discharge, such as leukorrhagia, irregular menstruation, uterine prolapse and amenorrhea, hence it is named 带脉 DaiMai.

【Location】Inferior to the free extremity of the 11th rib, at the level of the center of the umbilicus.

【Indications】①Irregular menstruation, red and white leucorrhoea; ②lower abdominal pain, hernia, pain of the waist and lateral costal region.

27 五枢 WuShu GB-27 (Meeting point of the Gall Bladder channel with the Belt vessel)

【Source】《黄帝明堂经》*Huangdi Mingtang Jing*

【Annotation】五 Wu represents five directions (east, west, south, north and center). Among the directions, 五 Wu locates in the center. 枢 Shu means the pivot for doors. This acupoint locates at the center of the five abdominal acupoints of the Gall Bladder channel, and in the center of the body as well. When a person turns his body or kneels with kowtowing to the ground, the acupoint locates precisely where the waist turns like the pivot for doors, hence it is named 五枢 WuShu.

【Location】3 cun inferior to the center of the umbilicus, medial to the anterior superior iliac spine.

【Indications】①Red and white leucorrhoea, irregular menstruation, hernia; ②lower abdominal pain, lumbago, pain of hip.

28 维道 WeiDao GB-28 (Meeting point of the Gall Bladder channel with the Belt vessel)

【Source】《黄帝明堂经》*Huangdi Mingtang Jing*

【Annotation】维 Wei means to maintain. 道 Dao refers to the vital traffic channels. This acupoint is the meeting point of the Gall Bladder channel with the Belt vessel. The Belt vessel, the only transverse channel in the meridian system, is the vital traffic channel to maintain other channels, hence the acupoint is named 维道 Wei Dao. It is usually used to treat disorders of menstruation and vaginal discharge, such as uterine prolapse, leukorrhagia and irregular menstruation.

【Location】0.5 cun anterior and inferior to the anterior superior iliac spine. Approximately 0.5 cun anterior and inferior to WuShu (GB-27).

【Indications】①Vomiting, poor appetite; ②edema; ③pain of the waist and leg.

29 居髎 JuLiao GB-29 (Meeting point of the Gall Bladder channel with the Yang Heel vessel)

【Source】《黄帝明堂经》 *Huangdi Mingtang Jing*

【Annotation】居 Ju means to squat. 髎 Liao refers to interosseous depression. This acupoint locates at the ilium, which forms a depression when people squat, hence it is named 居髎 Ju Liao.

【Location】At the midpoint of a line connecting the anterior superior iliac spine and the prominence of the greater trochanter.

【Indications】①Hernia, lumbago extending to the lower abdomen; ②pain of the waist and leg.

30 环跳 Huan Tiao GB-30 (Meeting point of the Gall Bladder and Bladder channels)

【Source】《黄帝明堂经》 *Huangdi Mingtang Jing*

【Annotation】环 Huan means annulus. 跳 Tiao means to jump. This acupoint locates at the hip. When selecting the acupoint, patients are always asked to lie on the side with the lower leg straight, and the knee and hip of the upper leg bent in a semicircular shape, like jumping, hence it is named 环跳 HuanTiao.

【Location】At the junction of the lateral one-third and medial two-thirds of the line connecting the prominence of the greater trochanter with the sacral hiatus.

【Indications】Pain of the waist and hip; flaccid obstruction and numbness of the lower limbs, hemiplegia.

31 风市 Feng Shi GB-31

【Source】《肘后备急方·治风毒脚弱痹满上气方第二十一》 *Zhouhou Beiji Fang:*

Zhi Fengdu Jiaoruo Biman Shangqi Fang the twenty-first

【Annotation】风 Feng means wind. 市 Shi means markets, and here refers to a gathering place. This acupoint is where the pathogenic wind of the lower limbs gathers. It is a key acupoint for dispelling wind and is mainly used to treat disorders like apoplectic hemiplegia, paralysis agitans, muscle spasms and dermatic pruritus, hence it is named 风市 FengShi.

【Location】7 cun superior to the base of patella, posterior to the iliotibial tract.

【Indications】①Hemiplegia, pain of the waist and leg, flaccidity and impediment of the lower limbs; ②pruritus.

32 中渎 ZhongDu GB-32

【Source】《黄帝明堂经》*Huangdi Mingtang Jing*

【Annotation】中 Zhong means middle. 渎 Du refers to great rivers. In the thigh, the three yang channels of the foot circulate parallelly like three great rivers. Furthermore, the Gall Bladder channel travels along the narrow depression formed by the vastus lateralis and the biceps femoris, in the middle of the Stomach and the Bladder channel, hence the acupoint is named 中渎 ZhongDu.

【Location】5 cun superior to the base of patella, posterior to the iliotibial tract.

【Indications】Flaccidity and impediment of the lower limbs, hemiplegia.

33 膝阳关 XiYangGuan GB-33

【Source】Presented as 阳关 YangGuan in《黄帝明堂经》*Huangdi Mingtang Jing* and as 膝阳关 XiYangGuan in《针灸学简编》*Zhenjiuxue Jianbian*.

【Annotation】膝 Xi refers to the knee. According to TCM theory, the lateral side of limbs belongs to 阳 Yang. 关 Guan means the joint. This acupoint locates in the depression on the lateral side of the knee, hence it is named 膝阳关 XiYangGuan.

【Location】Posterior and superior to the lateral epicondyle of the femur, in the depression between the biceps femoris tendon and the iliotibial tract.

【Indications】Swelling, pain and spasm of the knee and popliteal fossa; numbness of the lower leg.

34 阳陵泉 YangLingQuan GB-34 (*He*-Sea point, lower *He*-Sea point of the gallbladder, *Hui*-meeting point of Sinews)

【Source】《灵枢·邪气脏腑病形》*Lingshu: Xieqi Zangfu Bingxing*

【Annotation】陵 Ling means a hill. 泉 Quan refers to spring. This acupoint locates in the depression anterior and distal to the head of the fibula. The head of the fibula protrudes like a hill, and the acupoint is depressed like a spring. Opposite YinLingQuan (SP-9), it locates at the lateral side of the leg. According to TCM theory, the lateral side of the body belongs to yang, hence it is named 阳陵泉 YangLingQuan.

【Location】In the depression anterior and distal to the head of the fibula.

【Indications】①Pain of the lateral costal region, bitter taste in the mouth, vomiting, acid regurgitation; ②swelling and pain of the knee; numbness, flaccidity and impediment of the lower limbs.

35 阳交 YangJiao GB-35 (*Xi*-Cleft point of the Yang Linking vessel)

【Source】《黄帝明堂经》*Huangdi Mingtang Jing*

【Annotation】交 Jiao means to intersect. This acupoint locates at the lateral side of the leg, near the Bladder and the Stomach channels. Furthermore, it is the meeting point of the Gall Bladder channel with the Yang Linking vessel, hence it is named 阳交 YangJiao.

【Location】7 cun superior to the prominence of the lateral malleolus, posterior to the fibula.

【Indications】①Swelling and pain of the throat; ②fullness of chest; ③mania-depression, convulsions; ④flaccidity and impediment of the lower limbs, cramp.

36 外丘 WaiQiu GB-36 (*Xi*-Cleft point)

【Source】《黄帝明堂经》*Huangdi Mingtang Jing*

【Annotation】外 Wai means outer. 丘 Qiu refers to a hill. This acupoint locates at the lateral side of the leg. Meanwhile, it is on the same muscle as FengLong (ST-40), where the muscle is full like a hill, hence named 外丘 WaiQiu. Since the acupoint is level with YangJiao (GB-35) and both of them are *Xi*-Cleft points, it is used to treat emergencies such as acute pain of the head, chest, lateral costal region and other areas along the Gall Bladder channel.

【Location】7 cun superior to the prominence of the lateral malleolus, anterior to the fibula.

【Indications】①Distention and fullness of the chest and lateral costal region; ②mania-depression and epilepsy; ③flaccidity and impediment of the lower limbs.

37 光明 GuangMing GB-37 (*Luo*-Connecting point)

【Source】《灵枢·根结》*Lingshu: GenJie*

【Annotation】光明 GuangMing means bright. This acupoint is the *Luo*-Connecting point of the Gall Bladder channel, connecting to the Liver channel. It is mainly used to treat eye disorders such as pain of the eyes, nyctalopia and blurred vision, brightening the eyes, hence it is named 光明 GuangMing.

【Location】5 cun superior to the prominence of the lateral malleolus, anterior to the fibula.

【Indications】①Pain of the eyes, nyctalopia, myopia, corneal nebula; ②flaccidity and impediment of the lower limbs.

38 阳辅 YangFu GB-38 (*Jing*-River point)

【Source】《灵枢·本输》*Lingshu: BenShu*

【Annotation】辅 Fu refers to 辅骨 Fu Bone, which is the name of the fibula in ancient time. This acupoint locates at the lateral side of the fibula. Meanwhile, it is the *Jing*-River point of the Gall Bladder channel, which belongs to the fire according to the five-element theory. In TCM theory, both the lateral side of the body and fire belongs to yang, hence it is named 阳辅 YangFu.

【Location】4 cun superior to the prominence of the lateral malleolus, anterior to the fibula.

【Indications】①Swelling and pain of the throat; ②distention and fullness of the chest and lateral costal region, swelling and pain of the axillae, scrofula; ③flaccidity and impediment of the lower limbs.

39 悬钟 XuanZhong GB-39 (*Hui*–Meeting point for Marrow)

【Source】《黄帝明堂经》 *Huangdi Mingtang Jing*

【Annotation】悬 Xuan means hanging. 钟 Zhong refers to a clock. This acupoint is 3 cun superior to the lateral malleolus, from the acupoint to the lateral malleolus shaped like a hanging bell. The place is also where the foot bell is tied, hence the acupoint is named 悬钟 XuanZhong.

【Location】3 cun superior to the prominence of the lateral malleolus, anterior to the fibula.

【Indications】①Abdominal fullness, poor appetite; ②hemiplegia, flaccidity and impediment of the lower limbs, spasm and pain of the lower leg and foot.

40 丘墟 QiuXu GB-40 (*Yuan*–Source point)

【Source】《灵枢·本输》 *Lingshu: Benshu*

【Annotation】丘墟 QiuXu means a big hill. This acupoint is anterior and distal to the lateral malleolus, which protrudes like a hill, hence it is named 丘墟 QiuXu.

【Location】In the depression lateral to the extensor digitorum longus tendon.

【Indications】①Pain of the chest and lateral costal region, sighing, swelling of the neck, axillary swelling; ②malaria; ③blurred vision, corneal nebula; ④aching pain of the lower leg, swelling and pain of the lateral malleolus, foot drop.

41 足临泣 ZuLinQi GB-41 (*Shu*–Stream point, confluent point of the Belt vessel)

【Source】Presented as 临泣 LinQi in《灵枢·本输》 *Lingshu: Benshu and a*s 足临泣 ZuLinQi in《针灸资生经》 *ZhenJiu ZiSheng Jing*.

【Annotation】足 Zu refers to the foot. 临 Lin means looking down from a high place. 泣 Qi means to weep. This acupoint is on the dorsum of the foot. Its qi connects with the eyes and eyes are where the tears come out. Therefore, the acupoint can treat eye diseases such as redness and swelling, dizziness, and dryness, which are the same as TouLinQi (GB-15). Hence it is named 足临泣 ZuLinQi.

【Location】In the depression lateral to the fifth extensor digitorum longus tendon.

【Indications】①Migraine, dizziness; ②pain of the lateral costal region, scrofula; ③pain of knee, pain of foot; ④malaria; ⑤irregular menstruation, mastitis.

42 地五会 DiWuHui GB-42

【Source】《黄帝明堂经》*Huangdi Mingtang Jing*

【Annotation】There are two explanations for this name. Firstly, 地 Di refers to the ground. 五 Wu means five. 会 Hui means to meet. The Gall Bladder channel has five acupoints on foot. A collateral connects transversely TaiChong (LR-3) and this acupoint, like wood has roots underground, hence the acupoint is named 地五会 DiWuHui. Secondly, 地 Di also represents the earth qi. Wind, cold, heat and damp qi all meet on the ground, and those earth qi gather on foot. Therefore, the five toes are easily invaded by different earth qi, hence the name.

【Location】Between the fourth and fifth metatarsal bones, in the depression proximal to the fourth metatarsophalangeal joint.

【Indications】①Redness and swelling of the eyes; ②axillary swelling; ③mastitis; ④redness and swelling of the dorsum of the foot.

43 侠溪 XiaXi GB-43 (*Ying*-Spring point)

【Source】《灵枢·本输》*Lingshu: Benshu*

【Annotation】侠 Xia, an interchangeable word of 夹 Xia, means narrow. 溪 Xi refers to a stream. This acupoint locates in the crack between the fourth and fifth toes, which is like a narrow stream, hence it is named 侠溪 Xia Xi.

【Location】Between the fourth and fifth toes, proximal to the web margin at the border between the red and white flesh.

【Indications】①Febrile disease, headache, dizziness, swelling of the cheek; ②deafness, tinnitus, redness and swelling of the eyes; ③pain of the lateral costal region, pain of the knee and thigh, pain of foot; ④mastitis.

44 足窍阴 ZuQiaoYin GB-44 (*Jing*-Well point)

【Source】《灵枢·本输》*Lingshu: Benshu*

【Annotation】足 Zu refers to the foot. 窍 Qiao is understood as 空 Kong, meaning hollow. All three yang channels of the foot run from the head to the feet. Their *Jing*–Well points are like the end of yang and the beginning of yin. Yang is rooted in yin. This acupoint is the *Jing*–Well point of the Gall Bladder channel, which is rooted in qiao yin according to the theory of gen–root and jie–knot. This acupoint is mainly used to treat deafness, tinnitus, stiffness of the tongue, redness and swelling of the eyes, and headache. Its indications are similar to TouQiaoYin (GB–11), hence it is named 足窍阴 Zu Qiao Yin.

【Location】On the fourth toe, lateral to the distal phalanx, 0.1 cun proximal to the lateral corner of the toenail.

【Indications】①Headache, redness and swelling of the eyes, tinnitus, deafness; ②pain of the chest and lateral costal region; ③pain of foot.

Chapter 13
The Liver Channel Points of Foot Jueyin

1 大敦 DaDun LR-1 (*Jing*–Well point)

【Source】《灵枢·本输》*Lingshu: Benshu*

【Annotation】大 Da means big. 敦 Dun means thick, which is a metaphor for the big toe, because the big toe is the thickest one among toes, shaped like the large and thick ancient Chinese food containers called Dun, with a round cover. This acupoint is located at the big toe, 0.1 cun proximal to the lateral corner of the toenail, hence it is named 大敦 DaDun.

【Location】On the big toe, lateral to the distal phalanx, 0.1 cun proximal to the lateral corner of the toenail.

【Indications】①Hernia, swelling and pain of the testicles, pain of the external genitalia and lower abdomen, enuresis, retention of urine; ②irregular menstruation, uterine prolapse; ③infantile convulsion, epilepsy, loss of consciousness.

2 行间 XingJian LR-2 (*Ying*–Spring point)

【Source】《灵枢·本输》*Lingshu: Benshu*

【Annotation】行 Xing means to pass. 间 Jian means between. This acupoint is located between the first and second toes, at the border between the red and white flesh. The qi of the Liver channel passes between the two toes from DaDun (LR-1) to this acupoint, hence it is named 行间 XingJian.

【Location】On the dorsum of the foot, between the first and second toes, proximal to the web margin, at the border between the red and white flesh.

【Indications】①Hernia, pain of the lower abdomen and external genitalia, enuresis, retention of urine; ②irregular menstruation, leukorrhagia; ③redness and pain of the eyes, dry mouth, thirst, swelling and pain of the throat; ④pain of the lateral costal region, propensity to anger, sighing; ⑤epilepsy; ⑥swelling and pain of the foot and knee.

3 太冲 TaiChong LR-3 (*Shu*-Stream and *Yuan*-Source point)

【Source】《灵枢·九针十二原》《灵枢·本输》*Lingshu: Jiuzhen Shieryuan, Lingshu: Benshu*

【Annotation】太 Tai means large. 冲 Chong refers to important traffic channels. This acupoint is the *Shu*-Stream point and *Yuan*-Source point of the Liver channel. According to the TCM theory, the *Shu*-Stream point is often located behind the metacarpophalangeal or metatarsophalangeal joints, with the metaphor that this acupoint is the main passage of the Liver channel and the place where the original qi gathers, with a vigorous pulse, hence it is named 太冲 TaiChong.

【Location】On the dorsum of the foot, between the first and second metatarsal bones, in the depression distal to the junction of the bases of the two bones, over the dorsalis pedics artery.

【Indications】①Hernia, pain of the external genitalia and lower abdomen, retention of urine, enuresis; ②irregular menstruation, dystocia; ③jaundice, pain of the lateral costal region, distention of abdomen, nausea and vomiting; ④infantile convulsion; ⑤redness and pain of the eyes, dry throat, pharyngalgia; ⑥flaccidity and impediment of the legs, pain and swelling of the instep.

4 中封 ZhongFeng LR-4 (*Jing*-River point)

【Source】《灵枢·本输》*Lingshu: Benshu*

【Annotation】中 Zhong means between. 封 Feng refers to a mound. This acupoint is located between ShangQiu (SP-5) and QiuXu (GB-40), both of which have the meaning of a mound. Therefore, it is like standing between two mounds. Furthermore, 封 Feng can be interpreted as to seal. This acupoint is located at the anteromedial side of the ankle, and in the depression medial to the tibialis anterior tendon. Since it seems to be sealed by the sinew, the acupoint is named 中封 ZhongFeng.

【Location】On the anteromedial side of the ankle, in the depression medial to the tibialis anterior tendon, anterior to the medial malleolus. It can be selected between ShangQiu (SP–5) and JieXi (ST–41).

【Indications】Lumbago and pain of the lower abdomen caused by hernia, seminal emission, difficult urination.

5　蠡沟 LiGou LR–5 (*Luo*–Connecting point)

【Source】《灵枢·经脉》 *Lingshu: Jingmai*

【Annotation】There are two explanations for this name. Firstly, 蠡 Li refers to a worm that gnaws the wood. This acupoint is on the tibia, and when the filiform needle, whose tip looks like the mouthpart of a mosquito, is inserted into the acupoint, it looks like a worm gnawing on wood. Secondly, 蠡 Li can be understood as a gourd ladle, a tool for scooping water. This acupoint is 5 cun above the prominence of the medial malleolus, and the gastrocnemius muscle near this acupoint is shaped like a gourd ladle. 沟 Gou refers to a ditch. The medial border of the tibia is shaped like a ditch, hence it is named 蠡沟 LiGou.

【Location】On the anteromedial side of the leg, at the center of the medial border of the tibia, 5 cun proximal to the prominence of the medial malleolus.

【Indications】①Hernia, swelling and pain of the testicles, difficult urination, enuresis; ②irregular menstruation, red and white leucorrhoea, pudendal itch.

6　中都 ZhongDu LR–6 (*Xi*–Cleft point)

【Source】《黄帝明堂经》 *Huangdi Mingtang Jing*

【Annotation】中 Zhong means center. 都 Du means convergence. This acupoint is the *Xi*–Cleft point of the Liver channel, where the qi and blood of the Liver channel converge, and is located at the center of the medial border of the tibia, hence it is named 中都 ZhongDu.

【Location】On the anteromedial side of the leg, at the center of the medial border of the tibia, 7 cun proximal to the prominence of the medial malleolus. Divide the distance between the apex of the patella and the tip of the medial malleolus into half, the point can be selected at 0.5 cun inferior to the midpoint, at the center of the medial border of the tibia.

【Indications】①Hernia, lower abdominal pain, uterine bleeding, persistent flow of the lochia; ②diarrhea.

7 膝关 XiGuan LR-7

【Source】《黄帝明堂经》 *Huangdi Mingtang Jing*

【Annotation】膝 Xi refers to the knee. 关 Guan refers to the joint. This acupoint is located at the medial side of the knee joint, and is mainly used to treat knee disorders such as the swelling and pain of the knee, hence it is named 膝关 XiGuan.

【Location】On the tibial aspect of the leg, inferior to the medial condyle of the tibia, 1 cun posterior to YinLingQuan (SP-9).

【Indications】Hernia, lower abdominal pain, pain of the knee and thigh, flaccidity and impediment of the legs.

8 曲泉 QuQuan LR-8 (*He*-Sea point)

【Source】《灵枢·本输》 *Lingshu: Benshu*

【Annotation】曲 Qu means to bend. 泉 Quan means a spring. This acupoint is located in the depression above the medial end of the popliteal crease, which requires the knee to be bent during acupoint selecting. Meanwhile, this acupoint is the *He*-Sea and Water (five phases) point of the Liver channel, hence it is named 曲泉 QuQuan.

【Location】On the medial side of the knee, when the knee is flexed, the acupoint is at the medial end of the popliteal crease, posterior to the medial condyle of the femur, in the depression anterior to the tendons of semitendinosus and semimembranosus.

【Indications】①Hernia, pain of the external genitalia, lower abdominal pain, difficult urination; ②seminal emission, impotence; ③abdominal masses in women due to blood stasis, irregular menstruation, red and white leucorrhoea, uterine prolapse, pudendal itch; ④frighting-mania; ⑤swelling and pain of the knee, flaccidity and impediment of the legs.

9 阴包 YinBao LR-9

【Source】《黄帝明堂经》 *Huangdi Mingtang Jing*

【Annotation】包 Bao, an interchangeable word of 胞 Bao, refers to the genital organs such as the uterus in woman and essence chamber in man. This acupoint is located at the medial side of the thigh, and according to the yin–yang theory, the medial side of our body belongs to yin (阴). Furthermore, this acupoint is mainly used for treating diseases related to the uterus and essence chamber, such as irregular menstruation and lumbosacral pain extending to the lower abdomen, hence it is named 阴包 YinBao.

【Location】On the medial side of the thigh, between the vastus medialis and the sartorius, 4 cun proximal to the base of the patella.

【Indications】①Irregular menstruation, enuresis, difficult urination; ②lumbosacral pain extending to the lower abdomen.

10 足五里 ZuWuLi LR-10

【Source】Presented as 五里 WuLi in《黄帝明堂经》*Huangdi Mingtang Jing* and as 足五里 ZuWuLi in《针灸资生经》*Zhenjiu Zisheng Jing*.

【Annotation】足 Zu refers to the lower limbs. 五 Wu refers to the number five. 里 Li, an interchangeable word of 理 Li, means to manage. This acupoint is located at the lower limbs and is mainly used to manage diseases of the five viscera in the interior, which corresponds to ShouWuLi (LI-13), ShouSanLi (LI-10) and ZuSanLi (ST-36) (all of these acupoints can be used to treat internal diseases), hence it is named 足五里 ZuWuLi.

【Location】On the medial side of the thigh, 3 cun inferior to QiChong (ST-30), over the artery.

【Indications】Lower abdominal pain, difficult urination, uterine prolapse, swelling and pain of the testicles.

11 阴廉 YinLian LR-11

【Source】《黄帝明堂经》*Huangdi Mingtang Jing*

【Annotation】阴 Yin refers to the vulva. 廉 Lian generally means the edge or border and specifically refers to the groin here. This acupoint is located at the medial side of the thigh, in the groin next to the vulva, hence it is named 阴廉 YinLian.

【Location】On the medial side of the thigh, 2 cun inferior to QiChong (ST-30). To select this acupoint, let the patient flex the hip slightly, bend the knee, and abduct. The adductor longus is shown when the thigh abducts resisting drag force, and then select the acupoint at its anterior border.

【Indications】Irregular menstruation, infertility, lower abdominal pain.

12 急脉 JiMai LR-12

【Source】《素问·气府论》*Suwen: Qifu Lun*

【Annotation】急 Ji means torrential. 脉 Mai refers to the vessel. This acupoint is located at the position where the femoral artery pulses in the groin region, which is like a torrential current, hence it is named 急脉 JiMai.

【Location】In the groin region, at the same level as the superior border of the pubic symphysis, and 2.5 cun lateral to the anterior median line.

【Indications】Hernia, pain of the external genitalia, lower abdominal pain.

13 章门 ZhangMen LR-13 (Front-*Mu* point of the Spleen, *Hui*-Meeting point of the viscera, Meeting point of the Liver and Gall Bladder channels)

【Source】《黄帝明堂经》*Huangdi Mingtang Jing*

【Annotation】There are two explanations for this name. Firstly, 章 Zhang refers to a kind of ancient Chinese formal attire. 门 Men refers to a door or a key entrance. This acupoint is located on the midaxillary line, inferior to the free extremity of the 11th rib, where an ancient Chinese formal attire can be put on or taken off (like a door can be opened or closed). Secondly, 章 Zhang is an interchangeable word of 彰 Zhang, meaning conspicuous, and can extend to vigorous qi and blood. Being the Front-*Mu* point of the Spleen, this acupoint is a place where the qi and blood of the spleen gather and infuse into the abdomen. Meanwhile, as the *Hui*-Meeting point of the viscera, it is the entrance of the visceral qi, hence it is named 章门 ZhangMen.

【Location】On the lateral abdomen, inferior to the free extremity of the 11th rib.

【Indications】①Hernia, pain of the external genitalia, lower abdominal pain, vomiting; ②pain of the lateral costal region, abdominal masses, jaundice.

14 期门 QiMen LR-14 (Front-*Mu* point of the Liver, Meeting point of the Liver and Spleen channels with the Yin Linking vessel)

【Source】《黄帝明堂经》*Huangdi Mingtang Jing*

【Annotation】期 Qi means a cycle. 门 Men means a key entrance. The qi and blood of the twelve meridians circulate from YunMen (LU–2) to QiMen (LR–14) cyclically. Since it is the terminal acupoint of a circulation, where the meridian qi go back into, this acupoint is named 期门 QiMen.

【Location】In the anterior thoracic region, in the sixth intercostal space, 4 cun lateral to the anterior median line.

【Indications】① Masses in the lateral costal region, panting, hiccup, distension and pain of the chest and lateral costal region; ② vomiting, abdominal distention, diarrhea; ③ mastitis.

Chapter 14
The Governing Vessel Points

1 长强 **ChangQiang GV-1** (*Luo*-Connecting point of the Governing vessel, Meeting point of the Governing vessel with the Gall Bladder and Kidney channels)

【Source】《灵枢·经脉》*Lingshu: Jingmai*

【Annotation】长 Chang means long. 强 Qiang means strong. The vertebral column is long and strong, supporting the skull above and connecting to the hip bone below. In addition, the Governing Vessel governs all the yang channels, and the yang qi in this vessel is the strongest. This acupoint is the starting point of the Governing Vessel, hence it is named 长强 ChangQiang.

【Location】In the perineal region, inferior to the coccyx, midway between the tip of the coccyx and the anus.

【Indications】①Diarrhea, constipation, bloody stool, hemorrhoids, rectocele; ②mania-depression, infantile convulsion; ③lumbago, pain of the coccyx and sacrum.

2 腰俞 **YaoShu GV-2**

【Source】《素问·缪刺论》*Suwen: Miuci Lun*

【Annotation】腰 Yao means lumbar region. 俞 Shu, an interchangeable word of 输 Shu, means to transport. The Governing Vessel circulates from ChangQiang (GV-1) upward across the coccyx to this acupoint (at the sacral hiatus), where the meridian qi is transported from the inside to the outside and circulates in the midline of the lower back. In addition, this acupoint is mainly used to treat diseases of the lumbar region, whenever there is stiffness and pain in the lumbar region or an inability to flex and extend, hence it is named 腰俞 YaoShu.

【Location】In the sacral region, at the sacral hiatus, on the posterior median line.

【Indications】①Irregular menstruation; ②hemorrhoids; ③pain of the waist and back, flaccidity and impediment of the legs.

3 腰阳关 YaoYangGuan GV-3

【Source】Presented as 阳关 YangGuan in《素问·气府论》王冰注 *Suwen: Qifu Lun* (Wang Bing's notes) *and as* 腰阳关 YaoYangGuan in《针灸学简编》*Zhenjiuxue Jianbian.*

【Annotation】腰 Yao refers to the lumbar region. 关 Guan refers to a gateway. 阳关 YangGuan refers to the southern gateway from the Central Plains to the Western Regions in ancient times (the northern one is called 阴关 YinGuan). In the human body, YinGuan corresponds to GuanYuan (CV-4) and YangGuan corresponds to YaoYangGuan. GuanYuan (CV-4) is the meeting point of original yin and original yang of the abdomen, while YaoYangGuan is the projection of GuanYuan (CV-4) on the back. According to the yin-yang theory, the back belongs to yang. Meanwhile, the Governing Vessel is the sea of yang channels, hence this acupoint is named 腰阳关 YaoYangGuan, a key acupoint for treating lumbosacral disorders.

【Location】In the lumbar region, in the depression inferior to the spinous process of the fourth lumbar vertebra (L4), on the posterior median line.

【Indications】①Irregular menstruation, seminal emission, impotence; ②pain of the lumbosacral region.

4 命门 MingMen GV-4

【Source】《黄帝明堂经》*Huangdi Mingtang Jing*

【Annotation】命 Ming means life. 门 Men refers to a gateway. This acupoint is located between two kidneys, is the root of source qi and the life, and is the important gateway to life, hence it is named 命门 MingMen. This acupoint is a key acupoint for strengthening the body and treating deficiency diseases.

【Location】In the lumbar region, in the depression inferior to the spinous process of the second lumbar vertebra (L2), on the posterior median line.

【Indications】①Lumbago, pain of the lower abdomen, stiffness of the lumbar spine; ②red and white leucorrhoea, impotence; ③flaccidity and impediment of the legs.

5 悬枢 XuanShu GV-5

【Source】《黄帝明堂经》 *Huangdi Mingtang Jing*

【Annotation】悬 Xuan means dangling. 枢 Shu generally means the pivot for doors and specifically refers to the lumbar spine here. When a person is supine, the lumbar spine will be dangled for several cun (an ancient Chinese unit of length). The position of this acupoint is at the top of the dangling area, and is where the lumbar spine turns, hence it is named 悬枢 XuanShu.

【Location】In the lumbar region, in the depression inferior to the spinous process of the first lumbar vertebra (L1), on the posterior median line.

【Indications】①Pain of the abdomen, diarrhea; ②pain of the lumbar spine.

6 脊中 JiZhong GV-6

【Source】《黄帝明堂经》 *Huangdi Mingtang Jing*

【Annotation】脊 Ji refers to the spine. 中 Zhong means middle. The ancient Chinese believed that the spine consists of twenty-one vertebrae, including twelve thoracic vertebrae, five lumbar vertebrae, and four sacral vertebrae. The eleventh vertebra is the middle one of the twenty-one vertebrae. This acupoint is in the depression below the eleventh thoracic vertebra, next to the middle of the spine, hence it is named 脊中 JiZhong.

【Location】In the upper back region, in the depression inferior to the spinous process of the eleventh thoracic vertebra (T11), on the posterior median line.

【Indications】①Diarrhea, jaundice; ②epilepsy; ③pain of the waist and back.

7 中枢 ZhongShu GV-7

【Source】《素问·气府论》王冰注 *Suwen: Qifu Lun* (Wang Bing's notes)

【Annotation】中 Zhong means middle. 枢 Shu generally means the pivot for doors and specifically refers to the spinal bones here. The eleventh vertebra is the middle one of the twenty-one vertebrae. This acupoint is in the depression above the eleventh thoracic vertebra, next to the middle of the spine, hence it is named 中枢 ZhongShu, which is similar to the annotation of JiZhong (GV-6).

【Location】In the upper back region, in the depression inferior to the spinous process of the tenth thoracic vertebra (T10), on the posterior median line.

【Indications】Pain of the waist and back.

8 筋缩 JinSuo GV-8

【Source】《黄帝明堂经》*Huangdi Mingtang Jing*

【Annotation】筋 Jin refers to the sinew. 缩 Suo means contraction. This acupoint is in the depression below the ninth thoracic vertebra and is at the same level with GanShu (BL-18). Ganshu (BL-18) is the Back-*Shu* point of the liver. The liver governs sinews. If the liver is diseased, the muscles will contract, leading to symptoms of convulsion and spasm, such as clonic convulsions and stiffness of the spine. This acupoint can be used to treat such sinew diseases, hence it is named 筋缩 JinSuo.

【Location】In the upper back region, in the depression inferior to the spinous process of the ninth thoracic vertebra (T9), on the posterior median line.

【Indications】①Infantile convulsion, convulsions, mania-depression and epilepsy, upward staring eyes; ②stiffness and contraction of the spine.

9 至阳 ZhiYang GV-9

【Source】《黄帝明堂经》*Huangdi Mingtang Jing*

【Annotation】至 Zhi means extreme or peak. This acupoint is in the depression below the seventh thoracic vertebra and is at the same level with GeShu (BL-17). According to the yin-yang theory, the back of the human body belongs to yang, and the abdomen belongs to yin. Likewise, the part above the diaphragm belongs to yang, and the part below the diaphragm belongs to yin. Therefore, the part of the back below the diaphragm belongs to "yin within yang", and above the diaphragm belongs to "yang within yang" (where yang qi is at its peak). When the qi of the Governing Vessel travels up to this acupoint, it runs from "yin within yang" to "yang within yang", hence it is named 至阳 ZhiYang.

【Location】In the upper back region, in the depression inferior to the spinous process of the seventh thoracic vertebra (T7), on the posterior median line.

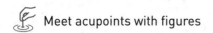

【Indications】①Jaundice; ②heavy body (the subjective heaviness sensation of the body with difficult movement); ③pain of the waist and back.

10 灵台 LingTai GV-10

【Source】《素问·气府论》王冰注 *Suwen: Qifu Lun* (Wang Bing's notes)

【Annotation】灵台 Lingtai refers to an ancient observatory, where the emperor offered sacrifices to gods or ancestors and granted an interview to feudal princes (dukes or princes under an emperor). The heart is an organ similar to the emperor. Therefore, LingTai is also known as the heart. This acupoint is in the depression below the sixth thoracic vertebra, a position that corresponds to the heart, hence it is named 灵台 Lingtai.

【Location】In the upper back region, in the depression inferior to the spinous process of the sixth thoracic vertebra (T6), on the posterior median line.

【Indications】①Cough, panting; ②pain of the spine, stiffness and pain of the neck.

11 神道 ShenDao GV-11

【Source】《黄帝明堂经》 *Huangdi Mingtang Jing*

【Annotation】神 Shen means spirit. 道 Dao refers to a channel. This acupoint is in the depression below the fifth thoracic vertebra and is at the same level with XinShu (BL-15). Therefore, it corresponds internal to the heart. The heart stores the spirit. This acupoint is the channel of the heart qi and is mainly used to treat heart diseases and mental disorders, such as heartache, fright palpitations, insomnia, and forgetfulness, hence it is named 神道 ShenDao.

【Location】In the upper back region, in the depression inferior to the spinous process of the fifth thoracic vertebra (T5), on the posterior median line.

【Indications】①Sadness and anxiety, fright palpitations, forgetfulness; ②chills and fever, headache, malaria; ③infantile convulsion; ④pain of the spine, stiffness of the spine.

12 身柱 ShenZhu GV-12

【Source】《黄帝明堂经》 *Huangdi Mingtang Jing*

【Annotation】身 Shen means the body. 柱 Zhu refers to a load-bearing pillar. This acupoint is in the depression below the third thoracic vertebra, on the midline between two scapulae. Since its position is like a load–bearing pillar for the scapulae, this acupoint is named 身柱 ShenZhu.

【Location】In the upper back region, in the depression inferior to the spinous process of the third thoracic vertebra (T3), on the posterior median line.

【Indications】①Cough, panting; ②fever, mania–depression, infantile convulsion, convulsions; ③pain of the waist and back.

13 陶道 TaoDao GV–13 (Meeting point of the Governing vessel with the Bladder channel)

【Source】《黄帝明堂经》 Huangdi Mingtang Jing

【Annotation】陶 Tao refers to an ancient pottery kiln. 道 Dao means a channel. The thorax is hollow like a pottery. This acupoint is located at the highest part of the thorax and is mainly used for treating bone–steaming tidal fever and fever and chills. With its capability of clearing yang heat, this acupoint is like the channel exit for the heat of a pottery kiln, hence it is named 陶道 TaoDao.

【Location】In the upper back region, in the depression inferior to the spinous process of the first thoracic vertebra (T1), on the posterior median line.

【Indications】①Chills and fever, malaria, bone–steaming tidal fever; ②stiffness of the spine.

14 大椎 DaZhui GV–14 (Meeting point of the Governing vessel with the six yang channels of the hand and foot)

【Source】《黄帝明堂经》 Huangdi Mingtang Jing

【Annotation】大 Da means big or prominent. 椎 Zhui means a vertebra. The spinous process of the seventh cervical vertebra is the biggest and the most prominent spinous process in the posterior region of the neck and the upper back region. This acupoint is in the depression below the seventh cervical vertebra, hence it is named 大椎 DaZhui.

【Location】In the posterior region of the neck, in the depression inferior to the spinous process of the seventh cervical vertebra (C7), on the posterior median line.

【Indications】①Febrile disease, malaria, chills and fever; ②cough, panting, bone–steaming tidal fever; ③spinal pain, stiffness and pain of the neck.

15 哑门 **YaMen GV-15** (Meeting point of the Governing and Yang Linking vessels)

【Source】《素问·气穴论》*Suwen: Qixue Lun*

【Annotation】哑 Ya means mute. This acupoint is mainly used to treat flaccid tongues with aphasia, and is a key acupoint for the treatment of inability to speak, hence it is named 哑门 YaMen.

【Location】In the posterior region of the neck, in the depression superior to the spinous process of the second cervical vertebra (C2), on the posterior median line.

【Indications】① Sudden aphonia, flaccid or stiff tongue with aphasia, epistaxis; ② headache, pain of the spine, stiffness and pain of the neck.

16 风府 **FengFu GV-16** (Meeting point of the Governing and Yang Linking vessels)

【Source】《素问·风论》《灵枢·本输》等 *Suwen: Feng Lun, Lingshu: Benshu*, etc.

【Annotation】风 Feng means wind. 府 Fu means convergence. 风府 Fengfu refers to the place where the pathogenic wind (a pathogenic factor characterized by its rapid movement, swift changes, and ascending and opening actions) converges. This acupoint is in the posterior region of the neck, which is the easiest part for wind pathogens to invade and accumulate, and is mainly used to treat wind diseases, hence it is named 风府 FengFu.

【Location】In the posterior region of the neck, directly inferior to the external occipital protuberance, in the depression between the trapezius muscles on both sides.

【Indications】① Swelling and pain of the throat, epistaxis, sudden aphonia; ② headache, dizziness, mania-depression; ③ wind stroke, stiff tongue with aphasia, hemiplegia; ④ pain of the spine, stiffness and pain of the neck.

17 脑户 **NaoHu GV-17** (Meeting point of the Governing vessel with the Bladder channel)

【Source】《黄帝明堂经》*Huangdi Mingtang Jing*

【Annotation】脑 Nao means the brain. 户 Hu refers to an entrance. This acupoint is in the depression above the external occipital protuberance, which is the entrance for the Governing vessel to the brain, hence it is named 脑户 NaoHu.

【Location】On the head, in the depression superior to the external occipital protuberance.

【Indications】①Mania-depression and epilepsy; ②dizziness; ③pain of the spine, stiffness and pain of the neck.

18 强间 QiangJian GV-18

【Source】《黄帝明堂经》*Huangdi Mingtang Jing*

【Annotation】强 Qiang means strong. 间 Jian means between. This acupoint is located between NaoHu (GV-17) and HouDing (GV-19), or more precisely, above NaoHu (GV-17) and below HouDing (GV-19). Meanwhile, it is near the lambdoid suture consisting of the parietal and occipital bones, the strongest part of the cranium, hence it is named 强间 QiangJian.

【Location】On the head, 4 cun superior to the posterior hairline, on the posterior median line.

【Indications】①Headache, mania-depression and epilepsy, convulsions; ②stiffness and pain of the neck.

19 后顶 HouDing GV-19

【Source】《黄帝明堂经》*Huangdi Mingtang Jing*

【Annotation】后 Hou means behind. 顶 Ding refers to the vertex. The vertex of the head (BaiHui) has one acupoint 1.5 cun in front of it and one acupoint 1.5 cun behind it. This acupoint is posterior to BaiHui (GV-20), hence it is named 后 顶 HouDing. Both QianDing (GV-21) and HouDing are used for treating cephalic and facial diseases, as well as mental disorders, with QianDing (GV-21) favoring the forehead and HouDing favoring the nape.

【Location】On the head, 5.5 cun superior to the posterior hairline (3 cun above NaoHu), on the posterior median line. It can be selected at 1.5 cun posterior to BaiHui.

【Indications】①Headache, dizziness, mania-depression and epilepsy; ②stiffness and pain of the neck.

20 百会 BaiHui GV-20 (Meeting point of the Governing vessel with the Bladder channel)

【Source】《黄帝明堂经》*Huangdi Mingtang Jing*

【Annotation】百 Bai, generally means hundreds and can be extended to numerous here. 会 Hui means to meet. Baihui, also known as 三 阳 五 会 SanYangWuHui. The head is a position where all the yang channels meet. This acupoint is located at the center of the vertex and is the meeting point of the Governing vessel with the Bladder channel. The hand and foot Shaoyang channels, as well as the Liver Channel also converge here. It has a wide range of clinical applications, leading to a statement that it can treat numerous diseases, hence it is named 百会 BaiHui.

【Location】On the head, 5 cun superior to the anterior hairline, on the anterior median line.

【Indications】①Headache, pain of the eyes, dizziness, tinnitus, nasal congestion; ②wind stroke, loss of consciousness, mania-depression and epilepsy, infantile convulsion, dementia; ③rectocele, uterine prolapse.

21 前顶 QianDing GV-21

【Source】《黄帝明堂经》*Huangdi Mingtang Jing*

【Annotation】前 Qian means front. 顶 Ding refers to the vertex. The vertex of the head (BaiHui) has one acupoint 1.5 cun in front of it and one acupoint 1.5 cun behind it. This acupoint is located in front of BaiHui (GV-20), hence it is named 前 顶 QianDing. Both QianDing and HouDing (GV-19) are used for treating cephalic and facial diseases, as well as mental disorders, with QianDing favoring the forehead and HouDing favoring the nape.

【Location】On the head, 3.5 cun superior to the anterior hairline, on the anterior median line.

【Indications】①Headache, dizziness; ②facial swelling, sinusitis; ③infantile convulsion.

22 囟会 XinHui GV-22

【Source】《灵枢·热病》*Lingshu: Rebing*

【Annotation】囟 Xin refers to the fontanel, which is the membranous part between the cranial bones of a fetus or newborn. 会 Hui means convergence. This acupoint is close to the anterior hairline and corresponds to the anterior fontanel, where the cranial bones converge, hence it is named 囟会 XinHui. The anterior fontanel generally closes at the age of 1–2 years, so infants are forbidden to use this point.

【Location】On the head, 2 cun superior to the anterior hairline, on the anterior median line.

【Indications】①Headache, dizziness, mania–depression and epilepsy; ②nasal congestion, epistaxis; ③infantile convulsion.

23 上星 ShangXing GV–23

【Source】《黄帝明堂经》*Huangdi Mingtang Jing*

【Annotation】上 Shang means upper. 星 Xing refers to a star. This acupoint is located at the top of the forehead, upper to the face, like a star hanging overhead. Meanwhile, it can relieve all the discomfort of the head and eyes, such as headache, dizziness, redness and pain of the eyes, and short sightedness. Its role is like a star in the darkness, hence it is named 上星 ShangXing.

【Location】On the head, 1 cun superior to the anterior hairline, on the anterior median line.

【Indications】①Sinusitis, epistaxis, pain of the eyes; ②headache, dizziness, mania–depression; ③febrile disease, malaria.

24 神庭 ShenTing GV–24 (Meeting point of the Governing vessel with the Bladder and Stomach channels)

【Source】《黄帝明堂经》*Huangdi Mingtang Jing*

【Annotation】神 Shen means the spirit. 庭 Ting refers to the forehead. This acupoint is vertical to the nose and close to the forehead. Since it is located at the head, which contains the brain, and the brain is the house of original spirit, hence it is named 神庭 ShenTing.

【Location】On the head, 0.5 cun superior to the anterior hairline, on the anterior median line.

【Indications】①Sinusitis, epistaxis; ②headache, dizziness, mania–depression and epilepsy; ③ vomiting.

25 素髎 SuLiao GV-25

【Source】《黄帝明堂经》 *Huangdi Mingtang Jing*

【Annotation】素 Su means white. 髎 Liao refers to a cavity. The nose is the orifice of the lung. According to the five-phase theory, it corresponds to white. This acupoint is located at the center of the nasal tip, corresponding to the cavities beside the nasal septum, hence it is named 素髎 SuLiao.

【Location】On the face, at the tip of the nose.

【Indications】Nasal congestion, sinusitis, epistaxis, nasal polyp, rosacea.

26 水沟 ShuiGou GV-26 (Meeting point of the Governing vessel with the Large Intestine and Stomach channels)

【Source】《黄帝明堂经》 *Huangdi Mingtang Jing*

【Annotation】水 Shui means water. 沟 Gou refers to a ditch. This acupoint is located at the philtrum. The philtrum is shaped like a ditch where the nasal mucus flows down, hence it is named 水沟 ShuiGou. This acupoint is also known as 人中 RenZhong. 人 Ren means human. 中 Zhong means between. Heaven qi communicates with the nose, and earth qi communicates with the mouth. The acupoint is located between the mouth and nose, hence it is named 人中 RenZhong. ShuiGou is one of the thirteen Sun Simiao Ghost points and is often used in the treatment of coma, epilepsy, and other mental illnesses, with its function of restoring consciousness. Therefore, it is an important acupoint of first aid treatment.

【Location】On the face, at the junction of the upper one-third and lower two-thirds of the philtrum.

【Indications】① Coma, syncope, wind stroke, epilepsy; ② deviated eye and mouth, salivation, lockjaw, nasal congestion, epistaxis; ③ wasting-thirst, edema; ④ stiffness and pain of the lumbar spine.

27 兑端 DuiDuan GV-27

【Source】《黄帝明堂经》 *Huangdi Mingtang Jing*

【Annotation 】兑 Dui, one of the divinatory symbols in《周易》*ZhouYi*, corresponds to the mouth. 端 Duan means upright and refers to the end of something as well. This acupoint is located at the middle end of the upper lip and is close to the end of the Governing vessel, hence it is named 兑端 DuiDuan.

【Location 】At the midpoint of the tubercle of upper lip.

【Indications 】①Toothache, bad breath; ②epilepsy, vomiting of foam, lockjaw.

28 龈交 YinJiao GV-28

【Source 】《黄帝明堂经》*Huangdi Mingtang Jing*

【Annotation 】龈 Yin means the gum. 交 Jiao means to meet. This acupoint is located at the upper gum, where the Conception vessel and the Governing vessel meet, and the teeth and lips meet here as well, hence it is named 龈交 YinJiao.

【Location 】At the junction of the frenulum of upper lip with the upper gum.Sit and lift up the head, lift the upper lip, and then select the acupoint at the junction of the frenulum of upper lip with the gum.

【Indications 】①Swelling and pain of the gums, gingival bleeding, nasal congestion, nasal polyp; ②infantile facial sores and tinea; ③mania–depression.

29 印堂 YinTang GV-29

【Source 】《针灸玉龙歌》*ZhenJiu YuLong Ge*

【Annotation 】The area between two eyebrows is called YinTang by astrologers. This acupoint is located on it, hence it is named 印堂 YinTang.

【Location 】In the depression of the midpoint between the medial ends of the eyebrows.

【Indications 】①Headache, dizziness; ②insomnia; ③sinusitis, epistaxis; ④infantile convulsion.

Chapter 15
The Conception Vessel Points

1 会阴 HuiYin CV–1

【Source】《黄帝明堂经》 *Huangdi Mingtang Jing*

【Annotation】会 Hui means to meet and cross. The anus is named posterior Yin, while the external genitalia and urethral orifice are named anterior Yin. This acupoint is located between the anterior and posterior Yin, hence the name 会 阴 HuiYin. Since the Conception, Governing, and Thoroughfare vessels all originate from the internal genitalia and go out through this point, the point can be used to treat diseases of the uterus, spermary, and genitalia.

【Location】At the midpoint of the line connecting the anus with the posterior border of the scrotum in males and the posterior labial commissure in females.

【Indications】① Genital diseases, difficult urination and defecation caused by the pain of the genital and anus; ② genital pain, genital itching, genital swelling, seminal emission, irregular menstruation; ③ hemorrhoids.

2 曲骨 QuGu CV–2 (Meeting point of the Conception vessel with the Liver channel)

【Source】《黄帝明堂经》 *Huangdi Mingtang Jing*

【Annotation】曲骨 QuGu refers to the pubic symphysis. This acupoint is superior to the pubic symphysis. Hence it is named 曲骨 QuGu.

【Location】Superior to the pubic symphysis, on the anterior midline.

【Indications】Inhibited urination, enuresis, testicular hernia, seminal emission, impotence, irregular menstruation, leukorrhagia.

3 中极 ZhongJi CV–3 (Front-*Mu* point of the Bladder, Meeting point of the Conception vessel with the Spleen, Liver and Kidney channel)

【Source】《黄帝明堂经》 *Huangdi Mingtang Jing*

【Annotation】中 Zhong means center. 极 Ji is used to describe something awesome. 中极 ZhongJi is the name of a star in the middle of the sky, governing all stars. Acupoints shine like stars, and this point is at the center of the human body. Hence the name 中极 ZhongJi.

【Location】4 cun inferior to the center of the umbilicus, on the anterior midline.

【Indications】①Irregular menstruation, flooding and spotting, prolapse of the uterus, genital itching, infertility, persistent flow of lochia, leukorrhagia; ②enuresis, inhibited urination, hernia, seminal emission, impotence.

4 关元 GuanYuan CV–4 (Front-*Mu* point of the Small Intestine, Meeting point of the Conception vessel with the Spleen, Liver and Kidney channels)

【Source】《素问·气穴论》《灵枢·寒热病》 *Suwen: Qixue Lun, Lingshu: Hanrebing*

【Annotation】关 Guan means being connected. 元 Yuan means original. This acupoint is on the lower abdomen where males store essence, and females store blood. It is a fortress where the original Yin and the original Yang converge. Hence it is named 关元 GuanYuan.

【Location】3 cun inferior to the center of the umbilicus, on the anterior midline.

【Indications】①Hernia, lower abdominal pain; ②dribbling and retention of urine, frequent urination, seminal emission, impotence; ③irregular menstruation, dysmenorrhea, leukorrhagia, uterine prolapse, persistent flow of lochia, infertility; ④diarrhea; consumptive disease.

5 石门 ShiMen CV–5 (Front-*Mu* point of the Sanjiao)

【Source】《黄帝明堂经》 *Huangdi Mingtang Jing*

【Annotation】Infertile women were called 石 女 ShiNv in ancient China. Ancient people considered that needling and burning moxa at this acupoint can cause infertility in women, hence the name 石门 ShiMen.

【Location】2 cun inferior to the center of the umbilicus, on the anterior midline.

【Indications】 ①Hernia, inhibited urination, enuresis, seminal emission, impotence; ②irregular menstruation, infertility, persistent flow of lochia, masses in the uterus; ③abdominal pain, diarrhea, edema.

6 气海 QiHai CV-6

【Source】《黄帝明堂经》 *Huangdi Mingtang Jing*

【Annotation】 海 Hai refers to a sea. 气海 QiHai refers to the sea where qi origins. Taoism calls it 丹田 DanTian, where the genuine qi is stored, like a sea of rivers. Moreover, this acupoint is mainly used to treat deficiency of visceral or genuine qi and all qi diseases that last long. Hence the name 气海 QiHai.

【Location】1.5 cun inferior to the center of the umbilicus, on the anterior midline.

【Indications】①Collapse syndrome, diarrhea, gripping pain in the abdomen, consumptive disease leading to weakness and thinness; ②hernia, abdominal pain; ③inhibited urination, enuresis, seminal emission, impotence; ④irregular menstruation, leukorrhagia, uterine prolapse, persistent flow of lochia.

7 阴交 YinJiao CV-7 (Meeting point of the Conception and thoroughfare vessels with the Kidney channel)

【Source】《黄帝明堂经》 *Huangdi Mingtang Jing*

【Annotation】交 Jiao means to meet each other. This acupoint is the meeting point of three yin channels, including the Conception and Thoroughfare vessels and the Kidney channel. Hence it is named 阴交 YinJiao. Therefore, it can treat abdominal diseases related to these three channels, such as periumbilical cold pain, diarrhea, and hernia.

【Location】1 cun inferior to the center of the umbilicus, on the anterior midline.

【Indications】①Irregular menstruation, leukorrhagia, infertility, diseases after labor, inhibited urination, hernia; ②abdominal pain; ③edema.

8 神阙 ShenQue CV-8

【Source】 Presented as 脐中 QiZhong in 《黄帝明堂经》 *Huangdi Mingtang Jing*, and as 神阙 ShenQue since《铜人腧穴针灸图经》*Tongren Shuxue Zhenjiu Tujing*.

【Annotation】神 Shen means the original spirit. 阙 Que means the palace. This acupoint is in the umbilicus. During pregnancy, a mother transmits nutrition to nurture the fetus through the umbilical cord, cultivating the fetus's innate spirit. Therefore, this point is like a palace of the original spirit. Hence the name 神阙 ShenQue.

【Location】In the center of the umbilicus.

【Indications】①Periumbilical pain, abdominal distention, borborygmus, diarrhea; ②edema, inhibited urination; ③apoplectic collapse.

9 水分 ShuiFen CV-9

【Source】《黄帝明堂经》*Huangdi Mingtang Jing*

【Annotation】水 Shui means water and fluid. 分 Fen means to separate. This acupoint can separate the clear and turbid moisture in the abdomen, promoting water and fluid to enter the bladder and the dross to the large intestine. Therefore, it is mainly used for treating edema and diarrhea. Hence it is named 水分 ShuiFen.

【Location】1 cun superior to the center of the umbilicus, on the anterior midline.

【Indications】①Pain, fullness, and hardness of the abdomen, abdominal distention leading to poor appetite; ②edema, inhibited urination.

10 下脘 XiaWan CV-10 (Meeting point of the Conception vessel with the Spleen channel)

【Source】《黄帝明堂经》*Huangdi Mingtang Jing*

【Annotation】下 Xia means lower. 脘 Wan means the stomach. This acupoint corresponds to the lower gateway of the stomach, the pylorus, hence it is named 下脘 XiaWan.

【Location】2 cun superior to the center of the umbilicus, on the anterior midline.

【Indications】①Vomiting after eating; ②abdominal distention, abdominal hardness, abdominal masses, poor appetite, thinness.

11 建里 JianLi CV-11

【Source】《黄帝明堂经》*Huangdi Mingtang Jing*

【Annotation】建 Jian, an interchangeable word for 健 Jian, means healthy and strong. 里 Li means to live. The spleen and stomach are the foundation of the postnatal constitution, generating essence to nourish five viscera and six bowels. During the stomach disorders and rehabilitation period, this acupoint can regulate and harmonize the spleen and stomach, strengthening our postnatal constitution to ensure the five viscera live and work in peace and contentment. Hence the name 建里 JianLi.

【Location】3 cun superior to the center of the umbilicus, on the anterior midline.

【Indications】Stomachache, vomiting, poor appetite, abdominal pain, borborygmus, abdominal distention, abdominal swelling.

12 中脘 ZhongWan CV–12 (Front–*Mu* point of the Stomach, *Hui*–Meeting point of the Fu–organs, Meeting point of the Conception vessel with the Small Intestine, Sanjiao and Stomach channels)

【Source】《黄帝明堂经》 *Huangdi Mingtang Jing*

【Annotation】中 Zhong means middle. 脘 Wan means the stomach. This acupoint corresponds to the middle part of the stomach, close to the lesser curvature of the stomach. It is located between XiaWan (CV–10) and ShangWan (CV–13), hence the name 中脘 ZhongWan.

【Location】4 cun superior to the center of the umbilicus, on the anterior midline.

【Indications】① Stomachache, abdominal distention, abdominal masses, diarrhea, constipation, poor appetite, vomiting; ② jaundice.

13 上脘 ShangWan CV–13 (Meeting point of the Conception vessel with the Small Intestine and Stomach channels)

【Source】《黄帝明堂经》 *Huangdi Mingtang Jing*

【Annotation】上 Shang means upper. 脘 Wan means the stomach. This acupoint corresponds to the cardia, the upper gateway of the stomach. Hence the name 上脘 ShangWan.

【Location】5 cun superior to the center of the umbilicus, on the anterior midline.

【Indications】Stomachache, vomiting, hematemesis, hiccup, poor appetite, abdominal distention, abdominal masses; epilepsy.

14 巨阙 JuQue CV-14 (Front-*Mu* point of the Heart)

【Source】《黄帝明堂经》*Huangdi Mingtang Jing*

【Annotation】There are two explanations for this name. Firstly, 巨 阙 JuQue is the most famous sword in ancient China[①]. This acupoint is located beneath the xiphoid process, mainly treating diseases caused by unseparated clear and turbid substances and restless minds, such as palpitation, mania-depression, heart pain, and vexation, like standing upright with a sword to eliminate violence and insurgency. Hence the name 巨 阙 JuQue. Secondly, 巨 Ju means huge, and 阙 Que means structures on both sides of a door. This acupoint is under the ribs, which resemble two huge structures beside the door. Hence the name.

【Location】6 cun superior to the center of the umbilicus, on the anterior midline.

【Indications】① Palpitation, vexation, heart pain, chest pain, panting; ② mania-depression, epilepsy.

15 鸠尾 JiuWei CV-15 (*Luo*-Connecting point of the Conception vessel)

【Source】《灵枢·九针十二原》*Lingshu: Jiuzhen Shieryuan*

【Annotation】鸠尾 JiuWei means a turtledove tail. The xiphoid process hangs like a turtledove tail, and the ribs on both sides resemble two stretched wings. This acupoint is named 鸠尾 JiuWei because it lies under the xiphoid process.

【Location】1 cun inferior to the xiphisternal synchondrosis, on the anterior midline.

【Indications】① Chest pain leading to back, panting; ② abdominal distention, hiccup; ③ mania-depression, epilepsy.

16 中庭 ZhongTing CV-16

【Source】《黄帝明堂经》*Huangdi Mingtang Jing*

【Annotation】中 Zhong means middle. 庭 Ting means courtyard. This acupoint is in the depression on the xiphisternal synchondrosis, and the sternum serves as a door. Meanwhile,

---

① According to Chinese legend, the Sword JuQue was cast by Ou Yezi, a famous sword maker in ancient China. It is said that King Goujian of Yue named this sword because it is so powerful that it can easily stab a huge iron pot and cut a carriage into two.

points on its sides are BuLang (KI–22), whose Chinese name means corridor. Therefore, the point is like a courtyard inside the door and between the corridors. Hence it is named 中 庭 ZhongTing.

【Location】In the middle of the xiphisternal synchondrosis, on the anterior midline.

【Indications】①Fullness of the chest and lateral costal region; ②dysphagia, vomiting.

17 膻中 DanZhong CV–17 (Front–*Mu* point of the Pericardium, *Hui*–Meeting point of the Qi, Meeting point of the Conception vessel with the Spleen, Kidney, Small Intestine and channels)

【Source】《黄帝明堂经》*Huangdi Mingtang Jing*

【Annotation】膻 Dan, an interchangeable word for 袒 Tan, means to be naked and expose one's breast. 中 Zhong means middle. This acupoint is in the middle of two breasts. Hence it is named 膻中 DanZhong.

【Location】Level with the fourth intercostal space, on the anterior midline.

【Indications】①Oppression in the chest, heart pain; ②cough, panting; ③dysphagia; ④insufficient lactation.

18 玉堂 YuTang CV–18

【Source】《黄帝明堂经》*Huangdi Mingtang Jing*

【Annotation】玉堂 YuTang is a laudatory title of a main hall, which here refers to the residence of a monarch. According to TCM theory, the heart is an organ similar to the monarch. This acupoint is above ZhongTing (CV–16), whose Chinese name means courtyard, and the monarch will enter the main hall after crossing the courtyard. Hence the name 玉堂 YuTang.

【Location】Level with the third intercostal space, on the anterior midline.

【Indications】①Cough, panting, oppression in the chest, chest pain; ②distending pain of the breast; ③vomiting.

19 紫宫 ZiGong CV–19

【Source】《黄帝明堂经》*Huangdi Mingtang Jing*

【Annotation】紫宫 ZiGong is an alternative name of 紫微 ZiWei[1], which is one of the fifteen stars in 紫微垣 ZiWei Yuan. It is the first of all stars and is known as the Emperor Star, corresponding to the residence of the monarch. This acupoint corresponds to the heart, like the monarch's bedroom, hence the name 紫宫 ZiGong.

【Location】Level with the second intercostal space, on the anterior midline.

【Indications】①Chest pain; ②cough, panting.

20 华盖 HuaGai CV-20

【Source】《黄帝明堂经》 *Huangdi Mingtang Jing*

【Annotation】华盖 HuaGai refers to a canopy cover on the ancient monarch's carriage, and traditional Chinese medicine compared the lung to a canopy. This acupoint levels with the first intercostal space, close to the upper edge of the lung. It is mainly used to treat chest and lung diseases, such as cough, panting, and chest pain. Hence it is named 华盖 HuaGai.

【Location】Level with the first intercostal space, on the anterior midline.

【Indications】Chest pain, cough, panting.

21 璇玑 XuanJi CV-21

【Source】《黄帝明堂经》 *Huangdi Mingtang Jing*

【Annotation】璇玑 XuanJi has the meaning of rotation[2], which was often used to describe fruity and smooth objects by the ancient. With the capacity of moistening and smoothening, this acupoint is mainly used to treat dry symptoms of the throat, such as pharyngitis, swollen throat, and painful pharynx. Hence the name 璇玑 XuanJi.

【Location】1 cun inferior to the suprasternal fossa, on the anterior midline.

【Indications】Chest pain, cough, panting; swelling and pain of the throat.

---

① In ancient Chinese astronomy, 垣 Yuan is a unit that divides the stars. Ancient Chinese divided the stars into many Chinese constellations, among which three constellations were called 三垣 SanYuan, namely 紫微垣 ZiWei Yuan, 太微垣 TaiWei Yuan, and 天市垣 TianShi Yuan.

② The second star of the Big Dipper is 璇 Xuan while the third star is 玑 Ji. The Big Dipper rotates, followed by 璇 Xuan and 玑 Ji.

22 天突 TianTu CV-22

【Source】《素问·气穴论》《灵枢·本输》*Suwen: Qixue Lun, Lingshu: Benshu*

【Annotation】天 Tian means the upper part of the human body, here refers to the chest. 突 Tu means prominent, here refers to a chimney which is prominent in a house. Qi from nature passes through the lung, and this acupoint serves as a chimney for the lung qi to enter and leave. Hence the name 天突 TianTu.

【Location】On the anterior midline of the neck, in the center of the suprasternal fossa.

【Indications】①Cough, panting, chest pain, hemoptysis; ②swelling and pain of the throat, loss of voice; ③fistula and tumor; ④dysphagia.

23 廉泉 LianQuan CV-23 (Meeting point of the Conception and Yin Linking vessels)

【Source】《黄帝明堂经》*Huangdi Mingtang Jing*

【Annotation】廉 Lian means edges and angles. The tip of the laryngeal prominence is shaped like an angle. This acupoint is in the depression above it, and beneath the point is the sublingual gland. Therefore, this acupoint can promote the body fluid to secrete like spring water gushing out, hence the name 廉泉 LianQuan.

【Location】On the anterior midline of the neck, above the tip of the laryngeal prominence, in the depression superior to the hyoid bone.

【Indications】①Aphasia after stroke, dysphagia, sluggish tongue, too much drool; ②swelling and pain of the throat or below the tongue.

24 承浆 ChengJiang CV-24 (Meeting point of the Conception vessel with the Stomach channel)

【Source】《黄帝明堂经》*Huangdi Mingtang Jing*

【Annotation】承 Cheng means to accept. 浆 Jiang means saliva. The ancient Chinese compared saliva to nectar and mouth to the Heaven Lake. This acupoint is inferior to the lips and exactly corresponds to the Heaven Lake storing nectar. Hence it is named 承浆 ChengJiang.

【Location】On the face, in the depression in the center of the mentolabial groove.

【Indications】 ①Deviation of the mouth and eye, lockjaw, swelling and pain of the teeth and gums; ②loss of voice; ③mania-depression, epilepsy; ④wasting-thirst with a desire to drink; ⑤pain and stiffness of the head and nape.